# VOCAL PATHOLOGIES

*Diagnosis, Treatment, and Case Studies*

# VOCAL PATHOLOGIES

## Diagnosis, Treatment, and Case Studies

**James Paul Dworkin, Ph.D.**
Professor
Department of Otolaryngology
Wayne State University
School of Medicine
Detroit, Michigan

**Robert J. Meleca, M.D.**
Assistant Professor
Department of Otolaryngology
Wayne State University
School of Medicine
Detroit, Michigan

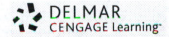
DELMAR
CENGAGE Learning

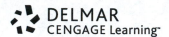
DELMAR
CENGAGE Learning™

**Vocal Pathologies:
Diagnosis, Treatment & Case
Studies and Protocols**
**James Paul Dworkin,
Robert J. Meleca**

For product information and technology assistance, contact us at
**Cengage Learning Customer & Sales Support, 1-800-354-9706**

For permission to use material from this text or product,
submit all requests online at **cengage.com/permissions**
Further permissions questions can be emailed to

Library of Congress Control Number: 96024941

ISBN-13: 978-1-56593-623-2

ISBN-10: 1-56593-623-X

**Delmar Cengage Learning**
5 Maxwell Drive
Clifton Park, NY 12065-2919
USA

Cengage Learning products are represented in Canada by Nelson
Education, Ltd.

For your lifelong learning solutions, visit
**delmar.cengage.com**

Visit our corporate website at **www.cengage.com**

**Notice to the Reader**

Printed in the United States of America
22 12 11 10

# Contents

# Preface

The field of laryngology has evolved considerably over the past 100 years. Assessment and treatment of laryngeal disorders have improved significantly with the introduction of videostrobolaryngoscopy, sophisticated computer software for acoustic and speech aerodynamic analyses, microlaryngoscopy, and microlaryngeal surgical instrumentation. With the advent of well equipped voice laboratories, often jointly directed by laryngologists and speech-language pathologists, these professionals have begun to redefine their respective clinical roles in the differential diagnosis and treatment of patients with voice disorders. This symbiotic relationship has spawned numerous coauthored textbooks and scientific papers. Some of these works are more current than others, but most offer very good information. The current project was designed as a unique alternative to these other references. This text includes thumbnail descriptions of voice disorders, laboratory methods of evaluation, surgical and non-surgical treatment techniques, video documentation of various laryngeal pathologies, numerous case studies, and companion audio CDs. The format and material presented should interest both practicing clinicians and students in training in the fields of speech-language pathology and otolaryngology, especially those who have limited experience in the study and treatment of voice disorders. Additionally, instructors of graduate courses in this subject area may be particularly pleased with the numerous case presentations and the accompanying CDs, which contains pre- and posttreatment voice samples of these patients for purposes of stimulating both clinical and academic discussions. Collectively, the introductory chapters and case studies offer the reader a comprehensive yet easy to follow sourcebook on differential diagnosis and treatment of voice disorders.

In Chapter 1, a brief overview of the anatomy of the larynx and physiology of phonation is provided. This chapter was not designed as an exhaustive account of this complex subject matter. Rather, it was written as a simple review for speech-language pathologists and laryngologists who may benefit from a refresher course on this topic and who aspire to treat patients with voice disorders. The schematic illustrations were selected to facilitate the flow of information. Chapter 2 outlines the methodology that may be followed to evaluate patients suffering from dysphonia. Both clinical appraisal and laboratory measurement techniques are described in detail, and the material is accented with numerous charts, tables, and illustrations for easy interpretation and future use by the reader. Videostroboscopic, acoustic, and speech aerodynamic examination procedures are discussed in detail, with special emphasis placed on differential diagnoses of various laryngeal pathologies. In Chapter 3, in-depth descriptions of these conditions are provided along with photographs illustrating various benign growths, malignant neoplasms, and neuromuscular abnormalities of the larynx.

Chapter 4 addresses surgical alternatives for all of these abnormalities. Focus is placed on procedures designed not only to improve voice, but also those that enhance swallowing function. Schematic illustrations augment the discussions. Chapter 5 is devoted to nonsurgical therapeutic options for many different types of voice disorders. Flow charts and illustrations are provided to facilitate appreciation of the differential clinical steps and procedures.

The final chapter offers numerous case studies that were selected to demonstrate the adverse phonatory effects of various laryngeal pathologies. Each case includes a description of the patient's history and findings obtained during the evaluation process. Results of the physical examination and voice laboratory measurements are detailed, followed by an explanation of the diagnosis. The treatment plan is provided, intervention outcomes are described, and pretreatment comparisons are drawn. The case presentation concludes with a discussion of the laryngeal

pathology exhibited by the patient. Photo-documentation of the appearance of the larynx prior to treatment is included for each case. When applicable, significant posttreatment effects are supported with additional photographs. The companion audio CD was designed to supplement each case study. When reviewing each presentation, the reader will be prompted to listen to CD samples. To experience the full benefit of this teaching format, these audio segments should be played in tandem with the case review.

In summary, this text was written as a practical guide to the evaluation and treatment of voice disorders. The information presented covers a broad range of topics with sufficient, but not exhausting, detail. This approach was purposely directed toward graduate students and busy practicing clinicians. Readers interested in more elaborate discussions on these subjects are encouraged to consult the suggested reading lists throughout the text.

# Acknowledgments

As with any major undertaking we are indebted to many individuals for their help with this project. First and foremost, we owe our greatest gratitude to our wives and children for their patience as we neglected their needs in favor of our commitment to complete this work in a timely manner. We are also grateful to Ilene Garfield for her technical advice and assistance in the construction of the tables and flow charts throughout the text. Thanks are due to Toni Merola for her secretarial support during different phases of manuscript preparation. Finally, special recognition must be focused on our patients, from whom we learn the most and for whom we continuously strive to improve our clinical skills.

# CHAPTER 1

# *Anatomy and Physiology of Phonation*

The larynx is a complex organ that functions as a biologic valve for regulation of phonation, respiration, and swallowing. Humans have developed a unique additional function by converting the sounds generated by the vocal tract into speech and song to communicate thoughts and emotions. This chapter provides a brief overview of laryngeal embryology, gross anatomy, and histology, followed by a discussion of the physiology of voice production. It is beyond the scope of this text to delve deeply into the anatomy and physiology of the phonation subsystem. There are numerous excellent references on this topic, some of which are listed at the end of this chapter. The material presented here is meant only as a brief review of this important subject. The complexity level was deliberately chosen to maintain the interest of readers with little or moderate knowledge of the subject. Those with an advanced understanding of the subject may wish to merely scan the chapter as a refresher exercise. The information provided builds a foundation to support and augment the material covered in the remaining chapters.

## EMBRYOLOGY

The larynx arises primarily from the paired branchial (visceral) arches III, IV, and VI, which contribute tissue of endodermal, mesodermal, and ectodermal origin (Table 1–1). Development of the respiratory system usually begins during the third week of embryonic growth as an endodermal outgrowth (respiratory diverticulum) from the foregut (Figure 1–1). The foregut differentiates into the pharynx, trachea, bronchi, and lungs, with the larynx serving as a conduit for air exchange between the pharynx and trachea.

The mesodermal layer provides muscles, blood vessels, lymphatics, bones, and cartilages of the larynx. Second arch mesoderm gives rise to the lesser horns (cornua) and upper portion of the body of the hyoid bone. The greater horns and lower part of the body of the hyoid, as well as the common and internal carotid arteries, originate from third arch mesodermal tissue. The thyroid and cuneiform cartilages, cricothyroid muscles, proximal subclavian artery on the

**TABLE I–I.** Branchial arch derivatives.

| Arch | Cartilage/Bone | Muscle | Nerve | Artery |
|------|----------------|--------|-------|--------|
| **first** | mandible | | | |
| **second** | hyoid (lesser cornu & upper body) | | VII | stapedial |
| **third** | hyoid (greater cornu & lower body) | | IX | carotid |
| **fourth** | thyroid, cuneiform | cricothyroid | X (superior laryngeal) | aorta (L) subclavian (R) |
| **sixth** | cricoid arytenoid corniculate | intrinsic muscles of larynx | X (recurrent laryngeal) | ductus arteriosus (L) pulmonary (R) |

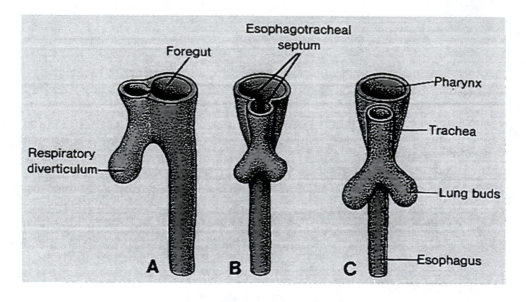

**FIGURE I–I.** Normal development of the human foregut and respiratory system. Lateral view at the end of 3 weeks (A). Ventral view during the 4th week (B, C). (From *Langman's Medical Embryology* by T. W. Sadler, 1985, 5th ed., p. 226. Baltimore: Williams and Wilkins. Copyright 1985 Williams and Wilkins. Reprinted by permission.)

right, and aorta on the left arise from fourth arch derivatives. The sixth arch contributes the cricoid, arytenoid, and corniculate cartilages, all of the intrinsic laryngeal muscles except the cricothyroid, the ductus arteriosus on the left, and the pulmonary artery on the right. Figure 1–2 illustrates structures formed by some of the cartilaginous components of the various pharyngeal arches.

From ectodermal tissues arise two primary branches of the tenth (vagus) cranial nerve, the superior and recurrent laryngeal

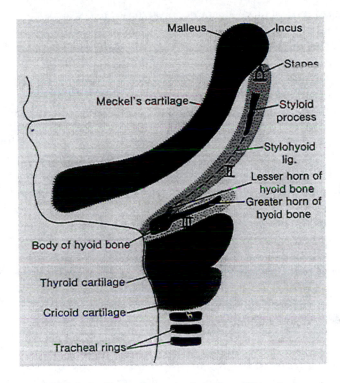

**FIGURE 1–2.** Pharyngeal arch derivatives. (From *Langman's Medical Embryology* by T. W. Sadler, 1985, 5th ed., p. 286. Baltimore: Williams and Wilkins. Copyright 1985 Williams and Wilkins. Reprinted by permission.)

nerves, derived from branchial arches IV and VI, respectively. The left recurrent laryngeal nerve is closely associated with its sixth arch vessel, the ductus arteriosus (ligamentum arteriosum), and is looped around this structure in the region of the aortic arch. The right recurrent laryngeal nerve does not loop around its sixth arch derivative. Instead, it courses further superiorly, looping around the right fourth arch vessel, the subclavian artery. The sixth arch disappears during fetal development. The intrathoracic course taken by the left recurrent laryngeal nerve, compared with the transcervical route of the right recurrent nerve, contributes to the higher incidence of left vocal fold paralysis secondary to injury of the recurrent nerve from intrathoracic disease or cardiothoracic surgery.

# LARYNGEAL GROSS ANATOMY

The larynx, lined with mucosal membranes that protect and lubricate the delicate vocal folds, is located within a rigid outer framework of bone and cartilage. This framework is suspended in the anterior neck region by a complex array of ligaments, muscles, and specialized joints. These interconnections work in concert to regulate laryngeal positioning and vocal fold vibratory dynamics during acts of respiration, deglutition, and voice production.

## Laryngeal Skeleton

The larynx is composed of three paired cartilages and three unpaired cartilages that interconnect to form the laryngeal skeleton. The thyroid, cricoid, and epiglottis are unpaired, and represent the largest cartilages. The arytenoid, corniculate, and cuneiform cartilages are paired, and are quite small in comparison. The hyoid bone, although not generally considered a component of the larynx, is connected to it by a series of membranes, ligaments, and muscles. Because of this linkage, the hyoid bone is instrumental in providing stability and influencing positioning of the larynx during swallowing and phonation. Figure 1–3 illustrates the anatomy of these cartilages.

Of the three unpaired cartilages, the thyroid is the largest, resembling the shape of a shield. It consists of two sides, or laminae, joined together anteriorly at an approximately 90° angle in males and 120° angle in females. This difference in angulation, coupled with a larger overall size, produces a prominence of the thyroid cartilage in males, called the thyroid notch or "Adam's apple." In females the most prominent structure in the neck is the cricoid cartilage because of the more obtuse angle formed by the thyroid alae. The thyrohyoid membrane interconnects the thyroid cartilage and hyoid bone, as shown in Figure 1–3A. The cricothyroid membrane (ligament) joins the cricoid and thyroid cartilages. The superior and inferior cornua, or horns, of the thyroid cartilage articulate with the hyoid bone and cricoid cartilage, respectively. The cricothyroid joint is diarthrodial; it is moveable and supported by ligaments and synovial (fluid secreting) membranes. The oblique line is a paired, diagonally oriented prominence of the thyroid cartilage which serves as a surface for attachment of the sternothyroid, thyrohyoid, and inferior constrictor muscles. These muscles are considered extrinsic laryngeal structures.

The cricoid cartilage is the only complete ring of the upper airway and is positioned between the inferior border of the thyroid cartilage and first tracheal cartilage, as illustrated in Figure 1–3. Its shape resembles a signet ring, with its ring-like structure, the arch, located anteriorly, and its broadened, signet portion, the posterior lamina, located posteriorly. The cricoid slopes upward from anterior to posterior, with the posterior lamina lying within the space created by the surrounding thyroid cartilage framework. The paired arytenoid cartilages articulate with the superior border of the posterior cricoid lamina, forming the cricoarytenoid joints. The cricoid cartilage serves as the origin of multiple paired muscles, including the cricothyroids, lateral cricoarytenoids, and posterior cricoarytenoids, as illustrated in Figure 1–4.

The arytenoid cartilages are shaped like pyramids. As previously mentioned, the base of the arytenoid, located inferiorly, articulates with the superior surface of the posterior cricoid lamina to form the cricoarytenoid joint. These paired synovial joints are critical contributors to phonation because their rocking and gliding movements directly influence vocal fold positioning and vibratory patterns. An anterior and medially directed projection, called the vocal process, serves as the posterior attachment of the vocal ligament and vocal fold musculature, as shown in Figures 1–3 and 1–4. A posterior and laterally directed muscular process of each arytenoid provides attachment for the posterior and lateral cricoarytenoid and interarytenoid muscles. These intrinsic muscles are vital to vocal fold activity during phonation. The apex and anterior surface of the arytenoids serve as attachment sites for the aryepiglottic folds.

The paired corniculate and cuneiform cartilages are found within the aryepiglottic folds and serve as structural supports for these otherwise nonrigid myoelastic tissues.

The epiglottis is an elongated, leaf-shaped cartilage. It contains secretory glands, distributed over its laryngeal surface, and multiple perforations through which tiny vessels pass from the laryngeal surface of the cartilage to the pre-epiglottic space. This transepiglottic vascular network provides the lymphatic channels that may account

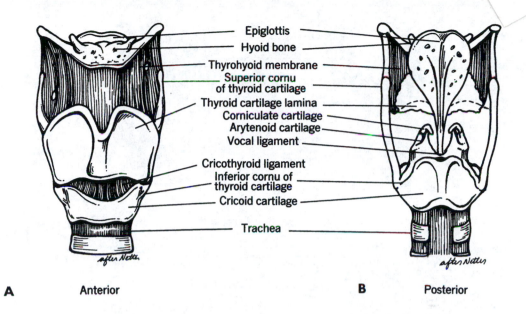

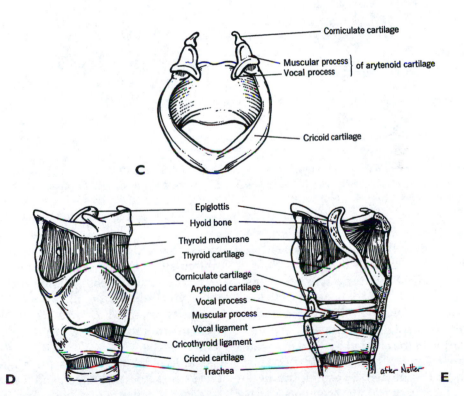

**FIGURE 1–3.** Anterior and posterior views of the larynx (A, B). View of the arytenoid as it articulates with the cricoid (C). Lateral view of the larynx (D). Midsagittal view of the larynx (E). (From *Professional Voice: The Science and Art of Clinical Care* by R. T. Sataloff, 1997, 2nd ed., p. 112. San Diego, CA: Singular Publishing Group. Copyright 1997 Singular Publishing Group, Inc. Reprinted with permission.)

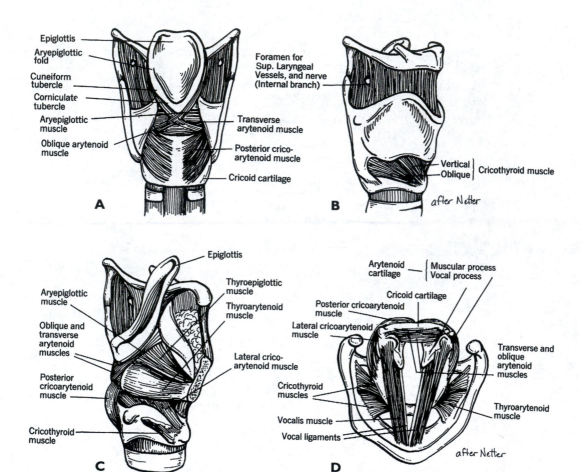

**FIGURE 1–4.** Intrinsic muscles of the larynx. Anterior view (A). Lateral view (B). Midsagittal view (C). Axial view (D). (From *Professional Voice: The Science and Art of Clinical Care* by R.T. Sataloff, 1997, 2nd ed., p. 112. San Diego, CA: Singular Publishing Group. Copyright 1997 Singular Publishing Group, Inc. Reprinted with permission.)

for the commonly encountered spread of glottic carcinomas into the pre-epiglottic space. The most inferior extension of the epiglottis, called the petiole, attaches to the inner surface of the thyroid cartilage by the median thyroepiglottic ligament. The upper portion of the epiglottis articulates with the inner surface of the hyoid bone by means of the median hyoepiglottic ligament. The glossoepiglottic ligaments attach the epiglottis to the base of the tongue on either side of the hyoepiglottic ligament. Mucosal-lined pouches are created between the midline hyoepiglottic and paired lateral

glossoepiglottic ligaments, known as the valleculae. The lateral free margins of the epiglottis attach to the anterior surface of the arytenoids by a wall of mucosa and obliquely oriented muscle fibers. These were referred to earlier as the aryepiglottic folds.

The hyoid bone defines the angle between the submental region and the anterior neck. It consists of a body and paired lesser and greater cornua, or horns. Its location in the neck is anteroinferior to the base of the tongue and superior to the thyroid cartilage. Several ligaments, tendons, and extrinsic laryngeal muscles attach to the hyoid bone. These structures suspend and stabilize the laryngeal skeleton in the anterior neck region and help produce many of the intricate laryngeal movements utilized during acts of respiration, deglutition, and phonation.

## Laryngeal Membranes and Ligaments

The conus elasticus is thick fibroelastic tissue that attaches in a horseshoe fashion along the superior and inner margin of the cricoid arch, as illustrated in Figure 1–5. Anteriorly, it runs from the cricoid arch to the inferior margin of the thyroid cartilage, forming the cricothyroid membrane. The ligament continues superiorly, in the midline, and attaches to the inner surface of the thyroid cartilage at the level of the vocal ligament. Posteriorly, the conus elasticus articulates with the vocal processes of the arytenoids. The thickened, free margins that are suspended between the anterior and posterior attachments form the vocal ligaments of the true vocal folds.

The quadrangular membrane is less well defined fibroelastic tissue, which attaches anteriorly along the lateral margin of the epiglottis. It runs posteriorly, within the aryepiglottic fold, to attach to the arytenoid and corniculate cartilages, just above the vocal processes. The free edge of the membrane, suspended between its anterior and posterior articulations, forms the vestibular ligament of the false (vestibular) vocal fold. These paired folds are composed primarily of fat and connective tissue, with muscle fibers from the thyroarytenoid complex located deep in these structures.

The thyrohyoid membrane is fibroelastic tissue that connects the superior surface of the thyroid cartilage to the hyoid bone. The lateral surface of the membrane is penetrated by the superior laryngeal vessels and internal branch of the superior laryngeal nerve.

## Laryngeal Joints

As previously mentioned, the cricothyroid and cricoarytenoid joints are true synovial articulations, supported by joint capsule ligaments. Contraction of the paired cricothyroid muscles approximates the anterior thyroid and cricoid cartilages. This increases the anteroposterior length of the glottis, therefore tensing the true vocal folds. This effect is shown in Figure 1–6. Technological advances in anatomic imaging, such as 3-D spiral computed tomography (CAT scan) and videolaryngoscopy, have greatly enhanced our knowledge of cricoarytenoid joint movement. Data obtained from these imaging modalities suggest that the primary action of the cricoarytenoid joint is a rocking motion of the arytenoid on the posterior cricoid lamina; tilting anteromedially for vocal fold adduction and posterolaterally for vocal fold abduction, as shown in Figure 1–7. There is little scientific data to

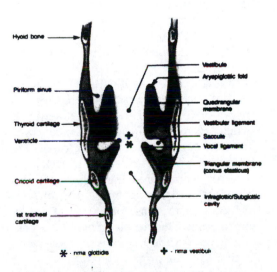

**FIGURE 1–5.** Coronal section of larynx demonstrating the quadrangular membrane and conus elasticus. (From *Neurologic Disorders of the Larynx* by A. Blitzer A., M. F. Brin, C T. Sasaki, S. Fahn, & K. S. Harris, 1992, p. 6. New York: Thieme Medical Publishers. Copyright 1992 Thieme Medical Publishers, Inc. Reprinted with permission.)

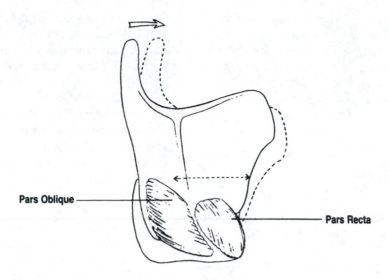

Pars Oblique

Pars Recta

**FIGURE 1–6.** Action of the cricothyroid muscle. (From *Clinical Voice Pathology* by J. C. Stemple, L. E. Glaze, & B. K. Gerdeman, 1995, p. 33. San Diego, CA: Singular Publishing Group. Copyright 1995 by Singular Publishing Group, Inc. Reprinted by permission.)

support classic textbook descriptions of rotary and gliding motions of the arytenoids during phonation or other valving activities. The anatomy of the joint is simply incompatible with the biomechanical demands of these motions.

## Intrinsic Muscles of the Larynx

The various pairs of intrinsic muscles of the larynx work harmoniously to open, close, tense, and relax the vocal folds during respiration, deglutition, and phonation activities. A discussion assigning only one of these movements to a given intrinsic muscle would be misleading because of the intricate and still poorly understood interactions of this muscle complex. That is, a specific intrinsic muscle may function to close (adduct) the vocal folds when the thyroid, cricoid, and arytenoid cartilages are held fixed in one position. This same muscle, however, may serve to tense or open (abduct) the vocal folds with slight

changes in positioning of these cartilages by other laryngeal muscles. For ease of review, the thyroarytenoid, lateral cricoarytenoid, and interarytenoid (transverse and oblique) muscles generally function as vocal fold adductors, as illustrated in Figure 1–8. The cricothyroid muscles are the chief tensors of the vocal folds. This action is particularly noticeable when phonating at extremely high pitches or high intensities. The posterior cricoarytenoid muscles are classically considered the only vocal fold abductors and the aryepiglottic muscles function primarily as sphincters of the laryngeal inlet. The muscle fibers of the ventricular vocal folds are not well understood relative to their origin, general course, or overall contribution to normal laryngeal function.

## Extrinsic Muscles of the Larynx

Extrinsic muscles of the larynx, illustrated in Figure 1–9, include the supra- and in-

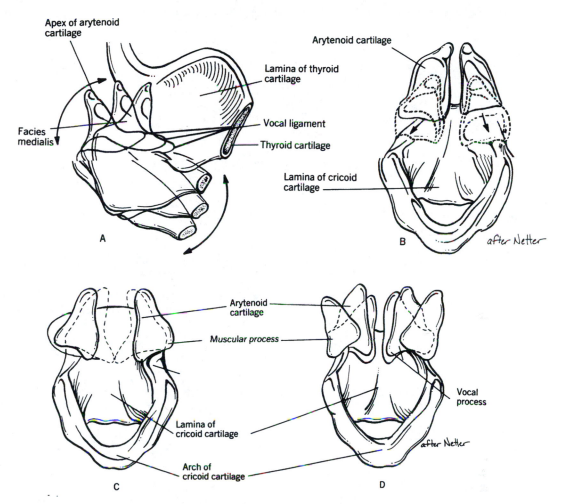

**FIGURE 1-7.** Schematic demonstrating tilting and gliding movements of the arytenoids (A-D). (From *Voice Surgery* by W. J. Gould, R. T. Sataloff, & J. R. Spiegel, 1992, p. 164. St. Louis, MO: Mosby. Copyright 1993 by Mosby Year-Book, Inc. Reprinted with permission.)

frahyoid muscles and the middle and inferior pharyngeal constrictors. In general, these muscles help to stabilize and alter the position of the laryngeal skeleton during respiration, deglutition, and swallowing.

The supra- and infrahyoid muscles, often called strap muscles, share a common insertion at the hyoid bone. The suprahyoid muscles attach above the hyoid bone, and with contraction, will pull the larynx superiorly. During the act of swallowing the suprahyoid musculature is instrumental in positioning the larynx upward and forward under the base of the tongue and retroflexed epiglottis, therefore providing airway protection from the food bolus. The infrahyoid group of muscles insert below the hyoid and act to lower the larynx. With phonation the laryngeal skeleton elevates with ascending pitch and lowers with descending pitch, resulting in changes in resting length and positioning of the intrinsic muscles. This dynamic interaction between the extrinsic and intrinsic muscu-

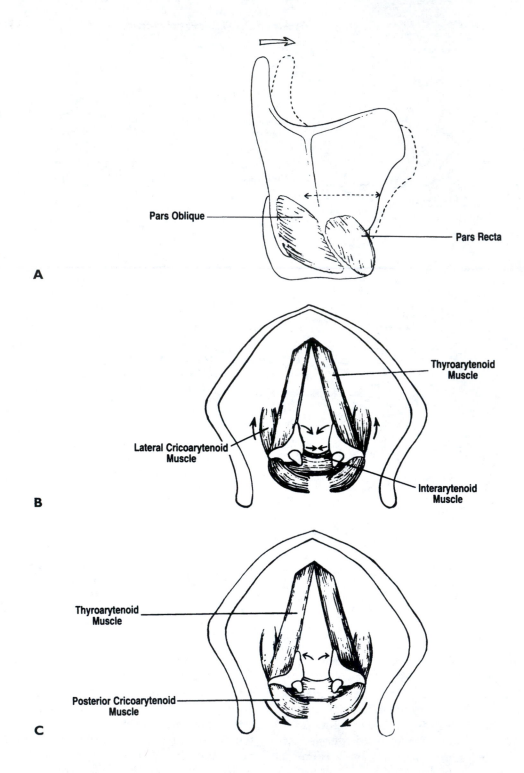

**FIGURE 1–8.** Intrinsic muscles of the larynx and their contributions to vocal fold movement. Action of the cricothyroid muscle (A). Action of the lateral cricoarytenoid and interarytenoid muscles during adduction (B). Action of the posterior cricoarytenoid muscle during abduction (C). (From *Clinical Voice Pathology* by J. C. Stemple, L. E. Glaze, & B. K. Gerdeman, 1995, pp. 33–34. San Diego, CA: Singular Publishing Group. Copyright 1995 by Singular Publishing Group, Inc. Reprinted by permission.)

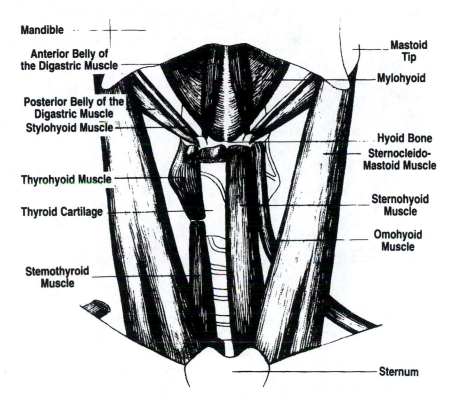

**FIGURE 1–9.** Extrinsic laryngeal muscles. (From *Clinical Voice Pathology* by J. C. Stemple, L. E. Glaze, & B. K. Gerdeman, 1995, p. 40. San Diego, CA: Singular Publishing Group. Copyright 1995 by Singular Publishing Group, Inc. Reprinted by permission.)

lature produces the many intricate vocal fold movements needed for phonation.

The middle and inferior constrictor muscles play a primary role during swallowing. Their movements assist in propulsion of the food bolus through the pharynx and into the esophagus.

## BLOOD SUPPLY OF THE LARYNX

Arterial blood supply to the larynx is contributed predominately by the superior and inferior thyroid arteries, as illustrated in Figure 1–10. The superior thyroid artery is the first branch from the external carotid artery. It branches to form the superior la-

ryngeal and cricothyroid vessels. The superior laryngeal artery gains access and supplies blood to the supraglottic larynx by penetrating the cricothyroid membrane and entering the piriform sinus along side the internal laryngeal nerve. The cricothyroid branch of the superior thyroid artery penetrates the cricothyroid membrane to provide blood supply to the subglottis. The inferior thyroid artery arises from the thyrocervical trunk and branches further to form the inferior laryngeal artery. This vessel travels with the recurrent laryngeal nerve, under the inferior constrictor muscle, to supply the subglottis.

Venous drainage parallels the arterial supply, with the superior thyroid vein draining into the superior and middle thy-

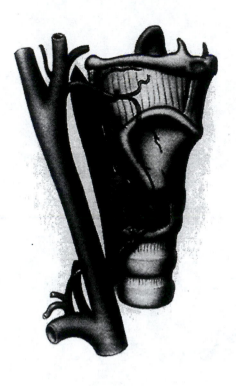

**FIGURE 1–10.** Superior and inferior thyroid arterial supply of the larynx. (From *Vocal Arts Medicine: The Care and Prevention of Professional Voice Disorders* by M. S. Benninger, B. H. Jacobson, & A. F. Johnson, 1993, p. 22. New York: Thieme Medical Publishers. Copyright 1993 by Thieme Medical Publishers, Inc. Reprinted by permission.)

roid vessels, and finally, into the internal jugular vein. The inferior thyroid veins empty into the middle thyroid vessel and directly into the left brachiocephalic trunk.

## LARYNGEAL INNERVATION

From a neurologic viewpoint, voice production requires an extremely complex and only partially understood interaction between the central and peripheral components of the nervous system, as shown in Figure 1–11. Speech production is initiated in a specialized region of the cerebral cortex, known as Broca's area. Information

from Broca's area is transmitted to the precentral gyrus (primary motor strip) of the motor cortex, which in turn transmits information to brainstem and spinal cord nuclei through corticobulbar and corticospinal tracts, respectively. Lower motor neurons from brainstem nuclei are transmitted as cranial nerves. Of all the cranial nerves, the tenth, or vagus, plays the most important role in phonation because it innervates the intrinsic laryngeal musculature. Lower motor neurons from spinal nuclei, or spinal nerves, are directed to supporting muscles used for phonatory breathing coordination. Of these nerves, the cervical third, fourth, and fifth, together forming the phrenic nerve, and 12 pairs of thoracic nerves are most important because they directly synapse with the diaphragm and chest and abdominal wall musculature, respectively. Auditory feedback from the ear to the cerebral cortex, as well as tactile stimuli from the throat and phonatory musculature, add vital information so that fine tuning of vocal output can be achieved. Sympathetic and parasympathetic interactions are also instrumental for performing autoregulatory functions of the larynx.

The vagus nerve originates in the medulla of the brainstem. Its motor nucleus, the nucleus ambiguus, receives input from the central nervous system and then transmits this information to the larynx via motor axons leaving the brainstem. The vagus nerve travels extracranially through the jugular foramen and immediately sends a branch toward the larynx, called the superior laryngeal nerve, as shown in Figure 1–12. The superior laryngeal nerve bifurcates near the tip of the greater horn of the hyoid into internal and external branches. The internal branch, traveling with the superior thyroid artery, penetrates the thyrohyoid membrane and provides sensation from the supraglottic larynx. The external division descends over the surface of the inferior constrictor muscles of the pharynx and pro-

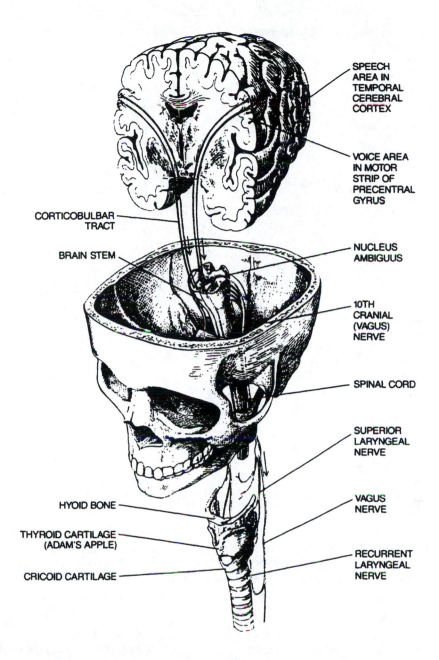

**FIGURE I-II.** Neurologic pathways for phonation. (From "The Human Voice." by R. T. Sataloff, *Scientific American*, 267(6), 108-115, reprinted with permission.)

vides motor innervation to this muscle, as well as to the cricothyroid muscle.

The recurrent laryngeal nerve branches from the main trunk of the vagus, lower in the neck. It loops around the right subcla- vian artery, from anterior to posterior, be- fore entering the tracheoesophageal groove. On the left side, this nerve runs lateral to the ligamentum arteriosum before ascend- ing the neck. Just before reaching the inferi-

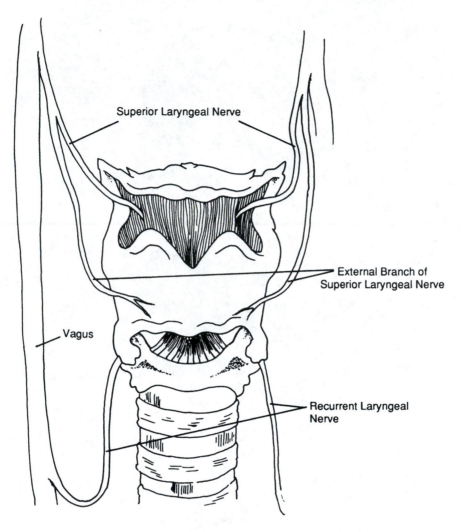

**FIGURE 1-12.** Superior and recurrent laryngeal nerve anatomy. (From *Introduction to Communication Sciences and Disorders* by F. D. Minifie, (Ed.), 1994, p. 489. San Diego, CA: Singular Publishing Group. Copyright 1994 Singular Publishing Group, Inc. Reprinted by permission.)

or border of the inferior constrictor muscle, the nerve divides, sending fibers that will ultimately anastomose with branches from the internal laryngeal nerve, known as Galen's anastomosis. The recurrent nerve then travels deep to the inferior constrictor and penetrates the larynx as it runs posterior to the cricothyroid joint. It provides sensation from and motor supply to the infraglottic larynx and all intrinsic muscles.

## LARYNGEAL MUCOSA

The tissue lining the laryngeal skeleton is referred to as respiratory mucosa. It is composed principally of pseudostratified, ciliated, columnar epithelium with interspersed goblet cells. Exceptions to this general rule include the lingual and apical surfaces of the epiglottis, free margins of the aryepiglottic folds, and the true vocal folds, which are composed of nonkeratinizing, stratified squamous epithelium. The junction between respiratory and squamous epithelium above and below the true vocal fold is known as the linea arcuata. The subglottis, trachea, and bronchi are lined with respiratory epithelium.

## THE VOCAL FOLDS

The human adult vocal fold consists of an overlying mucosa layer and a deeper thyroarytenoid muscle complex. The mucosa includes an outer stratified, nonkeratinizing squamous epithelium and an inner lamina propria, which can be further divided into superficial, intermediate, and deep layers. These components are illustrated in Figure 1–13.

The superficial layer of the lamina propria, often referred to as Reinke's space, consists mainly of amorphous material and few fibroblasts or elastic or cartilaginous fibers.

The intermediate and deep layers of the lamina propria form the thickened tissue located at the free edge of the conus elasticus, known as the vocal ligament. These deeper layers contain a higher density of fibroblasts and elastic and collagen fibers. This tissue matrix potentially increases the risk of scar formation after vocal fold surgery if the vocal ligament is disrupted and fibroblast proliferation occurs.

Based on an understanding of the layered anatomy of the vocal fold, Hirano (1975) described the cover-body concept of vocal fold vibration. The epithelium and superficial layer of the lamina propria represent the "cover," the intermediate and deep layers combine to form the "transition zone," and the vocalis muscle represents the "body." The gelatinous consistency of the superficial layer of the lamina propria allows for fluency of vibration of the epithelial cover over the vocal fold body. If movement of the cover over the body is studied in detail using stroboscopic imaging during normal phonation, the activity generated resembles travelling waves of mucosa (mucosal wave) from the inferior to superior surface of the vocal fold. Fibrotic, stiffened, adynamic vocal folds do not produce normal mucosal waves.

Most benign laryngeal pathologies, such as vocal fold polyps, nodules, and cysts develop in the superficial layer of the lamina propria. If large enough, they may cause a mass effect whereby fluency of vibration of the cover over the body is disrupted, resulting in perceived dysphonia. Laryngologists believe that precise dissection in the superficial layer of the lamina propria to remove benign vocal fold lesions, without disrupting the vocal ligament, will ultimately result in healing with significantly decreased scarring. Indeed, this philosophy is the impetus behind microlaryngeal surgery of the vocal fold as we know it today.

## FUNDAMENTALS OF PHONATION

The glottis can be divided into anterior and posterior compartments. The anterior glottis consists of the space created by and including the membranous true vocal folds. Its chief function is phonation. The posterior glottis includes the space between the arytenoids. It serves primarily as a conduit for respiration, but does provide a posterior glottic seal during phonation and swallowing. It should be noted that in some females with normal phonation a chink in the posterior glottis is observed during the closed phases of vibration. This gap has no apparent abnormal effect on vocal functioning.

The vocal folds produce a complex waveform which, if not shaped by the supraglottic resonators, sounds like a buzz. The supraglottic vocal tract transforms this primitive sound into the distinctive voice qualities that are perceived by a listener, referred to as timbre of voice production. The

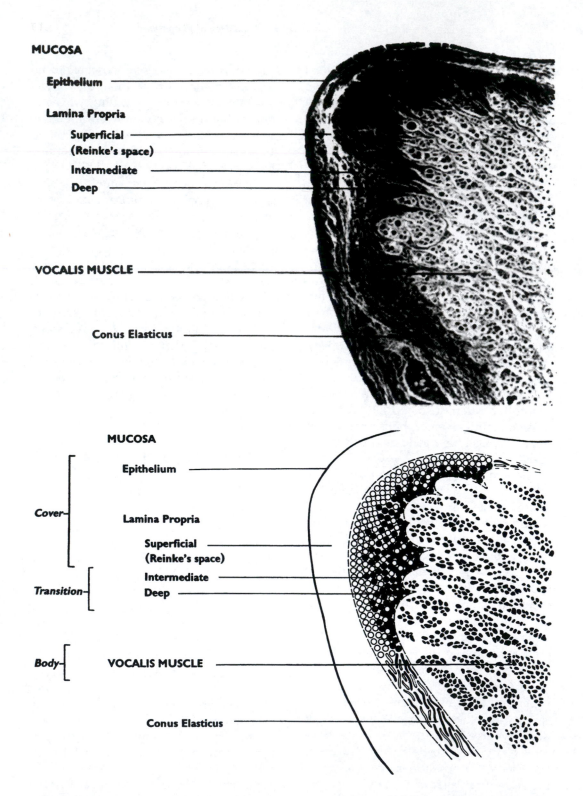

**FIGURE 1–13.** Photograph (A) and schematic (B) of the layered anatomy of the vocal fold. (From *Videostroboscopic Examination of the Larynx* by M. Hirano and D. M. Bless, 1993, p. 24. Copyright 1993 Singular Publishing Group, Inc. Reprinted with permission.)

supraglottic vocal tract includes the supraglottic larynx, oro- and nasopharynx, and oral and nasal cavities. Composed largely of muscle and connective tissue, the walls of this tract enhance, absorb, and reflect acoustic signals, thereby contributing substantially to the overall voice quality exhibited by an individual. Anatomic or physiologic abnormalities of any one or more of these structures, such as nasal congestion or tonsillar hypertrophy, may adversely affect the voice signal and result in significant dysphonic features, even if the vocal folds are unimpaired.

The infraglottic vocal tract includes the lungs, bronchi, trachea, diaphragm, abdominal, intercostal, chest, and back musculature. These respiratory subsystems function as a "power source" for phonation both by providing the aerodynamic supply for vocal fold vibration and by continually adjusting air pressure and flow during ongoing vocalization. Voice is produced when air from the lungs is propelled through the bronchi, trachea, and adducted vocal folds, thus producing vocal fold vibration. In preparation for speech, air is inhaled and tidal volume capacity achieved through the bellows action of the diaphragm. Sustained contractions by the abdominal musculature to provide support, combined with pulsatile contractions by the intercostal muscles, produce compressed puffs of air utilized for conversational speech. These complex motor behaviors, occurring automatically during nonspeech respiratory activity, are brought under voluntary control during conversational speech to allow for air pressure and air flow changes necessary for prosody variation (speech rate, rhythm, pitch, and loudness).

If breath support and air pressure through the closed vocal folds are diminished because of disease affecting the respiratory subsystem (i.e., chronic obstructive pulmonary disease, bronchial neoplasm, tracheal stenosis, phrenic nerve paralysis, abdominal surgery) or generalized respiratory muscle weakness from systemic illness, vocal fold vibration and voice quality will be altered, despite a normal functioning larynx. In addition, it is not uncommon for a patient with a voice disorder to exhibit poor breath support during speech efforts. This disturbance is usually not a result of respiratory subsystem disease, but rather, a compensatory respiratory pattern established to counteract the upstream glottic pathology. Respiratory subsystem and compensatory disorders, resulting in alteration of the infraglottic power source, will be discussed in more detail relative to individual case studies later in the text.

## Myoelastic-Aerodynamic Theory

Vocal fold vibration occurs when the infraglottic power source generates airflow through the closed vocal folds. Videostroboscopic visualization of the glottis, coupled with our understanding of laryngeal anatomy, have contributed significantly to the understanding of the physiology of vocal fold vibration. At the start of a vibratory cycle the true vocal folds are preset in a closed position in the midline of the glottis. Closure of the true vocal folds is achieved by contraction of the intrinsic adductor musculature, described earlier. Subglottic air pressure increases with volitional respiratory efforts to produce voice. When this pressure exceeds the resistance created by the closed vocal folds, the lower vocal fold margins will begin to open. Traveling mucosal waves with vertical and horizontal phase delays occur. This phenomenon is characterized by sequential opening of the vocal folds from their inferior to superior margins, as illustrated in Figure 1–14. The wave then continues from medial to lateral over the flat, horizontal surfaces of the vocal folds, in a rippling-like fashion. As the superior margins begin to open they emit a puff of air, which initiates the vacuumous Bernoulli effect. This results in rapid closure of the inferior margins of the vocal folds be-

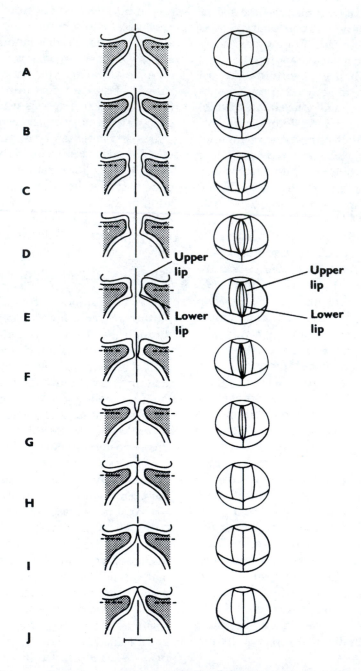

**FIGURE 1–14.** Normal vocal fold vibratory characteristics seen from a coronal view. Note that the vocal fold opens and closes sequentially from its inferior to superior lip margins. (From *Videostroboscopic Examination of the Larynx* by M. Hirano & D. M. Bless, 1993, p. 24. Copyright 1993 Singular Publishing Group, Inc. Reprinted with permission.)

fore the upper margins have completely opened. The Bernoulli force results from increases in the velocity of air molecules passing through the narrow glottic inlet, thus decreasing air pressure between the vocal folds and inducing glottic closure. Intrinsic laryngeal muscle closing forces and elastic properties of the upper vocal fold margins, combined with loss of air pressure as the puff of air passes beyond the glottis, result in closure of the upper margin to complete a glottal cycle. The ability to sustain vibration of the vocal folds during phonation is based on this myoelastic-aerodynamic interaction; that is, as long as infraglottic support of the air column continues, high enough infraglottic air pressures to overcome the muscular and elastic closing forces of the vocal folds will occur to sustain phonation.

## Parameters of Voice

There are three primary parameters of human voice: quality, loudness, and pitch. The quality, timbre, or overall pleasantness of voice is largely dependent upon the extent to which the vocal folds vibrate symmetrically and completely at the midline of the glottis. Any disturbance that adversely affects the synchrony or competency of vocal fold vibrations will likely distort the voice signal and the quality of sound produced. Excess noise is the consequence of escape of unphonated air through leaks in the glottis. When noise mixes with voice, the result is abnormal vocal quality. Terms such as hoarseness, breathiness, harshness, raspy, tremorous, and spasmodic are commonly used to describe quality disorders.

Vocal loudness, or intensity, is measured in decibels (dB) and is directly influenced by subglottal air pressure, glottal resistance force created by the myoelastic properties of the vocal folds, transglottal airflow rate, and amplitude of vocal fold vibration. Increasing these parameters will result in a louder voice. For example, to increase sub-

glottic air pressure, glottal compression force will increase owing to elevation of myoelastic tissue resistance of the vocal folds. As air molecules push through the constricted glottis, under these elevated respiratory and laryngeal forces, the amplitude of vocal fold vibration increases. This myoelastic-aerodynamic effect induces steep and forceful closing actions of the vocal folds, which result in louder voice. It is the briskness of vocal fold closure, which causes excitation of air in the vocal tract, that energizes the sound produced. These events are responsible for perceptual increases in vocal loudness.

Pitch, or frequency, is measured in cycles per second, or Hertz (Hz), and is directly influenced by alterations in the length, tension, and cross-sectional mass of the vocal folds. Cricothyroid muscle contraction results in lengthening of the vocal fold, which effects an increase in vocal fold tension and a reduction in cross-sectional mass. Under this condition the speed of vibration is faster than when the vocal folds are shorter, thicker, and more lax. Contraction of the thyroarytenoid muscle causes an increase in vocal fold body stiffness. Both increased tension and stiffness of the vocal folds result in increased velocity of vibration, which translates into higher vocal pitch. The vocal fold anatomical differences between males and females account for their fundamental frequency variations. Most males generate an habitual pitch of 128 Hz. Most females vocalize at twice this speed of vibration during normal phonation efforts.

Pitch can be characterized by concentration of sound energies at a particular fundamental frequency ($F_0$), as well as at several higher pitched harmonics of the fundamental. These harmonics can be enhanced or attenuated by increasing or decreasing sound energy levels at particular frequencies. Such alterations are dependent upon dynamic adjustments in the shape of the supraglottic larynx, pharynx, and oral and nasal cavities that occur during phonation. These enhanced frequencies are known as formants. They are partially responsible for the overall quality of voice. In fact, singers and professional voice users have a characteristic resonating voice that can usually be heard over background noise. This vocal quality is attributed to alterations of the shape of the supraglottic vocal tract, thus enhancing a harmonic occurring at approximately 3000 Hz. This harmonic is referred to as the singer's formant.

## CONCLUSION

In summary, laryngeal anatomy and physiology of phonation have been briefly reviewed. The laryngeal framework consists of nine cartilages, suspended in the anterior neck region by a complex array of ligaments, muscles, and specialized joints. Within this rigid framework rest the vocal folds. The extrinsic and intrinsic laryngeal muscles work in concert to regulate laryngeal positioning and vocal fold vibratory dynamics during acts of respiration, deglutition, and voice production. Blood supply to the larynx is provided by the superior and inferior thyroid arteries. The primary peripheral nerve supply to and from the larynx is the tenth cranial nerve, through its superior and recurrent laryngeal branches. The microscopic anatomy of the vocal fold permits fluency of vibration of the epithelial cover over the body, resulting in production of sound. This sound is altered by the infraglottic and supraglottic vocal tracts, imparting such characteristics as voice quality, loudness, and pitch. Pathology involving the vocal fold cover or body, respiratory vocal tract power source, or supraglottic vocal tract structures may all cause dysphonia. These pathologies will be discussed in greater detail in subsequent chapters.

## REFERENCES

Baer, T., Sasaki, C., & Harris, K. S. (1987). *Vocal fold physiology: Laryngeal function in phonation and respiration*. San Diego: College-Hill Press.

Bailey, B. J., & Biller, H. F. (Eds). (1985). *Surgery of the larynx*. Philadelphia: W. B. Saunders, Inc.

Benninger, M. S., Jacobson, B. H., & Johnson, A. F. (1994). *Vocal arts medicine: The care and prevention of professional voice disorders*. New York: Thieme Medical Publishing.

Cooper, D. (1988). The laryngeal mucosa in voice production. *Ear Nose and Throat Journal, 67*, 332–352.

Fawett, D. W. (1986). *A textbook of histology* (11th ed.). Philadelphia: W. B. Saunders, Inc.

Fink, B. R. (1975). *The human larynx: A functional study*. New York: Raven Press.

Ford, C. N., & Bless, D. M. (1991). *Phonosurgery assessment and surgical management of voice disorders*. New York: Raven Press.

Gould, W. J., Sataloff, R. T., & Spiegel, J. R. (1993). *Voice surgery*. St. Louis, Mosby.

Hirano, M. (1975). Phonosurgery. Basic and clinical investigations. *Otologia (Fukuoka), 21*, 239–442.

Hirano, M. (1981). *Clinical examination of voice*. New York: Springer-Verlag.

Hollinshead, W. H. (1982). *Anatomy for surgeons: Vol. I. The head and neck* (3rd ed.). Philadelphia: Harper & Row.

Isshiki, N. (1989). *Phonosurgery theory and practice*. Tokyo: Springer-Verlag.

Kent, R. D., & Vorperian, H. K. (1995). Development of the craniofacial-oral-laryngeal anatomy: A review. *Journal of Medical Speech-Language Pathology, 3*(3), 144–190.

O'Rahilly, R. (1986). *Anatomy: A regional study of human structure* (5th ed.). Philadelphia: W. B. Saunders.

Petcu, L. G., & Sasaki, C. T. (1991). Laryngeal anatomy and physiology. *The Clinics of Chest Medicine, 12*(3), 415–423.

Purser, S., Meleca, R. J., & Dworkin, J. P. (1996). Cricoarytenoid joint motion using 3-D reconstructions. Manuscript submitted for publication.

Sadler, T. W. (1985). *Langman's medical embryology* (5th ed.). Baltimore: Williams & Wilkins.

Sasaki, C., & Isaacson, G. (1988). Functional anatomy of the larynx. *The Otolaryngologic Clinics of North America, 21*, 595–611.

Sataloff, R. T. (1992). Office evaluation of dysphonia. *The Otolaryngologic Clinics of North America, 25*, 843–855.

Sataloff, R. T. (1995). Rational thought: The impact of voice science upon voice care. *Journal of Voice, 9*(3), 215–234.

Singh, W., & Soutar, D. S. (1993). *Functional surgery of the larynx and pharynx.* London: Butterworth-Heinemann.

Steinberg, J. L., Khane, G. J., Fernandes, C. M. C., & Nel, J. P. (1986). Anatomy of the recurrent laryngeal nerve: A redescription. *Journal of Laryngology and Otology, 100*, 919–927.

Titze, I. R., & Talkin, D. T. (1979). A theoretical study of the effects of various laryngeal configurations on the acoustics of phonation. *Journal of the Acoustical Society of America, 66*, 60–74.

Titze, I. R. (1980). Comments on the myoelastic-aerodynamic theory of phonation. *Journal of Speech and Hearing Research, 23*, 496–510.

Titze, I. R. (Ed.). (1993). *Vocal fold physiology frontiers in basic science.* San Diego: Singular Publishing Group.

Williams, P. L., Warwick, R., Dyson, M., & Bannister, L. H. (Eds.). (1989). *Gray's anatomy* (37th ed.). London: Churchhill Livingstone.

# CHAPTER

# 2

# *Evaluating The Patient*

This chapter reviews various office and voice laboratory examination procedures that may be employed to diagnose voice disorders. The techniques discussed highlight the methodology we routinely follow. Experienced laryngologists and speech-language pathologists may elect to retain the evaluation tools and steps that they have developed over the years. Others may discover that the approaches detailed here are worth adopting. The data for all case studies reported in this text were gathered according to these methods. To foster the flow of information presented, all supportive references have been deliberately withheld from the text and can be found in the list of suggested readings at the end of the chapter.

## ROLE OF THE LARYNGOLOGIST

The patient with persistent voice difficulties often visits an internist or general practitioner initially. This type of physician does not usually conduct more than a cursory or routine examination of the phonation subsystem. When laryngeal pathology is sus-

pected, a referral is made to a laryngologist for differential diagnosis and treatment.

The proper diagnostic workup for a patient with dysphonia should always begin with a thorough review of the history of the complaints, followed by a comprehensive physical examination of the head and neck region. Most laryngologists routinely include either an indirect mirror or fiberoptic endoscopic examination of the larynx in the initial assessment protocol. Based on the information obtained from the history taking and initial physical examination procedures, the laryngologist may either prescribe additional testing or specific treatment. For some patients, in-depth voice laboratory analyses are recommended to facilitate differential diagnosis. This may involve any combination of the following procedures: (1) high quality audiotape recordings for detailed perceptual analyses of voice abnormalities, (2) acoustic and speech aerodynamic measurements, (3) videolaryngostroboscopy, and (4) laryngeal electromyography.

For those with suspicious signs and symptoms, in addition to voice laboratory assessments, any of the following may be indicated: (1) head and neck CT scans, (2) chest x-rays, (3) blood tests, (4) thyroid scans, and (5) triple endoscopy and biopsies. Many patients do not require any ancillary evaluations, and may be effectively treated with various types of medications, brief periods of vocal rest, or both.

The laryngologist is responsible for analyzing all clinical, laboratory, and operating room data that were obtained from the patient. This investigative process usually leads to differential medical diagnosis and definitive treatment decisions, which may include recommendations for prescription drugs, surgery, and/or voice therapy. The laryngologist usually notifies the referring practitioner of the results obtained.

## ROLE OF THE SPEECH-LANGUAGE PATHOLOGIST

When the laryngologist consults the speech-language pathologist about a patient with voice difficulties, it is usually to obtain a comprehensive voice evaluation, and to institute a therapy program if requested and indicated. In some facilities, the speech-language pathologist also performs the videostroboscopy examination of the larynx. Data derived from this examination may be sought by the laryngologist to aid in the overall differential diagnosis of the laryngeal pathology initially identified.

The speech-language pathologist is responsible for preparing a detailed evaluation for the laryngologist, but should not proceed with voice therapy until the laryngologist authorizes initation of the program. For some patients, therapy alone may be considered by both the laryngologist and the speech-language pathologist to be the treatment of choice. Simultaneous administration of antireflux, antihistamine, nasal steroid, and/or antibiotic medication may be prescribed. For others, therapy may be indicated following laryngeal surgery. There are some patients for whom therapy may be contraindicated.

The speech-language pathologist and the laryngologist should work as a team with all patients who exhibit clinically significant voice disorders. Together, these practitioners offer patients a combination of skills that ensures the medical and therapeutic attention often necessary to resolve the problem. By keeping the laryngologist informed of progress in therapy and weekly interactions with patients, the speech-language pathologist provides continuity of care throughout the rehabilitation process.

Figure 2–1 is an algorithm that summarizes the role of the laryngologist and speech-language pathologist.

## HISTORY TAKING

The interview/history-taking process is of vital importance in the voice clinic because it enables the examiner to set the proper clinical mood, allows the patient to express important feelings and concerns, and provides the opportunity to explore numerous factors that may be causally related to the voice disorder. The astute clinician directs the line of questioning to avoid superfluous conversation, and usually permits the patient to do most of the talking during this segment of the examination. This strategy yields a good voice sample and at the same time allows for efficient extraction of valuable information regarding the presenting symptoms. Most experienced clinicians can obtain these important data without making the patient feel rushed or offended.

The interview should be conducted prior to formal examination of the patient. Its purpose is to explore, in as much detail as necessary, the medical and personal background that may relate to the reasons for the referral and evaluation. Normally, this exchange begins with a cordial greeting and is followed by a deliberate series of questions that probe these areas of importance. Good interviewers usually establish a friendly but professional atmosphere. Conducting a successful patient interview is an art that requires repeated practice before the process is mastered.

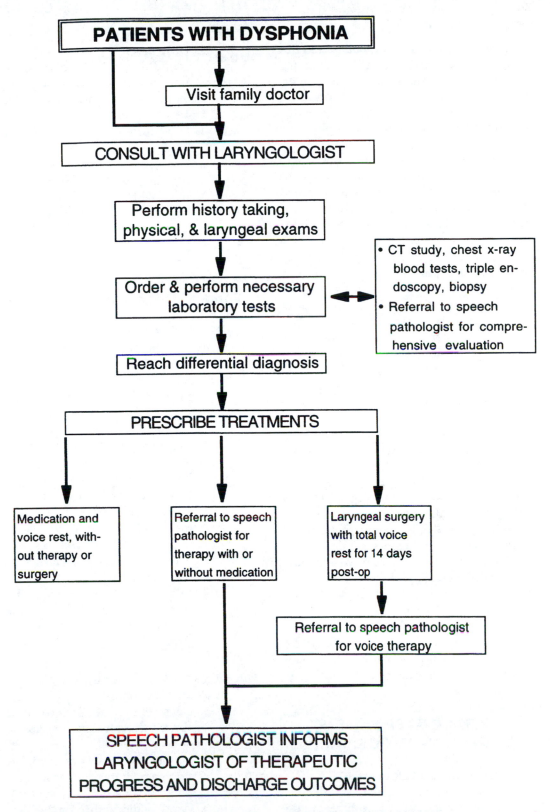

**FIGURE 2–1.** Algorithm that summarizes the roles of the laryngologist and speech-language pathologist in the evaluation and treatment of patients with voice disorders.

If the types of questions outlined in this chapter are routinely asked, and the patient's answers are guided by the interviewer so that specific information is obtained, the interview component of the evaluation should rarely exceed 10 to 15 minutes.

Although the style of questioning will vary from one practitioner to another, the information sought from all patients should remain relatively constant. Therefore, it is recommended that all of the categories discussed here be included in every initial interview. Answers to the questions posed in each area of inquiry should be recorded by the examiner. Table 2–1 illustrates a sample checklist form that can be duplicated for use during the interview process. Following the specific sequence listed here may prove beneficial, as this system was developed by the authors to ensure complete coverage of the patient's background using an easy-to-remember acronym: "I MADE A SPEECH."

Each letter in this mnemonic code represents in sequence 1 of the 12 separate interview steps described here. The "I" stands for Impressions of Dysphonia (Step I), the "M" symbolizes Medical-Surgical History (Step II), the "A" refers to Abusive Voice Patterns (Step III), and so on. Note that a scoring system is recommended, wherein certain abnormalities detected by the interviewer or described by the patient are checked and scored according to the perceived degree of severity. These ratings will facilitate writing the final report. Use of either this technique or another program designed for similar purposes is crucial to the overall evaluation process.

## TWELVE-STEP PATIENT INTERVIEW FORMAT

I. Impressions of Dysphonia
   A. Examiner Perceptions:
      1. What abnormal features are detected in the patient's voice?
      2. How severely abnormal does it sound? Do the voice characteristics vary throughout the interview, or are they relatively stable?
   B. Patient Responses:
      1. How long has the dysphonia persisted?
      2. Is it getting better, remaining constant, or has it progressively worsened?
      3. Are there times in the day when the voice is better or worse?
      4. Is the voice ever completely normal?

II. Medical-Surgical History/Medicine Usage
   A. Patient Responses:
      1. Has the patient undergone surgery requiring intubation anesthesia, which may causally relate to the onset of the voice disorder?
      2. Is there a history of trauma to the head and neck region that may explain voice changes?
      3. Are there any other salient medical problems for which the patient is under the care of other physicians? For example, is there a history of stroke or other neurologic disorders, thyroid disease, high blood presssure, diabetes, or lung disease?
      4. What types of medicine does the patient currently use, and for what conditions have they been prescribed?

III. Abusive Voice Patterns/Allergies
   A. Patient Responses:
      1. Does the patient admit to voice abuse behaviors at work, home, or play?
      2. Is the patient involved in singing activities, either in a local group or place of worship?
      3. What is the nature of the suspected voice abuse patterns?

**TABLE 2–1.** History-taking form, that may be used for listing salient abnormal characteristics during the history-taking examination.

---

**CASE HISTORY INFORMATION**

PLACE OF EXAMINATION

Patient's Name :          Sex:      D.O.B.

Address:

City:          State      Zip

Phone:    Home: (  )      Work: (  )

Date of Examination:      Examiner:

Presenting Complaint:

**SEVERITY SCORING KEY:**    1=Mild    2=Moderate    3=Severe    4=Profound

INSTRUCTIONS: Place √ next to the applicable choice(s) in each category of investigation. For each abnormal finding, either use the adjacent box to record a severity score (1-4) for the listing, or describe the specific problem.

1. **Impression of Patient's Voice**
   A. Quality

   | | | |
   |---|---|---|
   | a. Normal | b. Hoarse | c. Raspy |
   | d. Harsh | e. Strained | f. Breathy |
   | g. Whispered | h. Tremorous | i. Wet-Gurgly |
   | j. Hypernasal | k. Hyponasal | l. Variable |

   B. Pitch

   | | | |
   |---|---|---|
   | a. Normal | b. Reduced Range | c. Monotone |
   | d. Too High | e. Too Low | f. Shrill |
   | g. Pitchbreaks | h. Variable | i. Constant |

   C. Loudness

   | | | |
   |---|---|---|
   | a. Normal | b. Reduced Range | c. Monoloud |
   | d. Too Loud | e. Outbursts | f. Variable |

2. **Medical-Surgical History/Medications**

   A. Has patient had any type of surgery in past?   Yes _____    No _____
   If "Yes," list previous types of surgery and dates of intubation:

   _____

   B. Did the voice disorder coincide with head or neck trauma/injury?   Yes _____    No _____
   If "Yes," list when it occurred and the cause:

   _____

   C. Does patient report any of the following types of salient medical problems?
   Stroke _____ Date _____     Hypertension _____ Date of onset _____
   Other Neurological Disorders _____
   Diabetes _____ Date of onset _____ Thyroid Problems _____ Date of onset _____
   Heart Disease _____ Date of onset _____
   D. List present medications and purpose for use:

   _____

3. **Abusive Voice Patterns/Allergies**

   A. Does patient admit to abusive voice patterns? (e.g., yells at children, loud talk over noise at work, screams at ballgames, sings in choir.)   Yes _____ No _____
   If "Yes," describe specific types:   Loudness (1-4) [ ]    Talkativeness (1-4) [ ]

   _____

   B. Does patient complain of allergies? (e.g. hay fever, dust, animals.)   Yes _____ No _____
   If "Yes,"describe types: _____

   _____

**TABLE 2–I.** *(continued)*

4.   **Dysphagia/Aspiration**

   A.  Are there complaints of swallowing difficulties?     Yes _____     No _____

   If "Yes," describe specific symptoms:     Solids _____     Liquids _____

   B.  Is the patient aspirating liquids, solids, or both?     Yes _____     No _____

   If "Yes," describe complaints (e.g., coughing, choking): _____

   C.  Has the patient noticed wheezing sounds?     Yes _____     No _____

   If "Yes," describe features: _____

   D.  Has the patient experienced recent fevers?     Yes _____     No _____

5.   **Esophageal Reflux**

   A.  Is the patient suffering from any of the following types of reflux symptoms?

   If "Yes," check specific types.

   _____ Heartburn          _____ AM Sore Throat          _____ Throat Clearing from Excessive Phlegm

   _____ PM Sour Taste      _____ Globus Sensation        _____ Chronic Cough

   B.  Diet

   _____ Coffee-tea         _____ Chocolate               _____ Spicy Foods          _____ Citric Juice

6.   **Auditory Acuity**

   A.  Does the patient have a hearing loss?     Yes _____     No _____

   If "Yes," circle type (sensorineural/conductive/mixed)     Wears an aid? Yes _____     No _____

7.   **Shortness of Breath/Stridor/Speech Difficulties**

   A.  Is the patient short of breath?     Yes _____     No _____

   If "Yes," describe the symptoms and circumstances: _____

   B.  When the patient takes a deep breath are there audible vocal sounds (stridor)? Yes _____     No _____

   If "Yes," describe the severity, features, and inducing factors: _____

8.   **Purpose of Visit**

   A.  What is the primary reason for the patient's visit?     List the patient's responses: _____

9.   **Emotional Status of Patient**

   A.  Has the patient been under an unusual amount of emotional stress and anxiety in the recent past?

   If "Yes," describe the reasons: _____

10.  **ETOH (alcohol)/Tobacco Use**

   A.  Does the patient smoke or chew tobacco?     Yes _____     No _____

   If "Yes," what type, how much per day, and for how long? _____

   B.  Does the patient drink alcoholic beverages?     Yes _____     No _____

   If "Yes," what type, how much per day, and for how long? _____

11.  **Clearing of Throat/Coughing**

   A.  Does the patient admit to chronic throat clearing? Yes _____     No _____

   If "Yes," describe degree and date of onset: _____

   B.  Does the patient struggle with excess coughing?     Yes _____     No _____

   If "Yes," describe degree and date of onset: _____

12.  **History of Voice Difficulties**

   A.  Is there a past history of voice difficulties?     Yes _____     No _____

   If "Yes," describe what types, how they were treated, and whether they resolved.

4. Is there a positive past medical history of allergies, such as hay fever, allergic rhinitis, sinusitis, or abnormal food sensitivity?

IV. **Dysphagia/Aspiration**
   A. Examiner Perceptions:
   1. Does the voice sound wet-gurgly in quality?
   B. Patient Responses:
   1. Has the patient lost an undesired amount of weight in the recent past, owing to difficulty swallowing?
   2. Is the patient experiencing symptoms of aspiration, such as a chronic cough that is exacerbated when eating?
   3. Has there been a recent bout of pneumonia?

V. **Esophageal Reflux**
   A. Patient Responses:
   1. Are acid indigestion, heartburn, sour taste in the mouth, paroxysmal coughing when lying flat in bed, morning hoarseness or sore throat, or other forms of gastro-esophageal-reflux phenomena currently being experienced by the patient?
   2. If so, how long has this been going on, and what measures, if any, have been taken to combat these symptoms?
   3. What is the dietary history of the patient (i.e., coffee, tea, chocolates, colas, late night eating habits, etc.)?

VI. **Auditory Acuity**
   A. Examiner Perceptions:
   1. Does the patient appear to be struggling to hear the questions posed?
   B. Patient Responses:
   1. Does the patient report a history of hearing impairment?

2. If so, has an audiologic evaluation been conducted to assess the nature of the problem and the feasibility of fitting an aid?
3. What were the results of such examination?

VII. **Shortness of Breath/Stridor/Speech Difficulties**
   A. Examiner Perceptions:
   1. Does the patient exhibit any speech difficulties caused by neurologic deficits or anatomic anomalies that in any way might relate to the voice disorder?
   2. Is the patient significantly overweight?
   B. Patient Responses:
   1. Is the patient experiencing difficulty breathing during rest, play, or both?
   2. If so, are these symptoms accompanied by stridorous laryngeal behavior that can be detected during the interview or with use of a stethoscope?
   3. Is there a history of asthma, emphysema, or congestive heart disease?

VIII. **Patient's Perceptions of the Voice Difficulty**
   A. Patient Responses:
   1. What is the patient's reasons for making the appointment?
   2. On an equal appearing interval scale of 1 to 7, wherein a score of 1 represents normal voice and 7 indicates the most deviant from normal voice imaginable, what is the patient's own perceptions of the degree of voice difficulty exhibited?

IX. **Emotional Status of the Patient**
   A. Examiner Perceptions:
   1. Based on all of the findings accumulated for the patient at the

conclusion of the evaluation process, is there a strong and probable relationship between the dysphonia and any underlying tension-stress disorder?

B. Patient Responses:

1. Has the patient been under an unusual amount of stress or emotional anxiety in the recent past?
2. If so, what is the primary origin of the problem?

X. ETOH (Alcohol) Consumption and Tobacco Use

A. Patient Responses:

1. Is there a history of cigarette use, alcohol abuse, or both?
2. What are the specific details (e.g., amount per day and years of use)?

XI. Clearing of the Throat and Coughing Activities

A. Examiner Perceptions:

1. Does the patient clear the throat, cough, or both during the evaluation process?
2. If so, how severely?

B. Patient Responses:

1. Does the patient report excessive bouts of throat clearing, coughing, or both?
2. If so, how long has such difficulty been going on?
3. Does the problem occur on a daily basis?
4. How severe is it?
5. To what does the patient attribute these symptoms?
6. Is the patient struggling with symptoms and signs of post-nasal drip, or has there been a recent upper respiratory infection?

XII. History of Voice Difficulty

A. Patient Responses:

1. Is the presenting dysphonia unique to the patient's previous medical history, or have there been difficulties with voice ability in the past?
2. If so, what types?
3. Were treatments rendered at that time?
4. What were the outcomes?

## BACKGROUND HISTORY: AREAS OF INVESTIGATION

### The Discovery Process

The patient interview paves the way for the physical, laryngeal, and voice examinations. Before proceeding with the details of such testing, explanations for engaging the patient in this 12-step questioning paradigm are reviewed.

#### I. Impressions of Dysphonia

Describing the patient's voice characteristics using terms that are clear to the patient and other team members is an essential but arduous task. The descriptions and severity ratings generated in this segment of the evaluation are critical for various reasons. Most important, these data may be used at a later date to compare perceptual judgments of the patient's post-treatment voice parameters.

There are no universally accepted systems upon which we can rely for an accurate, unequivocal classification of the perceived voice difficulty. Because this process is wholly subjective and largely dependent upon the clinician's professional background and listening skills, esoteric descriptors should be abandoned in favor of clear and concise descriptions of the overall voice patterns. We prefer terms such as *hoarse, breathy, raspy, harsh, strained, gurgly, tremorous, high pitched, too loud,* and *variable* to describe the voice abnormality features. These expressions are, for the most part, self-explanatory. Certain alternative classifications suggested in the literature, such as *rough, thinness, asthenic,* and *plica ventricularis,* are considered confusing by many of our team members.

## II. Medical-Surgical History

Exploration of the patient's past medical problems and surgical experiences may reveal crucial background information that is causally related to the presenting dysphonia. Erythema, generalized edema, paresis, and paralysis of the vocal folds may occur either singly or in various combinations as sequelae to cerebral vascular accidents, neurologic disease or injury, neuropathic diabetes, prolonged intubation, surgery for thyroid gland or carotid artery abnormalities, laryngeal surgery, oral and pharyngeal cavity surgery, head and neck radiation therapy, lung disease, recurring upper respiratory infections, and laryngeal trauma. Strokes that involve the upper motor neuron system may result in spastic dysarthria and associated strained-strangled phonation. This is an especially difficult problem that does not usually lend itself to medical, surgical, or therapeutic methods of rehabilitation. Other abnormal neurologic conditions, such as Parkinson's disease, multiple sclerosis, dystonia, amyotrophic lateral sclerosis, Huntington's disease, cerebral palsy, muscular dystrophy, or myasthenia gravis, often cause phonation subsystem disturbances. The resulting voice difficulties and treatment options and outcomes vary among these populations.

Patients who have been intubated during recent surgery may present with diffuse laryngeal inflammation or signs of vocal fold trauma that adversely affect voice output. In many cases, no definitive medical-surgical or vocal exercise treatments are necessary. Carotid endarterectomy and thyroid gland surgical procedures may cause temporary (neurapraxia) or permanent vocal fold paralysis as a consequence of trauma to the trunk of the vagus nerve or resection of its recurrent laryngeal branch. With neurapraxia, return of vocal function is probable. At most, stimulative behavioral exercises may be recommended to facilitate such recovery. Patients who have suffered from intractable paralysis, owing to nerve transection, may benefit from phonosurgery to improve voice control and to protect the airway. In cases like these, reviews of the past medical histories and relevant surgical charts are of paramount importance to the development and implementation of effective treatment plans.

Wet-gurgly vocal quality is often a disabling side effect of ablative surgeries involving the oral and pharyngeal cavities. The patient whose larynx is shown in Figure 2–2 suffered from this problem following base of tongue and pharynx surgery for squamous cell carcinoma, staged as a T3N2M0 lesion. Associated weakness and paresis of the tongue pumping action and pharyngeal dysmotility in this case caused saliva and mucous secretions to accumulate in the hypopharynx, and then leak into the laryngeal inlet. These viscous substances disrupted vocal fold vibrations during voice efforts, resulting in wet and gurgly vocal quality. This problem was compounded by co-occurring aspiration and associated coughing behaviors, which irritated the vocal folds and exacerbated the dysphonia.

Lung diseases such as emphysema, tuberculosis, and asthma may threaten the airflow requirements for normal voice production. Volume may be weak, syllables per breath may be reduced, and vocal fatigue may occur as a consequence of such downstream disturbances. We have treated several patients in the recent past who developed profound ventricular fold dysphonia as secondary manifestations of emphysema. Figure 2–3 illustrates the larynx of a male patient who demonstrates this abnormal behavior. We suggest that he recruits the false folds as a supplemental voice generator to overcome an insufficient source of airflow. By employing the valving action of the false folds during vocal efforts he increases glottal resistance and reduces transglottal egress. Whereas this unnatural compensatory activity extends phonation time

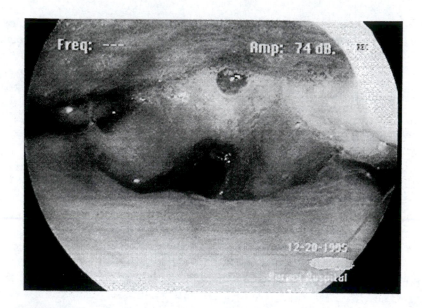

**FIGURE 2–2.** View of the laryngeal inlet of a patient who underwent ablative surgery of the base of tongue and pharynx for squamous cell carcinoma. Note the extensive amount of secretions pooling in the piriform sinuses, which leak into the glottis during inspiration. On the far right of the illustration note the presence of a Dobhoff feeding tube, which penetrates the piriform sinus enroute to the esophagus.

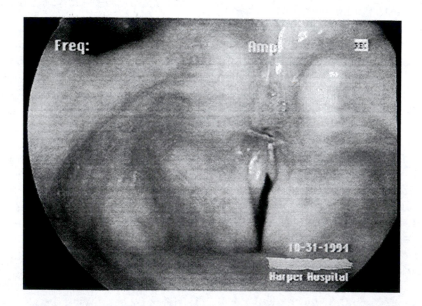

**FIGURE 2–3.** View of the laryngeal inlet of a patient with chronic emphysema who recruits the false vocal folds during all phonatory activity. Note that these folds virtually meet in the midline, obscuring views of most of the underlying true vocal fold mechanism.

and the number of syllables produced per breath, it also results in dysphonia characterized by hoarse-harsh quality and intermittent diplophonic features. Uncovering this pathophysiologic correlate helped the team members focus their attention not just on treating the patient's voice difficulties, but reassessing his current respiratory therapy protocol as well.

There are numerous other complicating illnesses that may be of etiologic significance in the management of patients with voice disorders. Invariably, these conditions influence the options for treatment and prognoses for improvement. Detailed descriptions and laryngeal photographs of patients who present with such medical backgrounds are provided in the case studies in Chapter 6.

### III. Abusive Voice Patterns

The most common cause of benign vocal fold pathologies such as diffuse polyposis Reinke's edema, Figure 2–4; hemorrhagic polyps, Figure 2–5; and nodules, Figure 2–6; is trauma to the mucosal coverings due to voice abuse or misuse. Yelling, screaming, excessive singing, protracted bouts of crying, chronically loud vocal habits, making motor noises, and so on, are the kinds of behaviors that children and adults with voice disorders are known to exhibit. These types of voice abuse patterns may be induced by the individual's personality, professional responsibilities, general lifestyle, hobbies, and home environment. Most of the time, definitive treatment involves behavioral modification therapy, including exercises to improve vocal hygiene. Even when surgery is performed for more advanced or chronic abnormalities, recurrence of the pathology and voice disorder is likely if the underlying abuse or misuse activities persist. For these reasons, exploration of this issue should be a routine policy during the history-taking process. Patients who convey little desire to change, or who demonstrate limited self-

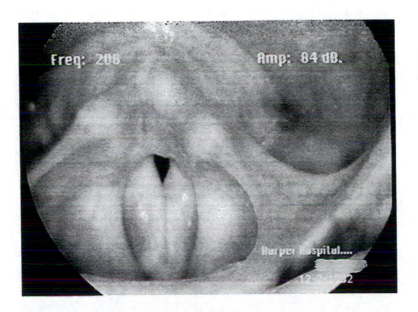

**FIGURE 2–4.** View of the laryngeal inlet of a young woman with bilateral polypoid degeneration of the true vocal folds. Note the triangular glottal chink in the posterior one-third of this mechanism. This is a characteristic feature observed in many patients with Reinke's edema.

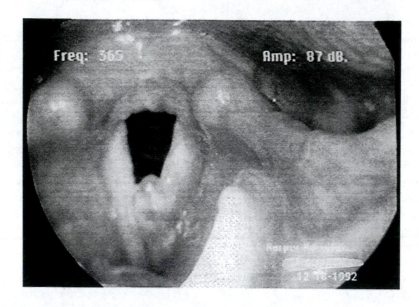

**FIGURE 2–5.** View of the laryngeal inlet of a young man with a hemorrhagic polyp emanating off of the anterior half of the left true vocal fold. Note the encroachment on the glottal space and the interference with glottal competency during phonatory effort. A large glottal chink in the posterior half of this mechanism causes profound breathy-hoarse dysphonia.

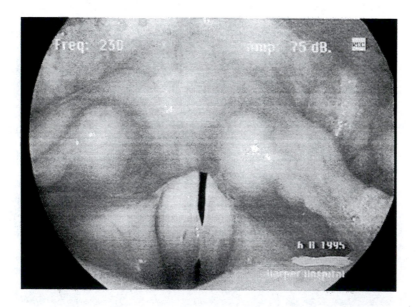

**FIGURE 2–6.** View of the laryngeal inlet of a young female nurse who frequently abuses her voice. Note the presence of a large edematous nodule on the middle one-third of the right true vocal fold and a small reactive nodule formation on the opposing fold. Also note the mild discoloration of the anterior half of both vocal folds caused by vascularity changes associated with voice abuse patterns.

control abilities, generally are not good candidates for any form of intervention that requires such cooperation to ensure satisfactory results.

## IV. Dysphagia/Aspiration

Adductor vocal fold paralysis will generally cause breathy-hoarse dysphonia early on, owing to midline glottal incompetency and coincident escapes of unphonated air during vocal efforts. With time, the uninvolved vocal fold may compensate by assuming a position across the midline of the glottis. This adjustment enables contact with the paralyzed fold, and an improvement of the glottal seal during phonation. When the paralyzed vocal fold hangs in the abducted position (Figure 2–7) the resulting dysphonia is usually worse than when it rests in the paramedian or median planes. In all cases, however, co-occurring dysphagia can be a problem because weak glottal valving threatens the airway during swallowing. Both liquid and solid food materials may be aspirated as a consequence of this condition, placing the lungs at risk for pneumonia. This risk increases in patients with bilateral paralysis, and in those with superior laryngeal nerve injuries, owing to loss of supraglottal sensation. Depending upon the etiology, and whether the condition is considered transient or permanent, definitive glottal reconstruction surgery, followed by voice and swallowing therapy, might be prescribed at the earliest possible date. If there is a chance that spontaneous recovery of the affected vocal fold might occur within a short period of time because of the nature of the underlying cause, and aspiration is not a problem, surgical management is usually delayed. In cases like this, behavioral exercise programs are ordinarily employed to stimulate rehabilitation

When the patient exhibits bilateral adductor paralysis, regardless of the cause,

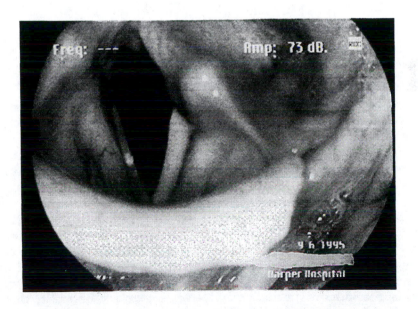

**FIGURE 2–7.** View of the laryngeal inlet of a middle-aged female with right vocal fold paralysis, which occurred several years after a complicated thyroidectomy procedure. Note that the paralyzed cord is atrophic and hangs in the abducted position. The patient's voice is profoundly breathy in quality and she struggles from episodic aspiration symptoms.

surgical medialization of one or both vocal folds is usually prescribed as the primary method of treatment, followed secondarily by therapy programs to improve voice and swallowing functions. Whereas a tracheostomy is usually required for this type of patient, at least in the beginning as a method of secretion control, it is not always necessary for the patient with unilateral paralysis. Phonosurgical intervention, such as medialization thyroplasty, may obviate the need for a tracheostomy.

Dysphagia and aspiration signs and symptoms may also be sequelae to vocal fold growths and lesions that significantly interfere with glottal closure dynamics. Malignant neoplasms, hemorrhagic polyps, nodules, submucosal cysts, traumatic scarring, and fibrotic stiffness of the vocal folds are examples of abnormal conditions that have been shown to be causally related to swallowing difficulties. Investigation of these types of complaints during the history-taking component of the examination is of utmost importance because the information gathered may significantly influence both testing and treatment decisions.

### V. Esophageal Reflux

This term has recently become popular in gastroenterology and otolaryngology clinics. The patient who complains about one or more of the following types of symptoms may be suffering from gastro-esophageal-reflux disease (GERD) and associated laryngitis and pharyngitis: (1) excessive belching, (2) acid indigestion, especially during sleep, (3) heartburn, (4) a sour taste in the mouth, (5) chronic sore throats, (6) persistent hoarseness without vocal abuse history, and (7) a globus (lump in the throat) sensation. The diagnosis of GERD is based both on clinical examination results, including exploration of the chief complaints of the patient, and an assortment of laboratory studies. For some patients, barium swallow examinations may prove helpful by highlighting overall esophageal motility and up-per and lower sphincter disturbances. For others, PH-monitoring and esophageal manometry evaluations offer definitive data regarding the presence and degree of GERD. Endoscopic study enables close anatomical inspection of the hypopharyngeal and esophageal mucosa for signs of acid regurgitation. Laryngologic examination may illustrate one or more of the following adverse effects of gastric acid on the mucosa lining the laryngopharynx: (1) edema and erythema of the arytenoids, vocal folds, postcricoid region, pyriform sinuses, and posterior pharyngeal wall, (2) ulcerations or granulation tissue over the vocal processes of the arytenoids, and (3) hyperplastic and redundant mucosa of the posterior commissure and interarytenoid regions.

Figure 2–8 illustrates some of these features in a 44- year-old male who admits to a hypertensive personality and late night eating binges. These anatomical anomalies may trigger abnormal vocal fold vibratory patterns and coincident degrees of dysphonia. For many patients, definitive treatment of these disturbances involves behavior modification strategies, such as changing the diet, establishing a weight loss program, and propping up the head of the bed to counter reflux potential during sleep. Other patients may not respond as well to such techniques without additional relief from medication. Whereas over-the-counter antacid liquids or chewable tablets may be of help for some individuals, the vast majority of these patients will require prescription-strength medication. The most common acid blockers used for such purposes include cimetadine (Tagamet), ranitadine (Zantac), and omeprazole (Prilosec). Reflux-induced laryngeal pathologies often resolve with effective behavioral modification, coupled with pharmacologic management when necessary. In cases of chronic, persistent, and relatively severe GERD, phonosurgery and voice therapy may be unavoidable. For these reasons, it is extremely important that the aforementioned signs and symptoms of GERD be discussed and

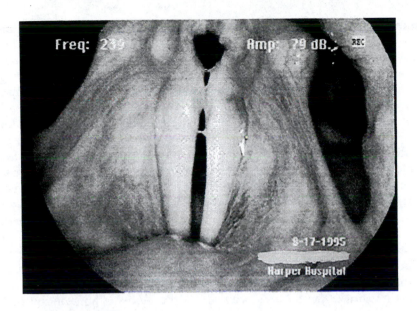

Freq: 239    Amp: 29 dB.    REC

8-17-1995

Harper Hospital

**FIGURE 2–8.** View of the laryngeal inlet of a middle-aged man with bilateral contact ulcerations on the medial surfaces of the vocal processes of the arytenoids. Also note the mild erythema in this location as well as pachydermal growth spreading into the interarytenoid region. This patient suffers from profound symptoms of gastro-esophageal reflux disease. His voice is mildly to moderately harsh-hoarse in quality

explored with every patient during the history-taking process.

### VI. Auditory Acuity

A conductive hearing loss may result in an abnormally soft voice. This occurs because the voice is heard through cranial bone conduction pathways without the feedback benefits of ongoing air conduction through the external and middle ear cavities. To the patient, the voice generated sounds quite loud as a consequence of this air-bone conduction imbalance. A sensorineural hearing loss may cause the patient to speak in an abnormally loud voice. This phenomenon occurs because bone conduction and neural transmission of the voice signal to the brain is faulty, and the patient inadvertently increases vocal loudness to compensate for the problem. Patients who are severely hard of hearing or deaf may abuse their vocal folds because of habitually loud, unmonitored voice behaviors.

Inquiring about hearing status during the patient interview is very important. Signs such as these, as well as indications that the patient is having a hard time hearing the questions posed, should be noted. Correlations between the types of voice difficulties exhibited and coexisting hearing loss should be considered. Full scale audiologic evaluations are necessary when hearing loss is suspected. Sometimes, fitting an appropriate hearing aid is sufficient to correct the associated voice disorder.

### VII. Shortness of Breath/Stridor/Speech Difficulties

Bulky vocal fold lesions can compromise transglottal airflow dynamics during speech production and nonspeech breathing activities. This interruptive effect may lead to shortness of breath, as the patient struggles to drive air through the glottal obstruction. Bilateral abductor paralysis often causes profound dyspnea. Figure 2–9 illustrates the larynx of a young man who underwent prolonged intubation following a closed head injury. Note that this photo depicts the profound degree of bilateral abductor paralysis of the vocal folds during deep inhalation efforts. Also observe the granulation tissue formation in the posterior glottal region, which likely developed as a consequence of emergency tube placement and extended dependence upon this artificial ventilation source. Curiously, for several weeks prior to this evaluation, the patient was treated for bronchitis because his internist had mistaken the stridorous breathing sounds as evidence of pulmonary wheezing. He was referred to otolaryngology service because of mildly hoarse vocal quality, not stridor. Results of the examination led to an emergency tracheostomy and

discontinuation of antibiotic therapy. Although the etiology of the paralysis was unclear, focal trauma associated with the emergency room intubation procedure was strongly suspected. In most instances, paralysis of this type is usually a temporary (neurapraxia) phenomenon. However, the length of time to full recovery is unpredictable, and may range from a few days to as long as one year. Definitive surgical repair, which may include laser cordotomy techniques, is normally delayed 9 to 12 months until no further improvements are likely to occur.

Both unilateral and bilateral adductor vocal fold paralysis may also result in shortness of breath. Stridor is not evident, as the glottis is abnormally wide and airflow is excessive, especially during vocalization. Because phonation time and the number of syllables produced per breath is reduced, the patient may recruit the respiratory subsystem to compensate for this

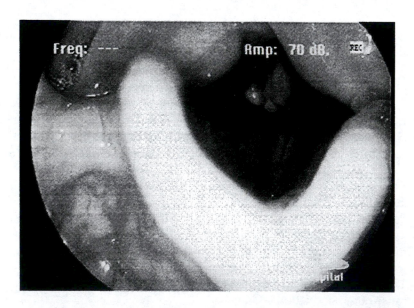

**FIGURE 2–9.** View of the laryngeal inlet of a young man with bilateral abductor vocal fold paralysis. Note the severe compromise of the airway during deep inhalation effort. Also note the moderate degree of granulation tissue in the posterior glottis region emanating from the arytenoid cartilages. These abnormal growths are likely sequelae to prolonged intubation.

problem. Frequent breaths and forceful expiratory patterns unfortunately tax the respiratory musculature. Patients who engage in these behaviors to overcome glottal incompetency often complain of shortness of breath, owing to associated pulmonary-respiratory weakness, and vocal fatigue symptoms. As mentioned earlier, patients who exhibit these types of signs and symptoms are at risk for aspiration pneumonia.

Pulmonary diseases such as emphysema, asthma, tuberculosis, neoplasms, and respiratory neuromuscular disturbances are well known causes of shortness of breath. Naturally, these conditions would not respond to the same treatments administered for laryngeal-induced breathing difficulties. The astute examiner understands these distinctions, and realizes the importance of including pulmonary function testing and chest x-rays for differential diagnosis.

Concurrent voice and speech difficulties may be of diagnostic importance. Such co-occurrence is often observed in patients with different types of dysarthria, owing to lesions involving the sensorimotor components of the central nervous system, peripheral nervous system, or both. The experienced examiner probes for pathophysiologic signs and symptoms that would implicate the nervous system and facilitate differential diagnosis of the overall communication disorder. Dysarthric patients usually exhibit varying degrees of phonation, resonation, articulation, and prosody subsystem disturbances, depending upon the lesion site and severity of involvement.

Invasive carcinoma involving the oral cavity and pharynx may also cause multiple speech subsystem breakdowns, including articulatory imprecision, slow speech rate, and hypernasality. Even if the larynx itself is free of disease, dysphonia may result from oropharyngeal secretion control problems. As mucous and saliva seep into the laryngeal inlet they trigger chronic coughing and throat clearing reflexes, which can irritate the vocal folds and cause benign inflammatory reactions and associated voice difficulties. Additionally, these secretions invariably mix with the sounds generated during phonation, giving the voice a wet-gurgly quality. Examiners should always listen for these multiple speech subsystem correlative abnormalities during the history-taking/interview session. Their presence usually compounds the subsequent diagnostic and treatment processes.

## VIII. Patient's Perceptions of the Voice Difficulty

Asking the patient to describe the voice difficulty usually provides important details about the perceived nature of the problem, and whether the characteristics have remained relatively stable or have progressively worsened. The data gathered can be compared to the examiner's impressions of the patient's voice for overall interrater reliability. Any discrepancies in the perceived dysphonia features can then be discussed and clarified. Requesting the patient to render an opinion about the problem demonstrates that the examiner is interested in hearing about the presenting complaints. This interchange reinforces the clinical rapport development process.

## IX. Emotional Status of the Patient

Stress may take many different forms: financial, marital, personal, professional, physical, mental, or emotional. Head and neck muscle tension symptoms are common sequelae to unusual and chronic degrees of stress. Hyperfunctional-hypertensive (true) and ventricular (false) vocal fold vibratory behaviors are often adverse side effects of underlying emotional anxiety associated with stress factors. The resulting voice disorder may be characterized by harsh-strained vocal quality and reduced pitch and loudness range. Probing the patient's emotional status for indications of increased stress factors may reveal causally related conditions that must be factored into the eventual treatment program.

### X. ETOH (Alcohol) Consumption and Tobacco Use

Chronic and excessive consmption of alcoholic beverages may result in systemic toxicity, with adverse effects on mental processes and functions of various body parts. Alcoholism is considered a disease, and has been shown to be causally linked to squamous cell carcinoma of the head and neck region. The use of tobacco products, especially cigarettes because they are inhaled, is highly correlated with the development of laryngeal cancer. Other, less serious conditions, such as leukoplakia or generalized erythema and edema of the vocal folds, are also frequently attributed to smoking behaviors. Even if the patient does not personally smoke, but is regularly exposed to secondary smoke in the workplace, at home, or in social settings, the larynx is still at risk for pathologic reactions. At the very least, those who smoke or who are exposed to smoke often exhibit chronic coughing activities that abuse the vocal folds and may result in diffuse edema and benign focal lesions such as nodules or hemorrhagic polyps. These individuals are also prone to respiratory difficulties, which can induce and exacerbate phonation subsystem disturbances. As a consequence of these common substance abuse problems, the ETOH consumption and tobacco use history of the patient should always be probed during the interview.

### XI. Clearing of the Throat and Coughing Activities

Perhaps the most abusive of all abnormal vocal fold behaviors are those associated with chronic throat clearing and coughing. Many patients suggest that these activities are triggered by excess mucous secretions and sinus drainage that accumulate in the hypopharynx and ultimately leak into the laryngeal inlet. Others may explain that clearing and coughing are uncontrollable reactions to a dry throat environment, which causes these hacking activities. Persistent coughing may be a side effect of asthma, often induced by exercise and physical stress, reflux laryngitis, and cigarette smoking. In many instances, throat clearing is merely a bad habit without other discernible explanations. Regardless of the cause, these behaviors result in violent forces of vocal fold contact and diffuse erythema and edema. Additional vocal fold pathologic changes may include the formation of benign growths and free edge deterioration. Figure 2–10 illustrates some of these adverse effects. The patient exhibits a mild to moderate degree of hoarse-breathy dysphonia, and lower than normal pitch features, owing to free edge glottal incompetency and underlying vocal fold edema.

Throat clearing and coughing behaviors are serious conditions that must be explored, explained, and extinguished. Antihistamine, antibiotic, nasal steroid spray, and bronchial dilator medications may help those patients who clear their throats and cough as a consequence of sinusitis, allergies, upper respiratory infections, or asthma. For others, behavioral modification therapy may be indicated to overcome these abnormal activities and improve phonation abilities.

### XII. History of Voice Difficulty

When interviewing a patient whose history is unfamiliar, it is important to ask whether or not there have been any previous voice difficulties. If the answer to this question is "yes," several additional questions must follow. It is essential to discover if the past disorder resembled the signs and symptoms of the current problem. It is equally necessary to learn about any evaluations that were conducted to determine the nature and cause of the dysphonia, and the types of treatments that may have been provided. Exploration of these factors will help determine whether the presenting disturbance is unrelated to the past vocal history, evidence of recurrence, or a sign of long-term persis-

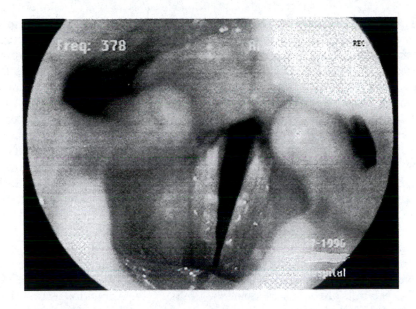

**FIGURE 2–10.** View of the laryngeal inlet of a middle-aged male who suffers from chronic throat clearing and coughing activities. Note the bilateral vocal fold edema and erythema. Also note the irregularity in the free edge anatomy of the right vocal fold. The patient suggested that the throat clearing and coughing activities are due to chronic postnasal drainage associated with allergies. His voice was moderately hoarse-breathy in quality with lower than normal pitch features.

tence of the same problem. The prognosis is usually guarded for the patient with a chronic or recurrent voice disorder, regardless of the etiology or treatment history.

## CLINICAL AND VOICE LABORATORY EXAMINATION PROCEDURES

This section focuses on the various instruments and examination techniques that may be employed to assess the anatomical and functional status of the phonation subsystem. Some of the procedures secondarily measure respiratory and overall vocal tract dynamics as well. Collectively, these procedures may yield important diagnostic information regarding these integrated systems. We consider each and every evaluation step listed here to be a critical component of the clinical examination process.

Results of some of these measurement techniques, however, may be subject to criticism because of the instruments used and the inherent limitations of the laryngeal pathologies studied. These drawbacks will be discussed subsequently.

Referrals to other laboratories and practitioners for ancillary testing often depend upon the results of the history-taking interview and voice laboratory examination. It is not uncommon to order CT and MRI scans, thyroid gland studies, chest x-rays, barium swallow analyses, and clinical evaluations by other specialists to facilitate a differential diagnosis and treatment plan.

### Audiotape Recordings

At the outset of the voice laboratory examination a high quality audiotape recording should be made for two primary reasons: First, capturing the voice and speech characteristics on tape permits convenient analyses and ratings by team members before treatment decisions are reached. Second, storing the pretreatment voice sample on tape ensures accurate posttreatment comparisons. Either a reel-to-reel or digital audiotape format should be implemented for these purposes. Standard cassette recorders, particularly those with built-in microphones, generate tapes with ambient noise that distorts the voice sample. Digital recorders are compact, produce CD quality tapes, and tag patients with ID numbers for easy file access and review. Although they may cost as much as $1,000.00 with speakers and a unidirectional microphone, they are well worth the investment in the long run. Reel-to-reel units are bulky, antiquated in design, and do not store patents by file number for easy location and review. They do, however, generate excellent quality recordings.

### Tape Samples

All recordings should be made in a relatively quiet room. Use of a unidirectional microphone will help shield some of the environmental noise from the recording. Maintaining a constant mouth-to-microphone distance of 12 to 15 cm ensures minimal degrees of signal distortion. Monitoring the loudness dial (VU meter) on the recorder is recommended throughout the recording. This procedure allows the examiner to adjust the distance of the microphone from the mouth of the patient if the voice is too loud or too soft. These modifications ensure consistent quality of recordings.

Note that for each task the examiner should judge whether it is necessary to have the patient repeat the performance one or more times to capture the true potential or disabilty. Begin the sample by requesting the patient to prolong the vowel /a/ for as long and steady as possible. During this performance the examiner should either silently count or use a stopwatch to determine the total number of seconds of vowel prolongation, which translates into the *maximum phonation* time score. Three attempts should be requested to obtain an average performance. Next, have the patient use the same vowel to sing up and down the scale several notes in each direction. For this task it may be necessary to demonstrate the behavior for some patients. Next, instruct the patient to cough sharply. Afterward, hand the patient a picture that illustrates an interesting scene involving people, and request a detailed, extemporaneous description of the events depicted. The "Cookie Theft" picture from the Boston Diagnostic Aphasia Examination serves this purpose very well. Finally, use a standard paragraph such as the "Rainbow Passage" or "My Grandfather" (see Appendix 2–1) and have the patient read it aloud. These samples usually do not take more than 5 minutes to collect. Analyzing the data, however, may take a significantly longer period of time.

### Acoustic Analysis

In the current world of high technology, use of a computer-driven program to analyze voice abnormalities objectively should not be viewed as excessive and unnecessary. Both laryngologists and speech pathologists are becoming more dependent upon and expert in the use of such instruments, in addition to their own perceptions, to characterize the parameters of voice disorders.

There are several types of commercially available systems designed exclusively for acoustic analyses. These instruments are all interfaced with computers and software programs that allow sophisticated data interpretations. Most of these systems have integrated spectrograph and waveform graphic capabilities for detailed displays of acoustic signals. Responsive to mouse and keyboard commands, these systems enable rapid data manipulation and numerous extrapolations. Although each system offers a unique blend of user friendly highlights and functions, they all provide the essential information sought by most laryngologists and speech pathologists. Recent research suggests that commercially available acoustical and speech aerodynamic analysis programs generally do not correlate highly with one another relative to the types of data they are designed to generate. These discrepancies are considered to be the result of the following interactive factors: (1) the different algorithms that have been employed by the program developers to analyze the speech samples, (2) the aperiodicity level of moderately to severely disturbed voice signals, which threatens the reliability and validity of perturbation, shimmer, and signal to noise ratio measurements, and (3) examiner biases when marking the cycle boundaries to be analyzed. Some clinical researchers have suggested that because of these inherent limitations, the values obtained during many of the acoustic and speech aerodynamic tests that are performed routinely may be invalid.

### Method of Data Collection

Voice samples should be obtained as the patient generates voice and speech at comfortable loudness levels. Unusually loud, soft, high pitched, or low pitched utterances should be discouraged so that the samples do not artificially skew the findings. Maintenance of a constant mouth-to-microphone distance of 12 to 15 cm is suggested. Begin by requesting the patient to prolong the vowel /a/ for as long and steady as possible. Before analyzing the signal, be certain to save it in its entirety. Most voice scientists then eliminate inital and final seconds of the recording, if the signal is long enough, to avoid voice onset and offset factors that may contaminate the analysis. A computer-generated printout of the acoustic features of this steady state signal include fundamental frequency, jitter, shimmer, and harmonic-to-noise ratio.

Depending upon the software used, these variables will be calculated according to slightly different formulas. Some programs provide normative baseline values for comparison and data interpretation. *Fundamental frequency* (Fo) refers to the average, most natural speed (cycles per second, or Hz) of vocal fold vibration during sustained phonation. Female and male adults average 256 and 128 Hz, respectively. The perceptual correlate of this measure is *pitch.*

*Jitter* values correspond to the degree of instability in the cycle-to-cycle (pitch) vibratory characteristics of the vocal folds. *Frequency perturbation* is a term used interchangeably with jitter. The frequency variability of a normal voice is usually less than 0.7% of the average pitch generated over the entire voice sample.

*Shimmer* is an index of vocal fold amplitude perturbation or instability. In normal phonation, the variation around the mean amplitude is not usually greater than 0.5 dB or 5% of the voice signal. Not unlike jitter values, mean shimmer is often higher in individuals with vocal fold pathologies, owing to adverse influences of such conditions on the stability of the ongoing vibratory patterns. Abnormally elevated jitter and shimmer levels are strongly correlated with perceived vocal quality disturbances. These measures are viewed by many voice scientists as important and sensitive indicators of vocal pathology. However, because jitter and shimmer are subject to contamination during testing, patients may adversely influence the results by using excessively loud, soft, high pitched, or low pitched phonation efforts. Hence, examiners need to structure the data collection process very carefully.

The *harmonic-to-noise ratio* (H/N) largely represents the amount of noise in the voice signal. All sounds generated by the larynx, both normal and abnormal, have random noise components because the vocal folds inherently vibrate aperiodically. This asymmetry of motion permits unphonated air to escape through the glottis during vocalization. The excess air-voice mixture causes noise in the signal over a broad frequency range. The H/N ratio is computed by dividing the energy levels at different sound frequencies by the underlying degree of noise. This equation is usually expressed in decibel units, and for those with normal voices the mean ratio is approximately +12.0 dB. Because patients with laryngeal pathologies generally produce increased amounts of vocal noise, their H/N ratios are typically very low. There is generally a very high correlation between the H/N ratio and perceptual ratings of the voice disorder.

Figure 2–11 illustrates the waveform and associated spectrogam of a sustained vowel produced by a patient with diffuse swelling of the vocal folds (Reinke's edema). Figure 2–12 provides a normal voice comparison. Note the differences in the appearances of the raw waveforms and spectrograms. Of particular importance is the obvious degree of noise in the voice signal, as can be extrapolated from the patient's high frequency streak artifacts on the spectrogram. This ab-

normal spectrographic feature correlates with the patient's acoustic analysis results, which suggested the presence of severe degrees of noise, jitter, and shimmr in the voice signal. Figure 2–13 was obtained from this same patient after 3 months of voice therapy (11 one-hour sessions). Note the moderate improvement in the regularity of the glottal pulses on the acoustic waveform tracing, and the reduction in the noise artifact features of the spectrogram. These changes were consistent with the patient's moderate gains in voice control and output.

Acoustic studies generate objective data regarding the functional integrity of the phonation subsystem. They are equally important measures at the completion of definitive treatment programs to assess the degree and nature of any improvements obtained. It

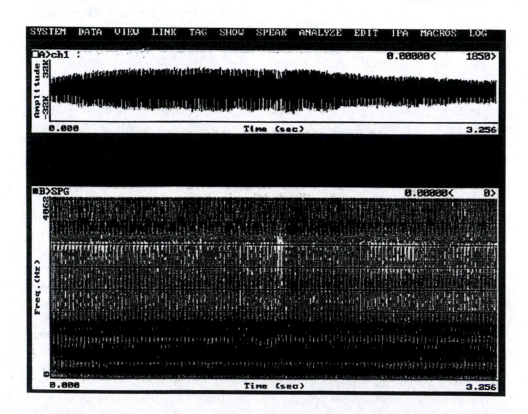

**FIGURE 2–11.** Acoustic waveform and spectrograph obtained from a patient with Reinke's edema. Note the high frequency noise artifacts on the spectrograph, which are illustrative of this patient's dysphonia.

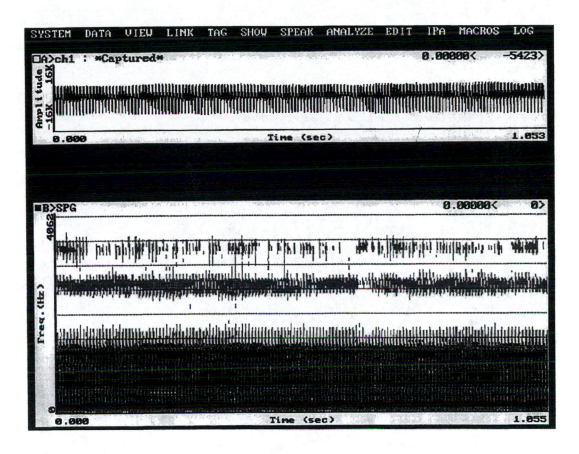

**FIGURE 2–12.** Acoustic waveform and spectrograph obtained from an individual with normal phonation. When compared to the patient in figure 2–11, these illustrations demonstrate the lack of noise and high frequency streak artifact frequently observed in patients with dysphonia.

should be remembered, however, that in cases of severe dysphonia these types of data are often unreliable. The degree of signal distortion may be so great as to elicit nonmeaningful acoustic values. Such results should be interpreted with extreme caution.

## Speech Aerodynamic Testing

### Subglottal Pressure

Air from the lungs serves as the source of energy or power for vocal fold vibration. The study of phonation would be incomplete without examination of how well this power supply is charged. Direct and indirect (noninvasive) measures of *subglottal*

*pressure* (Ps) accomplish this objective. In most clinical settings a noninvasive approach is utilized, wherein an estimate of Ps is derived from the degree of intraoral pressure that is generated during productions of vowel-consonant-vowel /ipi/ syllable trains. These measurements are made using an intraoral probe tube that is connected to a pressure transducer apparatus. The values obtained are calculated in cmH2O units. The minimal level of Ps needed to support vocal fold vibration is 5 cmH2O/5 sec. Patients with laryngeal pathologies, which cause either glottal incompetency and air wastage or airflow obstruction during phonation, often exhibit higher than normal Ps values. This occurs as a result of increased respiratory efforts to compensate

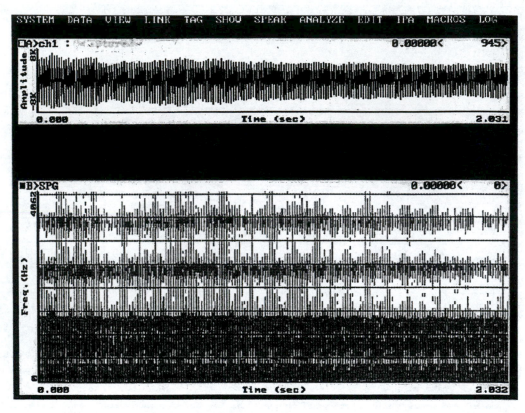

**FIGURE 2–13.** Acoustic waveform and spectrograph obtained from the same patient in Figure 2–11 after 11 sessions of voice therapy. Note the improved appearances of the acoustic waveform and spectographic spacing. Glottal pulsing is more regular and rhythmic and there is less noise and high frequency streak artifact in the voice signal.

for such difficulties. Patients who exhibit respiratry subsystem disturbances, such as asthma, emphysema, tuberculosis, cancer of the lungs, or neuromuscular abnormalities, struggle with low air pressure generating capabilities. As a consequence, phonation and conversational speech are usually compromised.

### Airflow Rate

The study of phonation would also be incomplete without examination of the amount of air that passes through the glottis and vocal tract during speech production. *Transglottal airflow* (FLOW g) is mea-sured in cc/sec, and mean values obtained from patients with voice disorders are usually strongly correlated with the degree of laryngeal dysfunction. Data collection is accomplished using a pneumotachograph, which is designed to transduce airflow through a face mask during various vocal tasks. During vowel prolongation at a comfortable loudness level, individuals with normal speech consistently generate about 100 cc/sec of airflow throughout the length of the utterance. Patients with hypofunctional laryngeal valves, owing to vocal fold paralysis or lesions that cause persistent chinks in the glottis during phonation, usually suffer from high transglottal airflow rates. Maximum phonation time is low in these patients, as the air supply that powers the voice is quickly wasted. Vocal and respiratory fatigue are common complaints because most patients attempt to compensate for the leakage by taxing the breathing mechanism.

Figure 2–14 is a schematic illustration of an apparatus that can be used to measure laryngeal airflow and intraoral air pressure dynamics, from which estimates of subglottal pressure and laryngeal resistance may be calculated.

Figure 2–15 illustrates the speech aerodynamic testing results of a patient with left true vocal fold paralysis, which was induced by a carotid endarterectomy surgical procedure on the ipsilateral neck. Mean air-

flow rate was measured at 1,026 cc/sec, roughly 10 times the normal degree. Voice was predictably breathy-hoarse, and the patient complained of limited syllable productions per breah and overall respiratory fatigue. This latter symptom was compounded by chronic aspiration of liquid foods and mucous secretions, which caused reflexive coughing and throat clearing activities.

Reduced transglottal airflow rates are often exhibited by patients with hyperfunctional glottal valving. This phenomenon is a common sequela of both adductor spasmodic dysphonia and spastic dysarthria. Both of these disorders are characterized by prominent forms of strained-strangled vocal quality. Vocal fa-

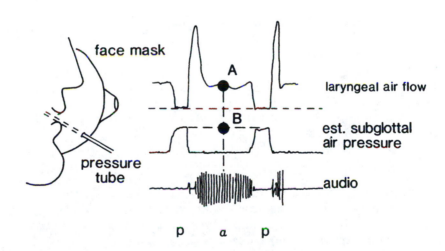

**FIGURE 2–14.** Schematic illustration of instrumentation that may be used for speech aerodynamic measurement. The waveforms seen were obtained from a person with normal speech repeating the syllable [pa] at a rate of approximately three syllables per seond. A and B signify the points of measurement for flow and pressure, respectively. Connected to the face mask at the left are both intra-oral pressure and transglottal flow transducers for these measurements. (*Source:* From "Laryngeal aerodynamics Associated with Selected voice Disorders" by R. Netzell, W. Lotz, A. Shaughnessy, 1984, *American Journal of Otolaryngology, 5,* pp. 397–403. Copyright 1984 by AJO. Reprinted with permission.)

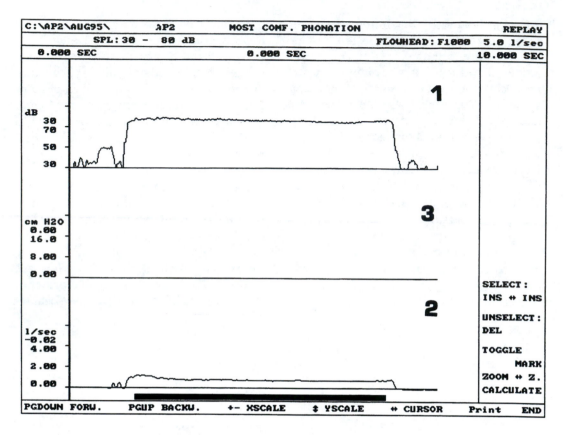

**FIGURE 2–15.** Airflow and voice signal waveforms obtained from a 62-year-old male patient with left true vocal cord paralysis. Note that during vowel prolongation excessive transglottal airflow is evident throughout the vocal effort. The numbers one and two mark the segments of the illustration for the audio signal and transglottal airflow, respectively. Section three on the illustration is blank because intraoral air pressure is negligible during the vowel prolongation task.

tigue and reduced syllables per breath are observed in patients with these conditions as well. Severe ventilatory and respiratory mechanism neuromuscular disorders also cause dramatically reduced airflow rate, which threatens phonation and overall verbal speech potential. Figure 2–16 highlights the low (20 cc/sec) flow dimensions in a patient with the harsh-strained vocal quality of adductor spasmodic dysphonia. Note the irregular airflow waveform characteristics, suggestive of intermittent rather than persistent levels of increased glottal resistance. Also observe the momentary arrest of phonation that occurred, characterized by a brief drop to baseline on the voice signal tracing.

### Glottal Resistance

The myoelastic-aerodynamic theory of phonation considers compression between the vocal folds to be a vital contributor to the onset and continuation of vibration. These *glottal resistance* (Rg) forces can be easily measured using Ohm's law, which specifies that resistance is the ratio of pres-

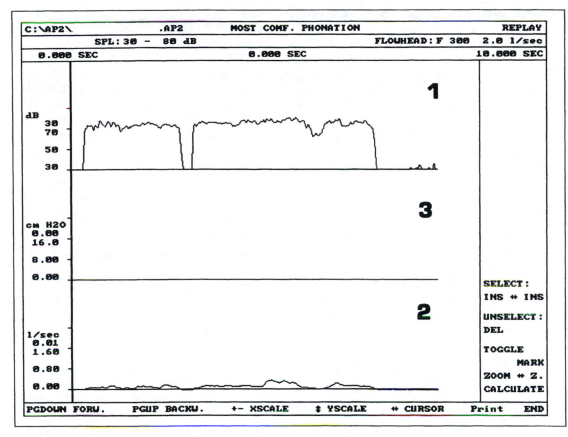

**FIGURE 2–16.** Transglottal airflow and voice signal waveforms obtained from a patient with adductor spasmodic dysphonia during speech aerodynamic measurements. Note the restricted transglottal flow throughout the entire vocal effort. Also note the arrest of phonation which occurred roughly one second into the vowel prolongation task, characterized by a drop to baseline on both the acoustic and airflow tracings. Also note that airflow was observed to cease momentarily during a profoundly strained segment of the continuous phonation task, near the end of the airflow tracing. The numbers 1 and 2 mark the segments of the illustration for the audio signal and transglottal airflow, respectively. Section 3 on the illustration is blank because intraoral air pressure is negligible during the vowel prolongation task.

sure to flow. During phonation, glottal resistance is equal to the ratio of the pressure drop across the vocal folds (Pg) over the degree of airflow through them, algebraically expressed as:

$$Rg = \frac{Pg}{Flow\ g}$$

The unit of resistance is cmH$_2$O/lps, wherein the pressure variable is measured by the degrees of water displacement and airflow rate is measured in liters per second (lps).

Individuals with normal phonation skills generate somewhere between 35 and 50 cmH$_2$O/lps of glottal resistance. Patients with hyperfunctional vocal fold activity, such as those with adductor spasmodic dysphonia, plica ventricularis, and generalized muscle tension dysphonia, usually exhibit significantly higher levels as a consequence of increased intraglottal compression forces. Those with vocal fold paralysis struggle with very low levels of Rg.

Please note that speech aerodynamic measurements may be contaminated in patients with fluctuating airflow dynamics. This may prove true when evaluating patients with spasmodic dysphonia, essential voice tremor, tremor associated with Parkinson's disease, and those with significant respiratory subsystem disorders, regardless of the etiology.

### Measurement Procedures

To obtain these types of data, differential pressure and flow transducers are ordinarily attached to a circumferentially vented pneumotachograph mask and interfaced with a computer workstation through a bridge amplifier network. The mask is usually held by the examiner and pressed tightly against the patient's face to prevent air leakage during testing. A 5 cm long rubber catheter is connected at its distal end to the intraoral pressure transducer, which is mounted on the outside of the airflow mask. This tube is passed through a fitting in the mask and the end is positioned in the patient's mouth approximately half way between the corner and middle portions of the right lip region. Two primary tasks are used during testing: sustaining the vowel /a/ for as long and steady as possible at a comfortable loudness level, and producing at least five contiguous repetitions of the /ipi/ vowel-consonant-vowel (VCV) syllable train. To ensure an adequate sample and to allow for human error factors each task should be repeated at least three times. Mean scores can then be calculated from the data generated.

Figure 2–17 illustrates speech aerodynamic waveforms obtained from a patient with a large hemorrhagic polyp emanating from the free edge of the left true vocal fold. In segment 2 of the graph, mean FLOW g was estmated to be 1,850 cc/sec. This result is roughly 18 times the amount that normally occurs during prolonged vowel production, and is suggestive of significant glottal incompetency (hypofunctioning). Segment 3 highlights the VCV repetitions. Note that peak estimates of Ps equaled 20 $cmH_2O$; Rg was calculated at 19 $cmH_2O/$lps. These findings were strongly correlated with the perceptual ratings of severely hoarse-breathy dysphonia, reduced pitch and loudness control, and excessive respiratory effort to vocalize. The patient's complaints of vocal and respiratory fatigue were easily explained using these aerodynamic data to augment the discussion. In our laboratory, we use the Kay Elemetrics Aerophone system for these measurements.

## Laryngo-Videostroboscopy

Figure 2–18 reveals the appearance of the laryngeal inlet during the typical mirror (indirect) examination. Note that the anterior commissure appears to point toward the patient's posterior pharyngeal wall. This is a mirror image distortion. Use of the mirror does not, however, alter the right and left anatomical landmarks; the right and left vocal folds appear in the mirror on their respective sides of the patient. It is important to remember these anatomical facts. When using either a mirror or a scope with a patient sitting in the examination chair, the right vocal fold always appears on the right side of the patient, but to the left from the examiner's point of view. The left vocal fold always appears on the left side of the patient, but to the right from the perspective of the examiner. When using a rigid or flexible endoscope to examine the larynx in the office setting (Figure 2–19), the anterior commissure is not reversed, as with the mirror exam.

Slightly different observations and anatomical relationships are realized during direct laryngoscopy in the operating room. The right vocal fold is always on the right side of the examiner, and vice versa for the left vocal fold. The anterior commissure always points to the interior of the thyroi cartilage, immediately below the notch.

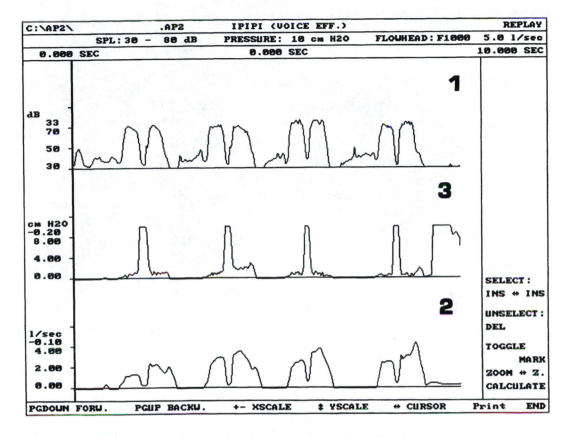

**FIGURE 2–17.** Numbers 1, 2, 3, illustrate the audio signal, transglottal airflow, and intraoral air pressure tracings, respectively. These were obtained from a patient with a left vocal fold hemorrhagic polyp during the repetitive productions of the vowel-consonant-vowel sequence /ipi/.

The use of stroboscopy has become widely accepted throughout the modern world as perhaps the most effective approach to the study of pathologic laryngeal anatomy and physiology.

### Stroboscopy Methodology

There are many different types of commercially available videostroboscopy instrument systems. They all function to provide essentially the same forms of data, though the specific features and quality of production vary from one manufacturer to the next. In our laboratory the Kay Elemetrics system (Model #9100) is used. All of the laryngeal photographs shown throughout this text were derived from patients examined with this equipment. We use a 70° rigid endoscope to view the larynx and surrounding soft tissue structures. When necessary, in approximately 25% of patients examined, an over-the-counter topical anesthetic spray (Hurricaine) is used to reduce gagging activity. This agent is very effective, and it is not long lasting. In most cases, however, its use is unnecessary, provided the approach to the examination is smooth, clinical rapport has been established, and the patient is positioned properly. Rubber gloves and 2 x 2 gauze are always used during this examination. To prevent fogging of the scope lens, an antifog solution can be applied or the scope

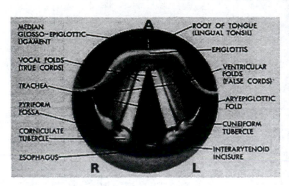

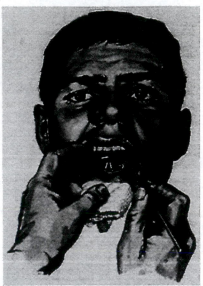

**FIGURE 2–18.** Illustration of the appearance of the larynx during mirror examination. R = right, L = left, A = anterior commissure. (*Source:* From "The Larynx" by F. Netter, 1964. *Ciba Pharmaceutical Corporation publication*, Plate V, p. 46. Reprinted with persmission.)

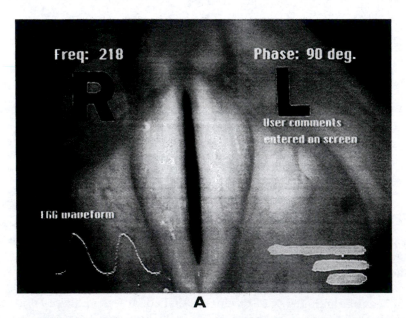

**FIGURE 2–19.** Illustration of the appearance of the larynx during rigid endoscope examination. R = right, L = left, A = anterior commissure.

tip can be dipped for a few seconds into a Hot Bead warmer. If the latter technique is employed, the examiner should check the temperature of the tip on the wrist area before proceeding with the examination. Figure 2–20 illustrates the best position of the patient for this exam. Use of a motorized chair facilitates the process. We have discovered that the best viewing angle with our 70° scope is when the patient is sitting upright, leaning forward, and extending the chin. The chair should be adjusted in height so that the examiner's eyes are at the level of the oral cavity opening of the patient.

The patient is requested to stick out the tongue so that it can be held steady by the examiner with gauze tissue. The gag reflex is often triggered when contact is made between the scope and either the soft palate, tongue, posterior pharyngeal wall, or all three. To help reduce this possible response, we have found that by resting the scope on the fingers holding the tongue the examiner is able to slide the tip into position for viewing without excitatory contact with these sensitive structures. Additionally, the examiner may wish to instruct the patient to begin phonating the vowel /i/ once the tip is in the vicinity of the uvula, but before contact is established. This vocal maneuver induces velar elevation and most often permits the tip of the scope to pass into the oropharynx without triggering the gag reflex. Maintaining or repeating this positioning technique throughout the examination is helpful, and seemingly less irritating to the patient, even though the scope remains in place and the uvula periodically drops onto the scope. Going through these extra steps can be very helpful if use of topical anesthesia can be avoided.

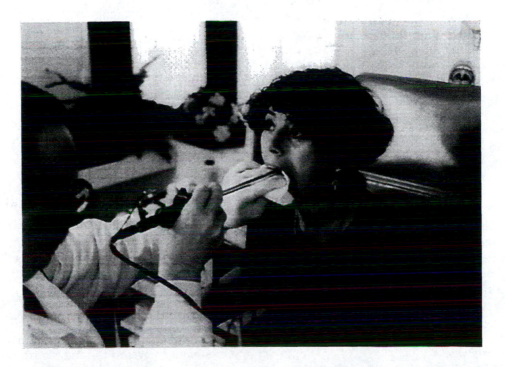

**FIGURE 2–20.** Use of a rigid endoscope interfaced with a videostroboscopy system to examine the larynx.

For data collection, the patient is requested to (1) prolong the vowel /i/, (2) use the same vowel to glide smoothly from low to high to low pitch, (3) repeat the vowel as rapidly and as evenly spaced as possible for at least 5 seconds (diadochokinesis), and (4) demonstrate quiet and deep breaths. These procedures are repeated at least three times to ensure an adequate sample. On many occasions it will be necessary to alter the steps followed, spend more time on a given step, readjust the position of the patient, scope, or both, and resort to a topical anesthetic spray to complete the examination.

Upon completion the videotape can be viewed and interpreted. Our system permits a variety of pausing and stop action options that afford in-depth analyses of the images obtained. A Mitsubishi color video processor is interfaced for the production of color photographs that capture single or multiple split frame images of the laryngeal inlet during the respiratory and ponatory tasks. These illustrations are important adjuncts to the patient's medical charts and all diagnostic and posttreatment reports.

The following parameters are generally analyzed, both with and without stroboscopy, when viewing these data: (1) overall laryngeal tissue appearance at rest, (2) laryngeal-respiratory biomechanics; that is, abductory and adductory motion of the vocal folds in association with cricoarytenoid joint integrity and mobility, (3) length, tension, and mass variability of the true vocal folds during pitch altering efforts, (4) glottal competency during the closed phases of vibration, (5) vibratory synchrony (phase symmetry), (6) amplitude of vibration, (7) presence of unusual activity of the supraglottic mechanism, most notably the ventricular folds, and (8) vocal fold mucosal wave dynamics. Most patients with voice disorders, regardless of the type or cause, exhibit disturbances in one or more of these categories.

Even if the patient's chief complaint is dysphonia, the examiner should not focus exclusively on the vocal folds when performing the endoscopy or when viewing the videotape results. Twisting and gentle repositioning of the depth and height of the scope in the oropharynx usually provides detailed views of the piriform sinuses, postarytenoid, postcricoid, valeculae, and lateral pharyngeal wall appearances. Additional diagnostic information may be gleaned from examination of these framework structures.

## The Mirror Examination of the Larynx

In our lab, mirror examination may be used initially to determine whether stroboscopy is indicated. Many laryngologists suggest that the mirror exam can be a valuable component of the overall test battery because it provides a quasi-three-dimensional view of the larynx, offers realistic depth of field images, and reflects the natural coloration or discoloration of the tissue studied. Also, this basic tool was used for many years by laryngologists as a reliable method of laryngeal appraisal long before endoscopes and stroboscopy technology appeared on the clinical scene. If for no other good reason, many laryngologists are very comfortable performing the mirror examination, and they are quite reluctant to relinquish the technique in favor of a less familiar approach such as stroboscopy. Differential diagnosis of a laryngeal lesion may, in fact, depend upon both the mirror and videostroboscopy examination results. Used in isolation, each technique may fall short of illustrating as completely as possible the associated anatomic abnormality and pathophysiology.

## Laryngeal Electromyography

Electromyographic testing is useful for differentiating vocal fold paralysis from arytenoid fixation, isolated superior laryngeal nerve paralysis from recurrent laryngeal nerve paralysis, transient (neurapraxia) paralysis from permanent vocal fold paralysis secondary to nerve degeneration, and psychogenic dysphonia from a pathophysiologic process. Data derived from such testing may influence treatment decisions based on prognosis for laryngeal nerve recovery. Stand-alone electromyography units may cost as much as $10,000.00, and hook-wire and needle electrodes are needed for the study of intrinsic laryngeal muscles. Thus, we call upon the EMG laboratory in the Department of Neurology to assist with this procedure. This association is cost-effective for us, and it ensures input from our neurologist colleagues regarding the differential diagnosis.

## Diagnosis and Discussion with Patient

### Malignant Neoplasms

When a lesion identified during the voice laboratory examination is suspected to be malignant many different ancillary tests and procedures are usually ordered and performed. With effective local anesthesia of the pharynx, larynx, and subglottal-tracheal region, accomplished with topical sprays and transtracheal/translaryngeal injections, a flexible endoscope can be used in the voice lab for close examination of the piriform sinuses, glottis, subglottis, trachea, and bronchial tree. The "trumpet" maneuver, wherein the patient is requested to place a thumb in the mouth and pretend to be blowing a trumpet, can be used during this examination to open the piriform sinus and post-cricoid region. This allows a closer and wider analysis of these areas than the traditional examination approach. Patients usually tolerate this technique without significant discomfort. If lesions are identified in these local areas, further support for the diagnosis of malignancy is obtained. This office procedure does not preclude boarding the patient for triple endoscopy and biopsy when malignancy is suspected. The findings, however, may strengthen the preliminary diagnosis and orient the surgeon with regard to the extent of the primary tumor.

Imaging studies, such as CT and MRI scans of the neck, may be useful for those patients with laryngeal malignancy. These tests aid in determining thyroid cartilage invasion by, or subglottal extension of, the tumor. In addition to these measurements, radiographic studies of the chest, including chest x-ray or chest CT, are indicated for detection of metastatic pulmonary disease. A variety of blood and urine tests, as well as an EKG and a general physical examination, are performed as probes for metastatic disease to bone or the liver. They are also important in evaluating the overall health of the patient, which may impact the treatment decision.

After the tumor has been properly staged, the patient's case is usually presented to a multidisciplinary tumor conference for determination of the most efficacious methods of treatment. These usually include a combination of the following alternatives: surgery, radiation therapy, chemotherapy, and speech and voice therapy. If metastases to the skull base, brain, lungs, or abdomen are identified, consultation with other medical specialists and surgeons is indicated for their recommendations and possible surgical cooperation.

In most hospital facilities, the tumor board team is composed of staff members from different disciplines: otolaryngology, radiology, radiation oncology, oncology, speech pathology, nursing, and social services. Typically, a head and neck surgeon is the team leader.

### Benign Laryngeal Pathologies

The term "benign" is somewhat of a misnomer. Although noncancerous by definition, certain benign lesions of the respiration-phonation complex may cause serious health problems. Earlier in this chapter examples were presented that illustrated the potential adverse effects of so-called benign pathologies of the vocal folds on airway protection during swallowing. Large nodules, polyps, cysts, degenerative changes, and adductor paralyses may result in glottal incompetency at the midline, placing the lungs at risk for aspiration pneumonia. Respiratory distress and vocal fatigue are common secondary manifestations of such lesions. These predictable and common sequelae are not benign difficulties. They often require therapeutic intervention(s) such as surgery and extensive behavioral therapy. Mass lesions may also compromise respiration activities by obstructing the glottis. Compensatory, labored breathing patterns may develop that place unusual stress on the respiratory subsystem. At times, emergency tracheotomy procedures are indicated, either prior to or concurrent with surgical removal of the lesion. Voice therapy is virtually unavoidable.

The laryngologist's initial focus is to differentiate a relatively benign laryngeal disorder from a malignant process. The patient's medical background and personal history, coupled with the videostroboscopy findings, are critical components of the differential diagnostic process. As previously mentioned, additional tests and lab work are ordered when cancer is suspected. In most cases, however, the laryngeal pathology observed is nonmalignant or benign and the need for ancillary evaluations varies from patient to patient. Data derived from thyroid gland, head and neck CT, Ph-monitoring, and swallowing function studies often prove indispensable for construction of a differential diagnosis and implementation of an effective treatment plan.

After all laboratory and clinical data have been analyzed and the diagnosis is determined, the laryngologist is charged with two primary tasks: first, the findings must be discussed with the patient, pertinent family members, and referring practitioners, and second, possible treatment options must be explained to these individuals. Relative to the latter issue, when the treatment of choice is considered to be relatively straightforward and uncontroversial it is generally easy to explain the recommendation. However, when alternative treatment options are suggested the decision process may be prolonged and occasionally complicated. The patient has the right and usually expects to receive as much information as possible about the test results, diagnostic implications, and treatment choices. Most patients follow the ultimate recommendations of the laryngologist. Some, however, may either seek other opinions or request additional time for consideration of alternatives before making a final treatment decision.

Both laryngologists and speech-language pathologists occasionally become frustrated with patients who fail to keep appointments, refuse necessary diagnostic evaluations, and ignore treatment recommendations. These individuals usually do not improve, regardless of their underlying disorder. Sometimes, establishing a very positive, friendly, and professional atmosphere during the history-taking and the clinical and voice laboratory examinations is the key to overcoming patient noncompliance and increasing the chance of a successful outcome.

In Chapter 3 the perceptual, acoustic, speech aerodynamic, anatomic, and pathophysiologic correlates of many different types of benign and malignant laryngeal abnormalities will be discussed in detail.

## SUGGESTED READINGS

Bielamowicz, S., Kreiman, J., Garrett, B. R., Douer, M. S., & Berke, G. S. (1996). Comparison of voice analysis systems for perturbation measurement. *Journal of Speech and Hearing Research, 39*, 126–134.

Bless, D. M. , & Abbs, J. H. (1983). *Vocal fold physiology: Contemporary research in clinical issues.* San Diego: College-Hill Press.

Baken, R. J. (1987). *Clinical measurement of speech and voice.* San Diego: College-Hill Press.

Borden, G. J., & Harris, K. S. (1984). *Speech science primer: Physiology, acoustics, and perception of speech.* Baltimore: Williams & Wilkins.

Colton, R. H., Woo, P., Brewer, D. W., Griffin, D., & Casper, J. (1995). Stroboscopic signs associated with benign lesions of the vocal fold. *Journal of Voice, 9,* 312–325.

Cudahy, E. A. (1988). *Introduction to instrumentation in speech and hearing.* Baltimore: Williams & Wilkins.

Finnegan, E. M., Luschei, E. S., Barkmeier, J. M., & Hoffman, H. T. (1996). Sources of error in estimation of laryngeal airway resistance in persons with spasmodic dysphonia. *Journal of Speech and Hearing Research, 39,* 105–113.

Gauffin, J., & Hammarberg, B. (1991). *Vocal fold physiology: Acoustic, perceptual, and physiological aspects of voice mechanisms.* San Diego: Singular Publishing Group.

Gelfer, M. P. (1995). Fundamental frequency, intensity, and vowel selection: Effects on measures. *Journal of Speech and Hearing and Hearing Research, 38,* 1189–1198.

Gould, W. J., & Korovian, G. S. (1994). The G. Paul Moore Lecture: Laboratory advances for voice measurements. *Journal of Voice, 8,* 8–17.

Hertejard, S., Geauffin, J., & Lindstead, P. (1995). A comparison of subglottal and intraoral pressure measurements during phonation. *Journal of Voice, 9,* 149–155.

Hirano, M., & Bless, D. M. (1993). *Videostroboscopic examination of the larynx.* San Diego: Singular Publishing Group.

Hixon, T., Hawley, J., & Wilson, J. (1982). An around the house device for the clinical determination of respiratory driving pressure: A note on making simple even simpler. *Journal of Speech and Hearing Disorders, 47,* 413–415.

Holmberg, E. B., Hillman, R. E., Perkell, J. S., Guiod, P. C., & Goldman, S. L. (1995). Comparisons among aerodynamic, electroglottographic, and acoustic spectral measures of female voice. *Journal of Speech and Hearing Research, 38,* 1212–1223.

Karnell, M. P. (1994). *Videoendoscopy: From velopharynx to larynx.* San Diego: Singular Publishing Group.

Karnell, M. P., Hall, K. D., & Landahl, K. L. (1995). Comparison of fundamental frequency and perturbation measurements among three analysis system. *Journal of Voice, 9,* 383–393.

Lieberman, P. (1977). *Speech physiology and acoustic phonetics: An introduction.* New York: Macmillan.

Netsell, R., & Hixon, T. (1978). Non-invasive method for clinically estimating subglottal air pressure. *Journal of Speech and Hearing Disorders, 43,* 326–330.

Orlikoff, R. F., & Baken, R. J. (1993). *Clinical speech and voice measurement.* San Diego: Singular Publishing Group.

Schutte, H. K. (1996). *The efficiency of voice production: An aerodynamic study of normals, patients, and singers.* San Diego: Singular Publishing Group.

Stemple, J. C., Stanley, J., & Lee, L. (1995). Objective measures of voice production in normal subjects following prolonged voice use. *Journal of Voice, 9,* 127–133.

Titze, I. R. (1994). The G. Paul Moore Lecture: Towards standards in acoustic analysis of voice. *Journal of Voice, 8,* 1–7.

# APPENDIX 2A.

## The Grandfather Passage

## My Grandfather

You wished to know all about my grandfather. Well, he is nearly ninety-three years old; he dresses himself in an ancient black frock coat, usually minus several buttons; yet he still thinks as swiftly as ever. A long, flowing beard clings to his chin, giving those who observe him a pronounced feeling of utmost respect. When he speaks, his voice is just a bit cracked and quivers a trifle. Twice each day he plays skillfully and with zest upon our small organ. Except in the winter when the ooze or snow or ice prevents, he slowly takes a short walk in the open air each day. We have often urged him to walk more and smoke less, but he always answers "Banana oil!" Grandfather likes to be modern in his language.

# CHAPTER 3

# *Pathologies of the Larynx: Voice Disorders*

This chapter comprehensively reviews many conditions that adversely affect laryngeal functioning. The chapter is divided into the following categories: etiologic factors associated with benign lesions, an overview of various types of nonmalignant disturbances of the vocal folds, and malignant neoplasms. Abnormaliies involving the subglottal and supraglottal regions that commonly impair phonation are also discussed.

## BENIGN LARYNGEAL PATHOLOGIES

### Etiologic Factors

The most common causes of benign dysphonias are self-induced voice misuse and vocal fold abuse. Examples of abuse and misuse, exhibited by both adults and children, include yelling, screaming, excessively loud speaking, protracted voice use, straining at phonation, making strange noises to mimic odd environmental sounds (e.g.,

children like to make motor noises and play war games by imitating the sounds of guns and heavy artillery), chronic throat clearing and coughing, mucosal irritation from cigarette smoke and air pollution, persistent gastro-esophageal reflux, recurrent upper respiratory infections, rhinitis, or sinusitis with postnasal drainage, and frequent use of caffeinated beverages with resultant drying of laryngeal secretions.

The individual's personality and psychological, intellectual, emotional, social, environmental, professional, and familial background influence the style and manner of habitual vocal expression. All of the aforementioned abnormal behaviors have been shown to induce, at the very least, transient and diffuse inflammation of the vocal folds as a consequence of increased vibratory compression forces. Chronic misuse of the voice may result in persistent and complex pathologic changes of the vocal folds, such as diffuse and focal polypoid swelling, increased vascularity and hemorrhaging, and formation of nodules and submucosal cysts. Recruitment of the ventricular (false) vocal folds to facilitate voice output is commonly exhibited to compensate for the adverse effects of these lesions on true vocal fold activity. Unfortunately, the results are usually counterproductive because this supraglottal mechanism does not vibrate efficiently. The voice produced is usually cacophonous, characterized by harsh-hoarse quality, low pitch, and reduced loudness control. Occasionally, the true and false vocal fods are driven to vibrate simultaneously during phonation efforts. However, as a consequence of irregular phase symmetry and asynchronous vibratory patterns, this abnormal combination may give rise to intermittent features of diplophonia, which compound the distorted voice signal.

The sounds generated during throat clearing and coughing activities are the result of abrupt and profound contact forces of the vocal folds. If these behaviors are protracted, as during the common cold, these hard glottal attacks will cause temporary erythema and edema of the entire laryngeal inlet. Because the laryngeal mucosa is inflammed from both infectious and irritative causes, a patient is at increased risk for submucosal hemorrhage of the vocal fold. When this occurs, acute dysphonia results, necessitating prompt medical attention. If these abusive activities become chronic and persistent, they may result in more serious vocal fold pathologies, such as nodules, hemmorrhagic polyps, and diffuse polypoid degeneration (Reinke's edema).

Allergic rhinitis, sinusitis, and postnasal drainage may cause pharyngitis, laryngitis, and associated voice disturbances. These signs and symptoms occur as sequelae to continuous postnasal secretions, which usually precipitate throat clearing and coughing reactions. This vicious cycle of events must often be broken with a combination of medical-pharmacologic and behavioral modification treatments.

Figure 3–1 illustrates the appearance of the vocal folds of a young man who had struggled with recurrent sinus infections

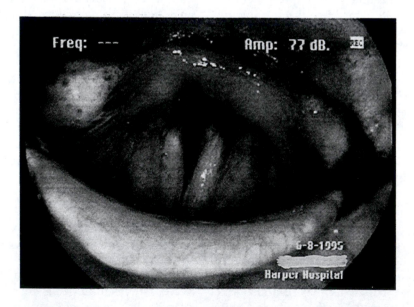

**FIGURE 3–1.** Appearance of the laryngeal inlet of a young man with chronic throat clearing and coughing behaviors. Note the diffuse erythema and edema of the vocal folds and soft tissue boundaries. Also note the persistent chink in the posterior half of the glottis during the closed phases of vibration associated with voice.

and intractable throat clearing activities for 9 months before he sought medical advice for these conditions. Note the diffuse inflammatory changes of both vocal folds, and the posterior glottal chink during the closed phases of vibration during phonation. The load effect of these mass alterations adversely affected vocal fold mucosal wave dynamics and phase symmetry by slowing their speed of vibration. This resulted in an abnormally low pitched (Fo = 87 Hz) voice. Pitch range and loudness variations were moderately impaired, owing to stiffness and noncompliance of the vocal folds. Of greatest concern to the patient was the severe hoarse-husky vocal quality that he exhibited. He tended to recruit the ventricular folds during vocal efforts, and this perverse activity merely compounded the dysphonia. The jitter (1.7%) and shimmer (0.93 dB) findings suggested a moderate degree of vocal fold vibratory instability. Mean airflow rate was 375 cc/sec, which represented roughly three times the normal degree of transglottal egress and hypofunctional vocal fold valving. Subglottal estimates exceeded 18 cmH2O and glottal resistance was measured at 20 cmH2O/lps. These results were interpreted as evidence of increased respiratory efforts and reduced compression forces between the vocal folds during vocalization. He was treated in several ways. First, allergy testing revealed profound sensitivities to pollen, ragweed, and mold. Nasal steroid and antihistamine therapy was instituted. A behavioral modification program was initiated, which included vocal exercises and educational instructions on the ill-effects of vocal abuse patterns such as throat clearing. Because swelling of the vocal folds did not resolve with these treatments alone, phonosurgery was performed. The vocal folds were stripped bilaterally to evacuate submucosal fluid accumulation. The patient was placed on 10 days of voice rest, and he returned for voice reevaluation and therapy, if indicated. No significant differences were evident between the pre- and postsurgical vocal fold appearances. Perceptual, acoustic, and speech aerodynamic measurements revealed virtually no improvements over the presurgical levels obtained. These results were considered failures, and they will be discussed in the broader context of phonosurgery and voice therapy alternatives later in the text.

Smoking cigarettes and chronic exposure to smoke in the workplace or social settings is dangerous to the health of the vocal tract in general, and the larnyx in particular. Other forms of environmental pollutants, such as dust particles and chemicals can also wreak havoc on the well-being of these structures. Smoke, dust, and chemical alterations of air quality have the potential to infiltrate nasal, oral, pharyngeal, laryngeal, tracheal, and pulmonary soft tissue. Hyperplasia and leukoplakia of the vocal folds, for example, are not uncommon biologic reactions to these types of irritating airborne substances. These pathologic changes are characterized by generalized inflammation and discrete white, thickened patches that develop on the vocal fold cover. The voice is usually low pitched and hoarse, because the irregular increases in vocal fold mass retard the cyclic speed and disturb the phase symmetry of vibration. Aperiodic chinks in the glottis during phonation result in leakage of unphonated air that mixes with the sound produced, causing excessive noise in the voice signal. Coughing and throat clearing may occur in response to these pollutants, which, as previously discussed, may exacerbate the dysphonia.

Figure 3–2 shows the larynx of a middle-aged female who had been smoking at least one pack of cigarettes per day for more than 30 years. Note the patchy leukoplakic abnormalities on the vocal folds and surrounding soft tissue boundaries of the laryngeal inlet. This patient's voice was indeed low pitched, hoarse-harsh in quality, and limited with respect to overall vocal range and power. These relatively benign lesions often progress into malignant neoplasms.

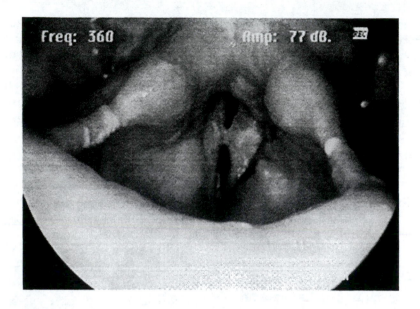

**FIGURE 3–2.** Appearance of the laryngeal inlet in a middle aged-female with a long history of cigarette smoking. Note the leukoplakic, white patchy lesions on the vocal folds, ventricular folds, and aryepiglottic folds bilaterally.

Noisy workplaces and social settings often require the use of greater vocal intensity to be effectively heard. Speaking above the noise for protracted periods of time may be harmful, as both compression forces between the vocal folds and underlying respiratory efforts are considerably greater during loud phonation. These behaviors may cause generalized edema and erythema of the vocal folds, inefficient vibratory activity, and resultant hoarse-harsh dysphonia. Patients with these types of difficuties frequently strain during phonation to overcome this mass effect reduction of vocal fold vibration. They will typically complain of vocal and respiratory fatigue. Symptoms of odynophonia (pain during voice usage) are not uncommon side effects, owing to the tenderness of the inflamed vocal fold tissue.

Gastro-esophageal-reflux disease (GERD) may cause destructive stomach acids to regurgitate through the upper esophageal sphincter and bathe the laryngeal inlet. This may result in symptoms and mucosal changes consistent with laryngitis. Chronic reflux may lead to laryngeal mucosa degenerative abnormalities, including ulcer-like formations or granulomas on the medial surfaces of the vocal processes of the arytenoid cartilages, hyperplasia and hyperkeratosis of the tissue of the interarytenoid region (pachydermia laryngis), and variable degrees of erythema and edema of the arytenoid apexes and aryepiglottic, ventricular, and true vocal folds. Figure 3–3 demonstrates such laryngeal abnormalities in a 36-year-old female who had been struggling with symptoms of GERD for several years without any form of pharmacologic intervention. These types of tissue changes are common sequelae to GERD, and they may be causally related to coexisting voice difficulties.

The use of Ph-monitoring devices to track and record reflux events is becoming a popular practice in both gastroenterology and otolaryngology clinics. Diet modification, combined with pharmacologic therapy to help reduce reflux, are standard therapeutic options.

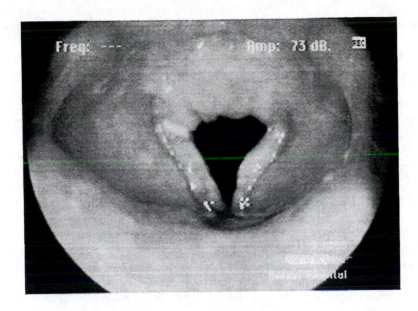

**FIGURE 3–3.** View of the laryngeal inlet of a patient with chronic and severe gastro-esophageal reflux disease. Note the widespread inflammatory and erythematous changes involving the vocal folds and interarytenoid region.

On average, the vocal folds normally vibrate at a speed of 125 Hz for adult males and 250 Hz for adult females. During connected discourse an enormous amount of thermal energy is created within the laryngeal inlet by these frictional vibratory activities. The larynx is richly invested with membranous tissue that secretes a protective mucous layer. This fluid serves to cool and lubricate the vocal folds and laryngeal inlet, thus protecting them from the potentially destructive heat-generating and traumatic mechanical effects of phonation.

Excessive consumption of diuretic beverages such as coffee, tea, and caffeinated soft drinks, without supplemental clear liquid intake, has the tendency to increase daily urinary output. This in turn may have a dehydrating effect on mucous membranes, including those of the larynx. If they are forced to vibrate within a dry, hot environment for prolonged periods of time, the vocal folds may undergo degenerative changes of their superficial layers. The laryngeal mucosa, in the early stages of this condition, may become bathed with abnormally viscous secretions that cling to the vocal folds and form mucous bands across them. This drying effect may cause a globus or itching sensation in the laryngopharynx, which necessitates throat-clearing activities as a way of scratching the itch. This vicious cycle of negative behaviors and pathologic changes is very difficult to break. Glottal competency and vibratory efficiency may be compromised along with voice functioning.

Diminishing the use of these types of beverages, combined with more frequent consumption of clear liquids to replenish body fluid levels, are routinely recommended strategies to combat this problem. This is especially important treatment for patients already diagnosed with vocal fold pathologies that adversely affect voice output. Excessive use of diuretics can compound the dysphonia and interfere with the objectives of the rehabilitation program.

Emotions and laryngeal functioning are inseparable behaviors. Many patients who exhibit benign voice disorders without histories of vocal abuse or misuse are struggling with psychoemotional disturbances. It is virtually impossible to conceal anger, despair, frustration, or happiness because these emotions become transparently evident during voice production. Vocal quivering and gulping, prolonged and unnatural pausing, harsh-raspy voice quality, and unusual pitch and loudness breaks are some of the most commonly associated speech and voice characteristics. The "apple in the throat" or "choking" sensations, which we have all experienced when confronted with high levels of stress, are not just imaginary. They usually result from tonic, involuntary contractions of the laryngeal musculature, both at rest and while speaking. These automatic responses are generally uncontrollable, and they adversely influence purposeful vocal efforts that may be superimposed upon the phonation subsystem at the same time. Protracted emotional difficulties, accompanied by chronic crying spells, for example, can lead to clinically significant voice disorders. Operating under increased muscle tension and compression forces for prolonged periods of time, the vocal folds may develop abnormal growths or lesions. Often, the initial treatments of choice involve psychological counseling combined with voice therapy. As discussed in Chapter 2, exploration of the patient's emotional status is an indispensable step in both the differential diagnosis and management of a voice disorder.

Conversion (psychogenic) dysphonia/aphonia varies from patient to patient with respect to presenting symptoms and underlying emotional or psychological causes. In all cases, however, there are no discernible pathologies of the vocal folds or surrounding soft tissues of the laryngeal inlet. The voice difficulties exhibited by the patient, therefore, cannot be attributed to organic causes (i.e., peripheral lesions or vocal fold growths). However, psychogenic dysphonia may cause organic vocal fold pathologies because of abnormal laryngeal function. Voice disturbances may range from only mildly hoarse in one individual to profoundly breathy, high pitched, and squeaky in another. Preservation of automatic, involuntary vocalizations is not uncommon in this population; laughter, crying, and biologic valving activities such as coughing all fall within normal limits of vocal quality, pitch, and loudness features. Intermittent signs of normal or near normal phonatory behaviors are frequently observed during conversational or automatic, reactive speech activities. These inconsistencies are very important indicators that the patient may indeed be suffering from some form of psychogenic or conversion dysphonia. The emotional and psychological history of the patient may offer revealing data as to the possible underlying reasons for the laryngeal disturbance. Pronounced anxiety, emotional despair, and personal conflicts are chief among the types of problems with which patients with conversion dysphonias are known to struggle. When the specific stressors escalate and cause intense emotional pain, this type of conversion disorder often is beyond the awareness of the patient, who may see the laryngologist after several weeks or months of persistent dysphonia, convinced of a bona fide laryngeal pathology that requires medical treatment. At most, examination of the larynx may reveal generalized hypertonicity and squeezing activities of the true and false vocal folds during phonation efforts. Accompanying these possible features may be intermittent anteroposterior compression forces of the entire soft tissue boundary of the laryngeal inlet. At rest, however, the vocal folds usually have a normal appearance.

Many patients with this suspected disorder complain of various combinations of chronic despair, recent hard times, feelings of failure, job-related distress, family or marital problems, and financial hardship. They also point to headaches and stiffness of the neck and shoulder regions as nagging symptoms of concern. Figure 3–4 was obtained from a 46-year-old woman who came to us with a 4-month history of

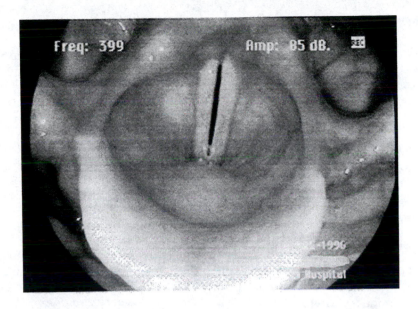

**FIGURE 3—4.** Appearance of the laryngeal inlet in a patient with psychogenic dysphonia. Note the frequency of voice was close to 400 Hz and the intensity was excessively high at 85 dB. Only the free edges were seen to vibrate against one another, causing a shrill, high pitched voice. No mucosal waves were evident as a consequence of this stiff, tension-ridden vibratory pattern.

bizarre, shrill, high-pitched voice patterns, not unlike that which one might hear from Minnie Mouse with laryngitis. She complained that her shoulders were extremely sore and that turning her head induced tenderness and pain. From an anatomical point of view, her head and neck and laryngeal examinations were virtually normal. Volitional phonation efforts were marred by tight lateromedial squeezing and anteroposterior strething forces of the true vocal folds. Only the free edges of the true folds were seen to vibrate, as there was a conspicuous stiffness of the entire laryngeal inlet. However, deliberate attempts to provoke laughter and coughing activities evoked more relaxed motion of the vocal folds, with fluid abductory and adductory dynamics. Discussion with the patient revealed that an office coworker with whom she had been arguing for days had recently attempted to strangle her. Fortunately, she did not experience any physical harm, as other associates intervened on her behalf al-most immediately. She pressed charges against the woman who attacked her, but was forced to continue to work by her side until the matter was settled legally. Her fragile personality could not take the stress of this work situation. She was unnaturally frightened for her life. Her voice problems were judged to be a conversion reaction, which actually served her well. She was dismissed from most of the usual working duties because she could not communicate effectively with customers. Instead, she was assigned to a different post, far away from the coworker she feared. Her dysphonia, which may have begun initially in response to increased emotional anxiety and tension associated with the office incident, progressed to a convenient disability that induced sympathy from her boss and others. After two sessions of voice therapy, which focused largely on muscle relaxation and easy voice onset exercises, and referral to a psychologist, the patient experienced a full recovery of voice.

When conversion dysphonias result in organic vocal fold pathologies, treatment becomes more complicated. In these cases, the underlying psychoemotional factors must be factored into the overall rehabilitation equation.

## OVERVIEW OF BENIGN LARYNGEAL PATHOLOGIES

This section provides overview of nonmalignant (benign) laryngeal pathologies that generally disrupt normal vocal fold vibratory activities and result in voice disorders. Information contained here should agment reviews of many of the case studies presented later in the text. To facilitate this discussion, the most common nonmalignant laryngeal pathologies have been subdivided into three basic categories, relative to underlying etiology.

### Category 1

In this category are patients whose voice difficulties are due to abnormal growths or lesions that have developed secondary to aggressive (hyperfunctional-abusive) vocal fold behaviors. Included in this group are those with vocal fold nodules, diffuse or focal swellings (polyps), contact ulcerations, and submucosal cysts. In most instances, these conditions are causally linked to excessive use of both the intrinsic and extrinsic laryngeal musculature during phonation. Bearing down on the laryngeal muscles through aggressive, strained vocalization habits are the usual triggers in many patients. Occasionally, the glottal incompetency that results from these types of vocal fold growths and lesions evokes hyperfunctional, compensatory contractions of the supraglottic false vocal fold mechanism. Unfortunately, recruitment of these relatively inefficient vibrators does not improve voice output in most cases.

### Category 2

Included in this group are patients whose voice difficulties are due either to abnormal growths and lesions, tissue degeneration, joint immobility, or fractures, which may have resulted from any one or more of the following conditions: vocal fold trauma induced by laryngeal surgery or intubation anesthesia, gastro-esophageal-reflux disease, chronic cigarette smoke inhalation, presbylaryngis, thyroid gland or systemic disease, upper respiratory infection, cervical rheumatoid arthritis, and external laryngeal trauma. Clustered within this category are many different types of benign pathologies, including: granulomas, webs, pachydermia laryngis, hyperplastic-leukoplakic lesions, cricoarytenoid joint fixation, bowing of the vocal folds, infectious laryngitis, degenerative vocal fold changes (e.g., myxedema, collagenous deterioration of sytemic lupus), and cartilaginous fractures.

### Category 3

Patients who exhibit neurogenic dysphonias compose this group. Their voice difficulties are not due to abnormal vocal fold growths or lesions, but rather are attributable to laryngeal neuromuscular impairments. The neuroanatomic site(s) of dysfunctioning may be within the central nervous system, peripheral nervous system, or both. Generic categorization of this group of patients might include all dysarthric and apractic patients, regardless of type or underlying etiology, who exhibit phonation subsystem disturbances.

It should be noted that patients may have complex anatomical and physiological laryngeal abnormalities that transcend these pathologic categories. For example, the patient with bowed vocal folds secondary to the aging process (presbylaryngis) may attempt to compensate for the resultant breathy-hoarse voice disorder by recruiting the ventricular folds. This activity may be performed to boost glottal valving, but usually exacerbates the dysphonia by superimposing strained vocalizations. What was initially a problem of vocal fold hypofunctioning may progress into a more complex disorder, with compounding hyperfunctional voice abuse features. Another mixed categorization example is the patient with flaccid paralysis of a vocal fold due to irreversible transection of the ipsilateral recurrent laryngeal nerve. At some point in time, usually no sooner than 6 months postonset, the involved vocal fold may atrophy. What began as a neurogenic pathology (Category 3), transformed into a mixed disorder with degenerative anatomic changes (Category 2). The associated dysphonic (and possibly dysphagic) features, which tend to worsen in concert with the disease progression, are especially challenging to evaluate and treat.

The focus here is to provide a brief overview of most of the aforementioned benign laryngeal pathologies. The suggested reading list at the end of this chapter provides excellent references for more comprehensive coverage of these subjects.

## Vocal Fold Nodules

By definition a nodule is a small densely packed collection of cells that appear distinctly different from neighboring tissue. Nodules commonly form on the vocal folds as a consequence of chronic voice abuse or misuse. The site of origin is usually in the superficial layer of the lamina propria, at the junction of the anterior and middle thirds of the fold. Initially, these lesions consist primarily of edematous tissue and collagenous fibers. Hoarse-breathy quality is usually the most predominant voice difficulty. The degree of dysphonia varies in concert with the severity of the pathology. In the early stage of development a single, small, hard or soft nodule may form on the free edge of one vocal fold, as seen in Figure 3–5. In cases like

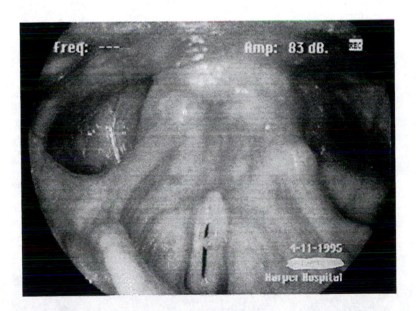

**FIGURE 3–5.** View of the laryngeal inlet in a 27-year-old female who abuses her voice. Note the presence of a small nodule on the middle one-third of the left true vocal fold. Observe the interference of this mass with complete glottal closure during voice output. Also note the mild degree of erythema involving the ventricular fold and arytenoid cartilage.

this, a mucosal wave will probably be evident along the nodule and involved vocal fold during phonation. Glottal incompetency and voice may only be mildly impaired. Bilateral, symmetric nodules are usually observed in chronic voice abusers, as seen in Figure 3–6. In these types of patients, generally the nodules are histologically more mature, with less water, and a greater density of inelastic, collagenous fibers. With increased stiffness of the vocal fold covers, the mucosal wave phenomenon becomes retarded or absent.

Early, immature nodules usually respond to voice therapy alone. The need for surgical removal applies almost exclusively to mature nodules; those that are fibrous, produce stiff vibratory patterns of the vocal folds, and evoke moderate to severe glottal incompetency and dysphonia. Voice therapy is always indicated postoperatively to address the underlying voice abuse patterns.

## Diffuse Vocal Fold Swelling

Polypoidal degeneration of the vocal fold is characterized by diffuse swelling, as illustrated in Figures 3–7 and 3–8. This occurs as Reinke's space (superficial layer of the lamina propria) becomes edematous, usually as a consequence of chronic misuse of the voice or repeated exposure to environmental irritants such as smoke or pollution. As a predominantly bilateral inflammatory reaction, the edematous vocal folds vibrate asymmetrically, aperiodically, at a slower than normal speed, and with a markedly reduced amplitude of horizontal excursion. The free edges are thickened, the covers become "flabby" (less stiff), and the normal, glistening, pearly white appearance of the folds is replaced by pale, grayish discoloration. These pathologic changes largely account for the hoarse-breathy, low pitch, and low intensity voice difficulties exhibited by most patients with Reinke's edema.

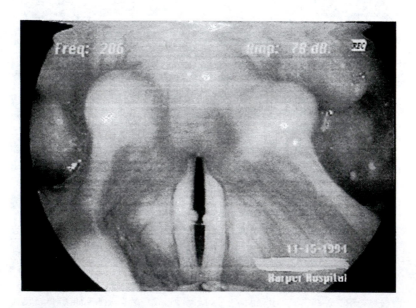

**FIGURE 3–6.** Appearance of the laryngeal inlet in a 52-year-old female with nodules on the middle one third of both true vocal folds. These masses cause the glottal chink to take on an hourglass configuration.

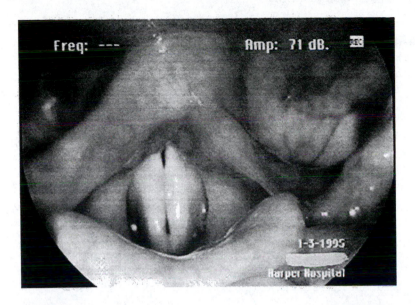

**FIGURE 3–7.** Laryngeal appearance of a 37-year-old female with bilateral polypoid degeneration (Reinke's edema) of the true vocal folds. This patient chronically abuses her voice both at work and in various social settings. Observe the mild hemorrhagic changes in the lateral vocal fold regions extending into the ventricle. Also note the mild erythema and granulation changes in the interarytenoid region. Full glottal competency is not possible during phonation as a consequence of the vocal fold swellings.

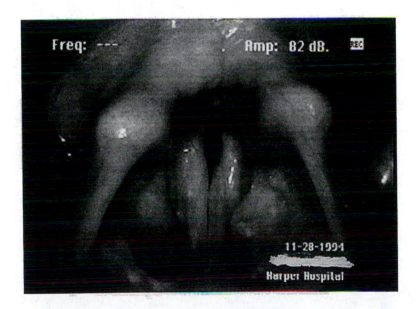

**FIGURE 3–8.** Laryngeal inlet of a 52-year-old male with chronic coughing and throat clearing activities associated with heavy smoking and alcohol consumption. Note the bilateral Reinke's edema and erythema of the vocal folds and surrounding soft tissue. The posterior glottal chink is commonly observed in patients with this pathology. Also note the mild hypertrophy of the left ventricular fold as a consequence of compensatory activity during phonation efforts.

Often, when the degree of bilateral swelling is profound and relatively uniform or symmetrical, complete glottal closure may be observed during phonation. Paradoxically, the quality of the voice signal may only be marginally impaired, and the H/N ratio may fall within normal limits. However, fundamental frequency is very low, intensity variations are markedly reduced, and jitter and shimmer correlates are often significantly abnormal.

## Vocal Fold Polyps

A polyp is a benign, circumscribed, fluid-filled outgrowth of tissue that rises from the superficial layer of the lamina propria. Though unilateral vocal fold lesions are more common, bilateral occurrences are not rare. Polyps are most often caused by an acute, violent episode of voice abuse. They can form anywhere along the length of the vocal fold, and they are generally broad based (sessile) growths. Occasionally, they may present as pedunculated lesions, possessing narrow stems. Hemorrhagic polyps are partially filled with blood, which accounts for their purple appearance, as shown in Figure 3–9. Fibrous polyps contain dense strands of connective tissue, as shown in Figure 3–10. Edematous polyps are generally smooth, soft, pliable, and translucent, as shown in Figure 3–11. During phonation efforts the vocal folds vibrate asymmetrically and aperiodically, owing to the load effect of the polyp. Incomplete glottal closure is a common problem, as the polyp deforms and laterally displaces the free edge of the opposing vocal fold during phonation, resulting in gaps around the mass. The quality of voice is typically hoarse-breathy, pitch is abnormally low, and volume range is substantially limited. The vibratory inertia caused by the polyp may inadvertently

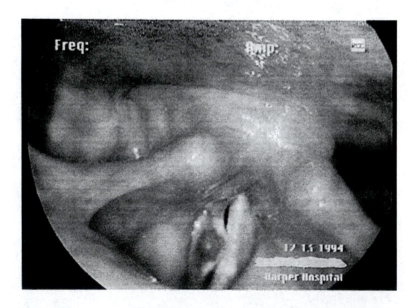

**FIGURE 3–9.** Laryngeal inlet appearance of a 47-year-old high school gym teacher who admitted to chronic loud voice behaviors. Note the presence of a unilateral hemorrhagic polyp on the middle one third of the right true vocal fold. This outgrowth causes deformation of the opposing cord and a persistent hourglass shaped chink in the glottis during phonation efforts.

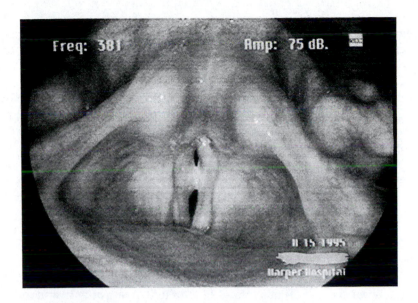

**FIGURE 3–10.** Appearance of the laryngeal inlet obtained from a 37-year-old female with a long history of voice abuse. Note the fibrotic, mature polyps on the middle one third of the true vocal folds. These masses cause an hourglass chink in the glottis during phonation, which accounts for the hoarse-harsh vocal quality exhibited by the patient. Also note the increased vascularity of both true vocal fold covers as a consequence of the voice abuse patterns.

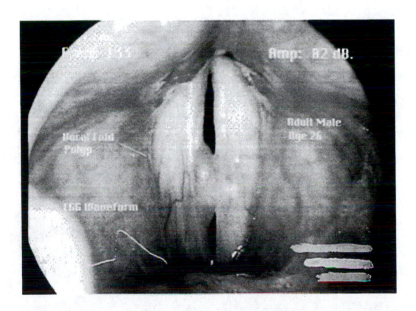

**FIGURE 3–11.** An edematous polyp on the middle one third of the right true vocal fold of a 27-year-old male salesman who admits to intermittent voice abuse patterns. Note the translucent gelatinous-like appearance of this mass.

lead to strained vocalizations to overcome such inefficiency. This behavior adds a harsh-rapsy overtone to the quality disturbance, and it taxes the respiratory subsystem as pleural and subglottal pressures are increased. If the ventricular folds are recruited to compensate for the leaky glottal valve, features of diplophonia may further complicate the voice disorder. From an acoustic viewpoint, (1) the H/N ratio is abnormally low, owing to excess noise in the voice signal, (2) the percentage of cycle-to-cycle vibratory instability (jitter) is increased, because of the mass and load effects, (3) the amplitude of vibration is unusually small and the excursions are generally irregular (shimmer), and (4) maximum phonation time is markedly reduced as a consequence of the glottal leak and increased airflow rate. Preservation or alteration of the mucosal wave phenomenon

largely depends upon the histology of the polyp. Generally, hemorrhagic and fibrous polyps interfere with the wave, and edematous ones do not.

On occasion a patient will exhibit a subglottic polyp; one that emanates from the cricoid ring or the inferior aspect of the lower lip of the vocal fold, as seen in Figure 3–12. Depending upon its size, interference with vocal fold vibrations and voice control may range from negligible to clinically significant. Most subglottic polyps are not visible during phonation. If the routine laryngoscopy examination includes deep breathing tasks, these types of (occult) growths will become observable as they tend to flap or flutter in and out of the glottis. When voice is impaired, the cause is usually disruptive impedance of airflow dynamics, rather than restriction of vocal fold mobility.

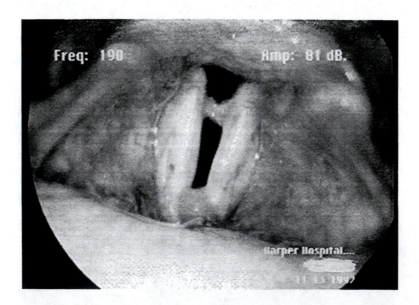

**FIGURE 3–12.** Appearance of the laryngeal inlet of a 49-year-old male who developed the anterior commissure and subglottal polyps shown during difficult intubation anesthesia for abdominal surgery. Also note the mild erythema and vascular changes on the free edges of the true vocal folds, as well as the surrounding soft tissue of the laryngeal inlet.

# LARYNGITIS (INFECTIOUS/NONINFECTIOUS)

We will use this term to categorize generalized inflammation of the vocal folds and laryngeal inlet. Most people have suffered from laryngitis in one form or another during an upper respiratory infection, following a shouting match, or after attending a sporting or musical concert event. Vigorous coughing and throat clearing activites, coupled with infectious mucosal involvement of the upper aerodigestive tract, are mostly responsible for the inflammatory-erythematous laryngeal reactions when one is struggling with a common cold. Yelling at a ballgame or during a heated argument are behaviors that are extremely traumatic to the delicate mucosa of the vocal folds and surrounding soft tissue. Increased vascularity (hyperemia) is evident beneath the covers of the folds in the form of well defined blood vessels, which are not normally visible. Generalized erythema and edema of the folds and neighboring structures are also common sequelae to voice misuse and abuse. The resultant dysphonia is characterized by variable degrees of hoarse-breathy vocal quality, low pitch, reduced volume control, and vocal fatigue, depending upon the severity of the pathology. In profound instances of laryngitis, patients will exhibit aphonia. Acoustic analysis usually strongly correlates with the perceptual impressions of the dysphonia; Fo is lower than normal, jitter and shimmer are abnormally increased, the H/N ratio is low, and maximum phonation time is reduced. Speech aerodynamic testing reveals excessive transglottal airflow rate, increased subglottal pressure, and reduced glottal resistance. These data are indicative of glottal incompetency and associated phonatory inefficiency, instability in the cyclic patterns of vocal fold vibration, increased noise in the voice signal, forceful expiratory efforts to vocalize, and weak compression forces between the vocal folds during phonation.

Videostroboscopy usually illustrates stiffness of the cover and limited mucosal wave activity as a consequence of the hyperemia and edema, which load the vocal folds and restrict the fluidity of vibration. Movements to and from the midline are predictably aperiodic and asymmetrical, most notably because the pathological vocal fold changes tend to be nonlinear, bilaterally. A persistent chink in the glottis may be evident, which would account for many of the aforementioned acoustic and aerodynamic abnormalities. The patient's history is of critical importance in making the correct diagnosis. Often complaints of odynophonia and odynophagia (pain when talking and swallowing, respectively) are registered by the patient.

Ordinarily, voice rest and occasional pharmacologic intervention (e.g., antibiotic, antihistamine, nasal steroid, and cough suppressant agents) are sufficient methods of management. Full recovery is expected within a 2-week period in most cases. For patients with persistent or chronically recurrent laryngeal symptoms, voice exercises and vocal hygiene techniques may be required adjuncts to this routine treatment regimen. Examples of these alternatives will be addressed in detail in the case studies in Chapter 6. The patient illustrated in Figure 3–1 also demonstrates some of these patholgical features.

## Ventricular Phonation

The false (ventricular) vocal folds are inactive during normal phonation. However, many patients with true vocal fold pathologies recruit these supraglottal structures in an effort to overcome underlying glottal incompetency. Some patients use false vocal fold voicing despite a (potentially) normal functioning larynx. This abnormal behavior may be of psychoemotional origin. To date, the anatomy and physiology of the false folds are not well understood. The segments most visible during laryngoscopy are composed largely of connective (membranous) and adipose tissue. Muscle fibers responsible for their movements are located deep to the body of the folds and lateral to the ventricles. These paraventricular muscles may arise from the thyroarytenoid muscle complex, which also forms the bodies of the true vocal folds. Hyperactivity of the ventricular folds during phonation efforts is most often classified as a musculoskeletal tension disorder. When these soft masses are brought closer together, apparently under voluntary control, they can wreak havoc with voice output, as was observed in the patient whose larynx is shown in Figure 3–13. This older woman developed ventricular phonation by straining during vocalization in an attempt to overcome glottal leakage caused by bowed vocal folds. Like most individuals who recruit the ventricular folds during phonation ("plica ventricularis"), voice quality was continuously harsh-raspy, pitch breaks were common with an overlay of diplopho-

nia, and intermittent strained-strangled features were evident. These types of dysphonic patterns may occur for several possible reasons: the false folds do not vibrate periodically and synchronously, their irregular and inefficient movements toward the midline contaminate the sound pulses generated below by the true vocal folds, the muscle tension responsible for hyperactivity of the false folds induces true fold stiffness as well, which compounds the vibratory difficulties and exacerbates glottal incompetency, and the voice produced by the ventricular folds themselves has a low pitched, raspy quality. Chronic recruitment, regardless of the cause, may lead to hypertrophy of the ventricular folds. This pathologic response often obscures views of the true vocal folds during laryngoscopy, making differential diagnosis of the potential primary condition very difficult.

Treatment of ventricular dysphonia can be challenging and frustrating for clinicians and patients. Coming to grips with the like-

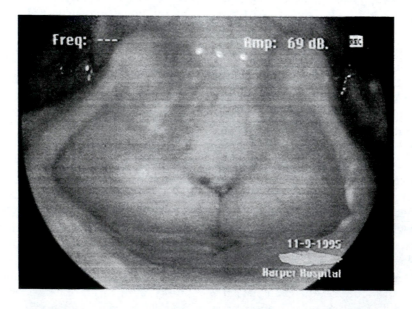

**FIGURE 3–13.** The laryngeal inlet of an older woman whose bowed vocal cords are likely responsible for the profound degree of ventricular fold hyperactivity during phonation. Note that action of these masses obliterates views of the underlying true vocal folds during voice activity.

ly etiology of this problem is critical to a comprehensive management program that includes methods to eliminate these secondary, disruptive behaviors and that also focuses on any underlying true vocal fold pathology. An interesting patient with such needs is presented in the case studies in Chapter 6.

## Contact Ulcers

As previously mentioned, chronic reflux of stomach acids into the laryngopharynx may cause inflammatory, necrotic lesions (ulcers) to form on the posteromedial aspects of the vocal folds. This region of the larynx is susceptible to the degenerative effects of reflux material because of its anatomic proximity to the upper esophageal sphincter. In some patients, generalized granulation (pachydermia laryngis) tissue develops, accompanied by overt erythema and edema involving the arytenoids, interarytenoid zone, and posterior one-third of the vocal folds. In others, ulcerative changes are focal to the mucosa coverings of the vocal processes of the arytenoid cartilages, to which the vocal folds attach posteriorly. On occasion, pronounced, odd-shaped granulomas may develop in this location, as illustrated in Figure 3–14. These types of pathologies are also observed in individuals who possess hard driving, "type A" personalities, with propensies toward bearing down on the vocal folds during phonation. The posterior vocal fold region is most vulnerable to the intense friction that results from such speaking patterns because the cyclic waves of vibration travel across the folds from back to front. If these abnormal and abrupt compression forces persist, inflammation may develop followed by contact ulcer formation.

Voice is typically characterized by hoarse-harsh quality, with a glottal fry overlay. Pitch may be too low, and volume, not unexpectedly, tends to be loud. Usually tracheal pressure and glottal resistance are in-

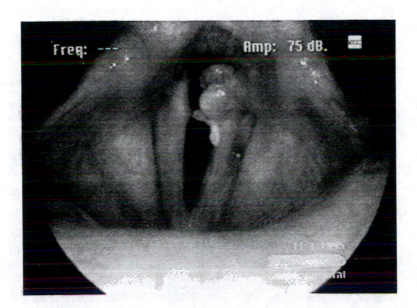

**FIGURE 3–14.** Contact granuloma formation on the posteromedial surface of the left arytenoid cartilage, owing to aggressive phonation behaviors and chronic gastro-esophageal reflux symptoms in a middle-aged industrial plant foreman.

creased, mean transglottal airflow rate is reduced, jitter is higher than normal, and a pronounced degree of noise is evident in the voice signal, together with a low H/N ratio. Videostroboscopy highlights the ulcerative lesions. Ruby red and inflamed arytenoid apexes and coexistent granulation changes in the interarytenoid region are suggestive of gastro-esophageal-reflux abnormality as a likely contributor to the contact ulcers. Powerful medial compression forces between the vocal folds, accmpanied by hard glottal attacks and prolongation of the closed phases of vibration, point to voice misuse as a probable cause. Not infrequently, both of these factors are culpable and must be considered in the treatment plan.

## Laryngeal Granulomas

Granulomas that occur in the larynx usually result from trauma induced by an endotracheal tube, as required in certain types of anesthesia, emergency room procedures for airway maintenance, and patients who are ventilator dependent. As the tube rubs against the posteromedial surfaces of the vocal folds and the adjacent interarytenoid region the mucosal coverings may slough and an ulcerative sore may form. Continuous irritation may convert this wound into small, rounded, fleshy granulation tissue, which can proliferate into larger masses called granulomas.

Laryngeal granulomas may be unilateral, bilateral, small, medium, or large. They may arise from the free edges of the vocal folds in the region of the vocal processes of the arytenoid cartilages, the anteromedial surfaces of the arytenoids, and the cricoid ring. Vocal quality disturbances vary from mildly to severely hoarse-breathy in patients whose granulomas interfere with glottal competency. Those who attempt to overcome the vibratory inertia by forcing the voice often superimpose strained-harsh dysphonic features. Figure 3–15 was obtained from a young woman who experi-

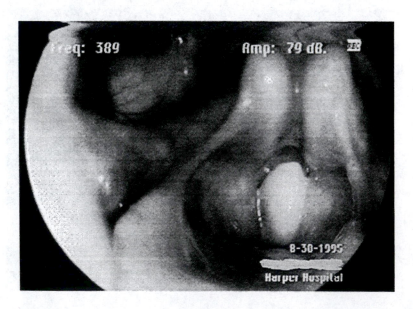

**FIGURE 3–15.** Note the large, egg-shaped granuloma extending off of the left ventricular fold across the glottis, obliterating views of the underlying true vocal folds.

enced complicated and prolonged intubation anesthesia many years earlier. She had been struggling with dyspnea and dysphonia since her operation, but did not seek medical attention for these symptoms until recently. Examination of the larynx revealed a large, smooth-textured, egg-shaped granuloma. This benign growth emanated from the ventricle of the left half of the larynx and extended across the glottis and right true vocal fold, but did not fuse with the surrounding soft tissue on that side. At no time during deep respiratory activities or vigorous phonation efforts were the true vocal folds visible for examination. The patient was extremely dyspneic and stridorous. Her voice was hoarse-harsh in quality, with pronounced muffling characteristics.

## Presbylaryngis/Bowing of the Vocal Folds

The aging process may alter the anatomy and physiology of the larynx. The most common changes include variable combinations of the following: ossification of the laryngeal cartilages, arthritis of the cricoarytenoid and cricothyroid joints, degeneration of all layers of the vocal folds, with generalized thinning of the covers and atrophy of the bodies, shrinkage of the mucous glands, with fatty infiltration of the epithelium, and concommitant bowing of the vocal folds as sequelae to underlying weakness, mucosal and muscle wasting, and hypotonicity. Pathologic lung-thorax changes and pulmonary disease, such as emphysema, may compound the effects of presbylaryngis. The general physical condition of the individual is a factor that has been shown to influence the degree of dysphonia that may result from these abnormalities. The patient who is elderly, and in good health and who exercises regularly usually exhibits better voice than another individual who is ill and out of shape. Formal vocal training is also believed to be beneficial in thwarting the adverse effects of aging on laryngeal functioning.

In general, presbylaryngis is characterized by these types of perceptual voice disturbances: higher than normal pitch, owing largely to vocal fold thinning, hoarse-breathy quality, secondary to vocal fold atrophy and bowing, trembling quality with occasional pitch breaks, as manifestations of tremorous laryngeal muscle contractions, and raspy-harsh quality, due to supraglottic hyperactivity. Voice laboratory studies may yield the following types of data: (1) increased jitter and shimmer values, (2) as sequelae to inherent instability in the cyclic vibratory patterns, (3) reduced H/N ratio, indicative of increased noise in the voice signal, abnormally elevated subglottal pressure, as a consequence of increased respiratory effort to overcome glottal incompetency, (4) increased transglottal airflow rate, owing to glottal leakage, (5) reduced glottal resistance, and (6) aperiodic and asymmetrical vocal fold vibratory activity, accompanied by a persistent chink in the glottis, retarded mucosal wave dynamics, and excessive false vocal fold activity.

Bowing of the vocal fold occurs when its myoelastic tension is diminished, causing an unnatural concavity from the midline of the glottis. This condition may result from the aforementioned types of laryngeal degenerative changes associated with the aging process. It may also be caused by weakness and hypotonicity of the vocal fold musculature following damage to either the recurrent laryngeal nerve, superior laryngeal nerve, or both. Figure 3–16 was obtained from a 74-year-old man suffering from both the aging process and neuropathic diabetes.

Bilateral bowing usually induces more severe voice, swallowing, and respiratory-phonatory fatigue than unilateral involvement. The patient who exhibits a bowed vocal fold may also exhibit hoarse-breathy dysphonia. Vocal fatigue is a common complaint because of air wastage through the incompetent glottis during phonation. There may be a harsh-strained vocal quality component that compounds the dyspho-

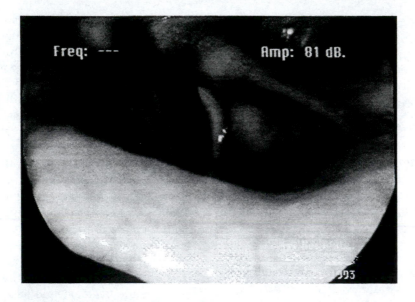

**FIGURE 3–16.** Laryngeal appearance of a 74-year-old man suffering from the aging process and neuropathic diabetes. Note that the left true vocal fold was moderately paretic, resting in the paramedian position during deep inhalation. Also observe the concave bowing of this vocal fold, which exacerbates the dysphonia exhibited. Voice is breathy-hoarse in quality and the patient complains of episodic aspiration on thin liquid materials.

nia profile, as the patient may recruit the ventricular folds to facilitate glottal closure. Of chief concern is the potential for aspiration pneumonia in this patient. Inquiries regarding swallowing difficulties are critical in determining the need for additional diagnostic testing and aggressive surgical management.

## Neurogenic Vocal Fold Pathologies

Most patients with dysarthria and some with apraxia of speech also exhibit dysphonia as a component of the overall motor speech disorder. It is beyond the scope of this book to describe in detail the different types of dysarthria and apraxia. Only a brief overview will be offered, with particular emphasis on the characteristic phonation disturbances associated with these disorders. Generally, dysarthric and apractic patients may be clustered into two primary groups relative to the types of voice difficulties they exhibit: those who suffer from consistent and predictable perceptual/ acoustic abnormalities, and those whose features of dysphonia vary, fluctuate, and are unpredictable. Spastic, flaccid, and hypokinetic dysarthric patients usually belong to the former group. Ataxic and hyperkinetic dysarthric patients compose the latter group. Within and between these primary groups there are clinically significant differences in the basic dysphonic features exhibited by each subpopulation.

### Spastic Dysarthria

Spastic dysarthric patients have strained-strangled vocal quality, periodic arrests of phonation, reduced maximum phonation time and transglottal airflow, and increased jitter, shimmer, subglottal pressure, glottal resistance, and noise in the voice signal (low H/N ratio). These perceptual, acoustic, and speech aerodynamic disturbances result from weakness, paresis, hypertonicity, and hyperadduction of the vocal folds, owing to bilateral lesions involving the corticobulbar tracts of the pyramidal system. Videostroboscopy may reveal ostensibly normal appearing vocal folds and surrounding soft tissue. During respiratory tasks, movements to and from the midline may be mildly to moderately slow-labored, but breath support is not compromised as a consequence. Phonation events are characterized by prolonged glottal closure time and squeezing, hyperactive supraglottal activities. The mucosal wave is usually retarded due to underlying muscle stiffness. Coexistent articulatory, resonatory, and prosody subsystem impairments are the rule rather than the exception.

### Flaccid Dysarthria

Flaccid dysarthric patients who suffer damage of the Xth cranial nerve (vagus) anywhere along its path from the medulla to the larynx have voice difficulties as a result of vocal fold paralysis. The type and extent of dysphonia largely depends upon the lesion site, and whether the damage is unilateral, bilateral, partial, or complete. Bilateral complete lesions, involving both the superior and recurrent laryngeal branches of the nerve, result in total weakness, hypotonicity, atrophy, and paralysis of the vocal folds. The patient is aphonic, and the risk for aspiration pneumonia is very high. Electromyography (EMG) demonstrates that all intrinsic laryngeal muscles are silent in response to complete involvement of all of their motor units. This condition usually requires a tracheotomy, at least temporarily, for pulmonary evacuation. Phonosurgery may be indicated to medialize at least one vocal fold to improve phonation, deglutition, and laryngeal-respiratory biomechanics. Bilateral incomplete lesions often cause partial paralysis of the vocal folds. Breathy-hoarse, wet-gurgly vocal quality, increased

jitter and shimmer values, and low H/N ratios are predictable. Shortness of breath and vocal fatigue are common presenting symptoms, as glottal incompetency and reduced glottal resistance results in air wastage during phonation and taxing respiratory compensation. EMG studies reveal reduced electrical activity. Bilateral lesions of the recurrent laryngeal nerves only, as may occur following head and neck surgery or trauma, often produce bilateral abductor paralysis, wherein the vocal folds are fixed in the median position and cannot be abducted. This occurs as a consequence of the tonal stretching and adducting effects of the cricothyroid musculature, which is innervated by the extrinsic branch of the superior laryngeal nerve. In these patients, voice features are often near normal, as are swallowing abilities. However, the airway at the glottic level is compromised due to the midline position of the paralyzed vocal folds. These patients exhibit inspiratory stridor and dyspnea, and they require a tracheotomy for respiratory relief.

Unilateral recurrent laryngeal nerve paralysis causes hoarse-breathy voice quality, as the affected vocal fold usually hangs motionless in the paramedian position. Glottal incompetency results, accompanied by excessive translottal airflow rate during phonation, increased degrees of (pitch) jitter, (loudness) shimmer, and subglottal pressure, reduced glottal resistance, and a low H/N ratio. These findings are pathognomonic of a large glottal chink due to vocal fold paralysis. Once atrophic changes take place, the free edge of the affected fold thins out and becomes bowed. During videostroboscopy, the vocal folds are observed to vibrate asymmetrically and aperiodically. Excursions away from the midline on the side of involvement are usually limited, and the mucosal wave may be completely absent. However, pulmonary airflow causes the paralyzed vocal fold to flap like a flag in the wind during phonation efforts. This activity alone should not be misconstrued as evidence of incomplete paralysis.

The patient whose larynx is shown in Figure 3–17. experienced a brainstem stroke and multiple cranial nerve lesions. Intramedullary damage to the left vagus nerve resulted in ipsilateral vocal fold paralysis and bowing. Also note the excessive pooling of saliva in the piriform sinus region due to dysphagia, exacerbated by lingual weakness and unilateral paralysis, secondary to left hypoglossal nerve damage.

If damage occurs high in the trunk of the vagus nerve, or at the nuclei of origin in the medulla, all branches that supply the larynx and the velopharynx are at risk for disturbed functioning. The previous patient also exhibited velopharyngeal dysfunctioning for this reason. Denervation of the cricothyroid musculature, because of superior laryngeal nerve involvement, coupled to the aforementioned signs of recurrent laryngeal nerve damage, results in pronounced flaccidity of the vocal fold. Loss of the adductory, stretching forces of this musculature causes the vocal fold to hang motionless in the abducted position. Associated glottal incompetency and resultant dysphonia and dysphagia are usually severe. In this type of patient, coexistent hypernasality is predictable, owing to weakness and paralysis of the velopharyngeal musculature on the side(s) of involvement.

Figure 3–18 was obtained from a 68-year-old female who was diagnosed 3 months earlier with Guillain-Barré syndrome, an acute infective polyneuritis condition of viral origin. She was wheelchair bound because of severe axial musculature weakness, and her voice was profoundly breathy-hoarse, owing to bilateral paresis and bowing of the vocal folds. A percutaneous endoscopic gastrostomy (PEG) was performed for tube feeding purposes be-

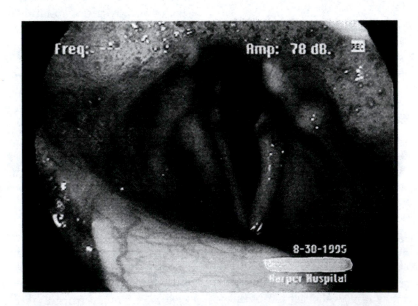

**FIGURE 3–17.** Appearance of the laryngeal inlet of a 64-year-old male who suffered a brainstem stroke with multiple cranial nerve lesions. Note that the left vocal fold is paralyzed in the paramedian position. Also observe the moderate degree of bowing caused by vocalis muscle weakness. There is a profound amount of saliva that pools in the piriform sinus and pre-epiglottal region, which seeps into the airway during breathing. The patient has had three bouts of pneumonia over the past 8 months. His voice is moderately breathy-hoarse in quality.

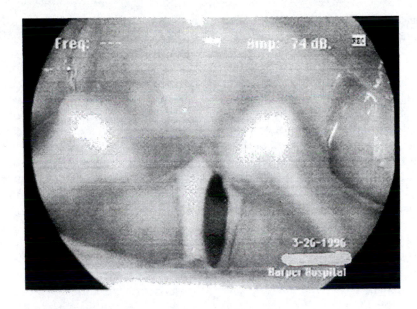

**FIGURE 3–18.** Laryngeal appearance of a 68-year-old female with Guillain-Barré syndrome. She exhibited bilateral vocal fold paralysis, with consequent glottal incompetency and bowing of the true vocal folds. Note the large elliptically shaped glottal chink during vigorous vocal effort. The patient suffered from profound vocal fatigue and transglottal airflow leakage during phonation. Also observe that the left ventricular fold has become mildly hypertrophic, partially obscuring views of the underlying true vocal fold. The patient has developed a moderate degree of hyperventricular activity to compensate for this problem.

cause the patient was aspirating all food items and her own secretions. Gelfoam injection into the left true vocal fold was recommended to improve glottal competency for both phonation and swallowing activities. Because the prognosis for partial or full recovery is usually good in these types of patients, a more permanent phonosurgical treatment approach, such as medialization thyroplasty, was considered unnecessary in this early stage of the disease process.

### Neuropraxia of Phonation

This condition results from reversible trauma to the vagus nerve, as may occur in certain head and neck surgical procedures such as thyroidectomy and carotid endarterectomy. When the nerve is retracted or compressed, it becomes inflamed and impulse activity is suppressed. The ipsilateral vocal fold presents with signs and symptoms that may mimic the paralytic effects of irreversible nerve damage. Knowledge of the patient's history is of paramount importance in differentiating these similarly appearing conditions. Laryngeal neurapraxia may also be observed, for unclear reasons, in patients who have suffered a severe upper respiratory virus. In most cases, full recovery can be expected within a few months following onset. Occasionally, the healing process can take as long as a year. It is the rare patient who fails to improve with time. Definitive treatment in the beginning usually involves stimulative behavioral therapy that incorporates glottal valving exercises. If the patient is at risk for aspiration, temporary gelfoam injection of the affected vocal fold may be performed to augment glottal competency, which may aid both swallowing and phonation during the recovery process.

### Hypokinetic Dysarthria

Patients with hypokinetic dysarthria usually suffer from Parkinson's disease, which is caused by degeneration of the upper brainstem substantia nigra complex and its dopamine-rich cells. Widespread hypertonicity and rigidity of muscle movements are the hallmark pathophysiologic features of this disease. Most patients with Parkinson's disease exhibit hoarse-harsh vocal quality, with limited pitch and volume range, because of laryngeal musculature involvement. Although the appearance of the vocal folds may be within normal limits, recruitment of the ventricular folds is not uncommonly observed during laryngoscopy. Speech aerodynamic testing reveals decreased levels of glottal resistance and increased transglottal airflow rate, owing to underlying weakness of vocal fold compression forces.

### Ataxic Dysarthria

Ataxic dysarthric patients typically struggle with uncontrollable loudness and pitch outbursts. They may occasionally exhibit a coarse vocal tremor overlay as a consequence of clumsy, uncoordinated, and tremorous laryngeal musculature contractions. Laryngoscopy may reveal mild to moderate tremors of the laryngeal inlet upon phonation, but not at rest. No discernible anatomical abnormalities are evident when examining the status of the vocal folds. This motor speech disorder occurs secondary to lesions of the cerebellum.

### Hyperkinetic Dysarthria

Although there are quick, slow, and tremor forms of hyperkinetic dysarthria, each is partially characterized by fluctuating voice difficulties. Only the latter two forms will be addressed here. Focal laryngeal dystonia is a slow movement disorder, which commonly results in spasmodic dysphonia, of which there are three types: adductor, abductor, and mixed adductor/abductor. The adductor type is most prevalent. Its signs and symptoms include strained-strangled vocal quality, periodic arrests of phonaion, and limited pitch and volume control. Glottal resistance measures may reveal three to four times the normal degree of vocal fold compression forces during phonation efforts. Reduced transglottal airflow rate and increased subglottal pressure are predictable findings. Prolonged vocal fold closure time, reduced amplitude of vibration, and limited mucosal wave dynamics are often, but not always, evident during videostroboscopy. At times, vibratory patterns appear to be within normal limits, and the overall features may vary from patient to patient. Mild to moderate vocal tremors may be superimposed upon the predominant spasmodic features. The abductor type occurs in approximately 25% of all cases. It is characterized by intermittent breathiness, owing largely to spasms of the posterior cricoarytenoid muscles. Increased transglottal airflow rate and subglottal pressure and reduced glottal resistance are not uncommon signs of this condition. Vocal fatigue is a common complaint, owing to laryngeal valving inefficiency and chronic air wastage, especially during contextual speech. The mixed form of this disorder is uncommon. When it occurs, features of both subtypes are present and either one may be predominant. The etiology and site of lesion responsible for spasmodic dysphonia are not well understood, though extrapyramidal system abnormalities have been implicated.

The well-known voice and head shaking characteristics exhibited by the legendary actress Katherine Hepburn are excellent examples of the effects of essential tremor syndrome. The organic voice tremor component can be quite crippling to communication efforts, as quavering of intonation patterns, fluctuations or rhythmic alterations in loudness, monopitch, and intermittent strained-harsh quality are perceptually distracting. These vocal characteristics occur as a result of synchronous tremors of the abductory-adductory laryngeal musculature during phonation and at rest. Orofacial, head, and limb tremors frequently co-occur.

## Leukoplakia/Hyperkeratosis of the Vocal Folds

This is considered a premalignant condition that occurs as a result of hyperplastic thickening of the epithelial cover of the vocal fold. This lesion may involve the superficial layer of the lamina propria. Invasion into the vocal ligament will not occur unless it has undergone malignant degeneration. When the affected epithelial cells display atypia, the lesion is called epithelial dysplasia. It can occur unilaterally or bilaterally, and frequently causes irregularity of the free edge anatomy and asymmetry of vibration. Of critical importance in the differential diagnosis is the lack of mucosal wave activity over the lesion site, which may signify malignant transformation of the lesion. Glottal incompetency may result from increased stiffness and mass of the vocal fold cover(s) and the associated load effect on vibratory periodicity. Vocal quality ordinarily is hoarse-harsh, pitch is lower than normal, and volume is reduced. Chronic exposure to tobacco products and other vocal tract irritants, gastro-esophageal-reflux material, and general voice misuse patterns have all been causally linked to this pathology. Figure 3–19 illustrates laryngeal dysplasia that ultimately evolved into moderately differentiated invasive squamous cell carcinoma. This patient's laryngeal cancer was staged as T4N1M0, for which he underwent a total laryngectomy and right radical neck dissection. Note the edema and erythema of the postcricoid, arytenoid,

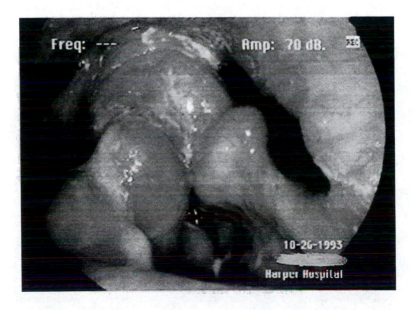

**FIGURE 3–19.** This laryngeal photograph illustrates widespread edema, erythema, and leukoplakia involving the laryngeal inlet, arytenoid cartilages, and postcricoid regions in a 54-year-old man. Unfortunately, this disease process evolved into squamous cell carcinoma, resulting in a total laryngectomy.

and aryepiglottic, ventricular, and true vocal fold regions, bilaterally. Also observe the disseminated leukoplakic lesions in these locations. This 54-year-old man was a heavy smoker and an alcoholic for 30 years. His voice was severely hoarse-harsh in quality.

## Laryngeal Papilloma

This neoplastic condition usually has its onset in the early childhood years, and it is considered nonmalignant. Papillomas have a wart-like appearance, and they tend to grow in clusters. Histologically, they are composed of stratified squamous epithelium with connective tissue cores. Papillomas are thought to occur as a consequence of viral infection of the involved tissues. These extrusive tumors have a strong tendency to multiply and rapidly recur after excision. They may spread within the larynx as well as extrinsically to the oropharynx, trachea, and bronchi. The voice is profoundly impaired in patients with papilloma of the larynx, as the growths interfere with glottal closure and vibratory symmetry. The amplitude of movement and mucosal wave over the lesion site are virtually absent, owing to increased cover stiffness and abnormal load effects. The patient with severe papilloma may be aphonic. Although $CO_2$ laser surgery is still considered the treatment of choice, recent experimentation with drugs injected directly into the tumors has been moderately successful.

Figure 3–20 illustrates laryngeal papilloma in 28-year -old female with moderate to severe hoarse-breathy and low pitched voice features. To date, she has undergone eight surgical procedures over the course of 2 years for this recurring condition.

## Vocal Fold Cysts

By definition, a cyst is a sac of tissue that contains a liquid or semisolid substance. Epidermoid and retention cysts are the

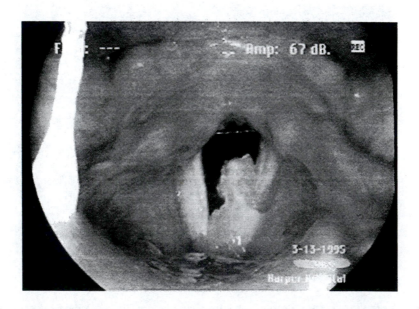

**FIGURE 3–20.** Laryngeal papilloma in a 28-year-old female. Note the gross invasion of the left true vocal fold with extension into the glottis. The patient suffers from severe dysphonia as a consequence of this massive lesion.

most common types that affect the vocal folds. Usually unilateral, these pebble-like growths rise submucosally from the superficial layer of the lamina propria. When viewed during videostroboscopy they may be embedded in the cover of the fold without extension to the medial border. From a mechanical viewpoint, cysts produce stiffer and more asymmetrical vibratory patterns than nodules or polyps. The mucosal wave phenomenon is most often significantly retarded or absent on the affected side, and the amplitude or lateral vibratory excursions are markedly limited. Glottal incompetency is responsible for the hoarse-breathy vocal quality exhibited by patients with vocal fold cysts. The etiology is unknown, but these benign growths have been ascribed both to faulty developmental factors and trauma. Not unlike nodules and focal polyps, cysts have a tendency to recur.

Figure 3–21 demonstrates a submucosal vocal fold cyst in a young man who is aspiring to be a professional singer. In this case, trauma to the epithelial layer of the vocal fold was induced by chronic abuse and misuse factors. Invagination of cells into the submucosal space occurred, which later developed cystic properties. His voice was moderately hoarse-breathy, with limited pitch and volume range.

## Laryngeal Web

Webs of the larynx usually form at the level of the anterior commissure of the vocal folds. They may be congenital, but most often they develop as thin, interconnecting bands of membranous tissue following bilateral vocal fold surgery. Webs may obstruct the airway and cause dyspnea. These abnormal growths also have a tendency to tether vibrations of the folds, and result in shrill vocal quality and high pitch. Figure 3–22 illustrates a web that formed shortly after bilateral vocal fold surgery for small, hemmorrhagic polyps in the region of the anterior commissure. For this reason, many

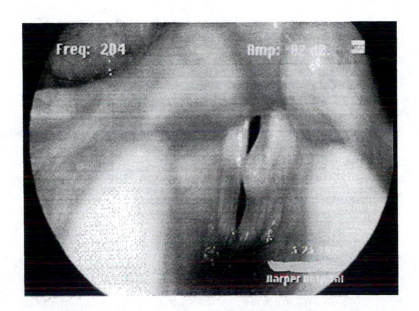

**FIGURE 3–21.** Appearance of a submucosal cyst involving the middle one third of the left true vocal fold. Note the hourglass shaped glottal chink caused by this bulbous mass. Also observe the moderate degree of increased vascularity on the covers of both true vocal folds, likely sequelae to voice abuse behaviors.

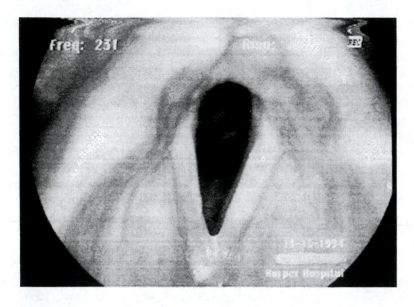

**FIGURE 3–22.** Laryngeal web formation in the anterior commissure region following bilateral vocal fold surgery. Note the thick, erythematous, membranous band interconnecting the two vocal folds in this location.

laryngologists elect to stage surgical procedures involving both vocal folds to allow time for adequate healing of one before operating on the other. Fortunately, this middle-aged female patient developed near normal phonation skills following surgery and a brief stint of voice therapy, notwithstanding the web formation. Videostroboscopic examination of vocal fold vibratory patterns, however, illustrated restricted amplitudes of excursion and stiff mucosal wave characteristics. Male patients may suffer more from these abnormal side effects, as the pitch of voice tends to be higher than normal, with an overlying asthenic quality.

## MALIGNANT NEOPLASMS

Roughly 10,000 new cases of laryngeal malignancy are identified in the United States each year. Most of these patients (93%) exhibit either poorly, moderately, or well differentiated squamous cell carcinomas. Much less common histologic types include other carciomas of epithelial origin, such as verrucous carcinoma or melanoma, glandular malignancies, such as adenocarcinoma, salivary gland malignancies, sarcomas, lymphoreticular cancers, and metastatic lesions to the larynx, usually from melanomas or renal cell or breast carcinomas.

## TNM Classification System

Laryngeal cancers are categorized as either supraglottic, glottic, or subglottic, and they are staged according to the "TNM" classification system. Table 3–1 outlines this laryngeal staging system. The "T" rating is based largely on the site(s) of involvement and status of vocal fold mobility. Four stages are used to classify the severity of disease: T1, T2, T3, and T4. The "N" stands for the presence, location and size of metastatic nodal neck disease. There are six locations or levels of the neck in which positive lymph nodes may be detected. Figure 3–23 illustrates these regional compartments. The "M" symbolizes the presence of distant metastasis from the primary site of disease

**TABLE 3–1.** System commonly used to stage laryngeal tumors.

| LARYNGEAL TUMOR "STAGING SYSTEM" | |
|---|---|
| **Site Stage** | **Tumor Characteristics** |
| **Supraglottis** | |
| $T_1$ | Confined to [1] subsite of supraglottal region: normal cord mobility |
| $T_2$ | Involvement of surpaglottis and other subsite(s) (i.e., glottis); normal cord mobility |
| $T_3$ | Fixation or extension to post cricoid, medial pyriform, or preepiglottal region |
| $T_4$ | Cartilaginous invasion; extrinsic spread |
| **Glottis** | |
| $T_1$ | Limited to one cord (T1a); both cords (T1b) - normal mobility |
| $T_2$ | Cord hypomobility; supraglottal or subglottal extension |
| $T_3$ | Confined to larynx; one or both cords fixed |
| $T_4$ | Spread beyond larynx or invading cartilage |
| **Subglottis** | |
| $T_1$ | Limited to suglottal region |
| $T_2$ | Extension to cord; with or without impaired mobility |
| $T_3$ | Confined to larynx; one or both cords fixed |
| $T_4$ | Cartilaginous invasion; extrinsic spread |

in the larynx. Table 3–2 illustrates the nodal-distant metastasis classification criteria using the TNM staging system. A laryngeal malignancy can be further categorized into Stage I through Stage IV disease. Table 3–3 highlights the distinctions between these severity ratings.

Whereas the assignment of a TNM rating is largely based on results of the clinical and endoscopic examinations, with malignancy confirmed by the pathologist, the treating physician may also turn to computerized axial tomography (CAT) scans and magnetic resonance imaging (MRI) for additional, supportive information related to extent of local, regional, and distant disease. Signs of cartilaginous destruction and metastatic spread are often very difficult to assess without these ancillary examinations. Because T1, T2, and T3 staging is primarily dependent on clinical perceptions of the degree of vocal fold mobility, the accuracy of such impressions is of critical importance. In reality, patients with laryngeal carcinoma do not always exhibit clear-cut disturbances of vocal fold mobility. More often, questions arise during laryngoscopy regarding the actual degree of immobility. Without detailed appraisal of the activities of the vocal folds during various phonation

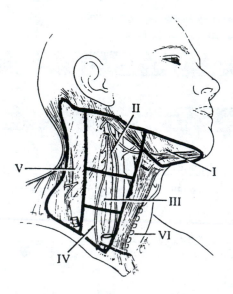

**FIGURE 3–23.** Lymph node compartments of the neck:[1]
  I.  Submandibular;
  II.  Upper Jugular;
  III.  Middle Jugular;
  IV.  Lower Jugular;
  V.  Posterior Triangle;
  VI.  Anterior Compartment.

  1. *Source:* From "Standardizing Neck Dissection Terminology" by K. T. Robbins, J. E. Medina, G. T. Wolfe, P. A. Levine, R. B. Sessions, and C. W. Pruet, 1991, *Archives of Otolaryngology,* 117 (6), pp. 601–605. Copyright 1991 by *American Medical Association.* Reprinted with permission.

and respiration tasks it is virtually impossible to appreciate the subtle differences between a mildly hypomobile cord (T2) and one that is vibrating within normal limits (T1). Distinguishing a fixed cord (T3) from one that is severely hypomobile is equally challenging. Perceptual errors along these lines may result in incorrect staging of the underlying disease, which may lead to questionable treatment decisions and outcome interpretations.

With the advent of highly sophisticated voice laboratory instruments, as discussed in the preceding chapter, analyses of vocal fold vibratory patterns have become considerably more reliable and accurate. Attempting to stage a laryngeal carcinoma based on the results of a mirror examination alone

may result in an inaccurate diagnosis, as this type of indirect laryngoscopic procedure fails to reveal the intricate behaviors of vocal fold motion. Today, laryngologists and voice pathologists rely heavily on rigid and flexible endoscopes, with camera and videotape recording capabilities, to evaluate the adverse effects of suspicious laryngeal lesions. Many practitioners equip their laboratories with videostroboscopic instrumentation for even more elaborate and definitive evaluations.

The patient illustrated in Figure 3–24 exhibited moderately differentiated squamous cell carcinoma of the larynx, which was staged as a T2N1M0 glottic lesion. The left vocal fold was judged to be hypomobile as a consequence of this large lesion, which

**TABLE 3–2.** System used to stage regional lymph nodes and distant metastasis in patients with laryngeal carcinoma.

| REGIONAL NODE & METASTASIS STAGING | |
|---|---|
| **Site Stage** | **Characteristics** |
| Lymph Nodes (neck) | |
| $N_0$ | No regional (positive) nodes |
| $N_1$ | (1) positive node on ipsilateral side; <3 cm |
| $N_{2a}$ | (1) positive node on ipsilateral side; 3-6 cm |
| $N_{2b}$ | Multiple nodes on ipsilateral side; <6 cm |
| $N_{2c}$ | Bilateral nodes; <6 cm |
| $N_3$ | Node(s) > 6 cm |
| Metastasis | |
| $M_0$ | No distant metastasis |
| $M_1$ | Positive distant metastasis |

encroached upon the anterior commissure. Upon clinical examination of the left neck, a single node was rated as grossly enlarged (2.0 cm), but mobile. A laryngeal preservation protocol was administered as the method of treatment. This included full course [6600 cGy (200 X 33 treatmens)] radiation therapy. The patient responded well. Figure 3–25 was obtained approximately 4 months after completion of this therapy program. At present, this 74-year-old woman remains disease free and is very active. Her voice, however, is mildly harsh-hoarse in quality, with a persistence of reduced pitch and loudness controls. Although this posttherapeutic outcome represents only a minimal gain in functional voice ability, the patient is very pleased that she still posseses her larynx and does not have a tracheotomy.

Figure 3–26 shows the laryngeal inlet of a 35-year-old male whose past medical history includes chronic use of hard drugs, tobacco, and alcoholic beverages. His voice was profoundly breathy-hoarse in quality with an overlay of severe harshness, as he was prone to strain at phonation. He complained of vocal fatigue and shortness of breath. Maximum phonation time was less than 5 seconds, transglottal airflow rate averaged greater than 1,000 cc/sec, and jitter and shimmer values were markedly abnormal (3.6% and 1.4 dB, respectively). These pretreatment examination findings led to direct laryngoscopy, which revealed verrucous cell carcinoma. This disease accounts for less than 2% of all patients with malignant laryngeal neoplasms. The tumor was staged T3N2A (Stage IV), because of left vocal fold fixation and metastatic neck disease. The patient elected radiation therapy alone as the method of treatment. His complete history will be detailed in a case study in Chapter 6.

Figure 3–27 illustrates the laryngeal inlet of a 73-year-old male. The lesion shown

**TABLE 3–3.** Staging system used to categorize the overall severity of the disease in patients with laryngeal carcinoma.

| OVERALL STAGE GROUPING - LARYNX | | |
|---|---|---|
| **Stage** | **T N M GROUP** | |
| I | $T_1$ $N_0$ $M_0$ | |
| II | $T_2$ $N_0$ $M_0$ | |
| III | $T_3$ $N_0$ $M_{0,\ or}$ | |
| | $T_{1-3}$ $N_1$ $M_0$ | |
| IV | $T_4$ $N_{0-1}$ $M_{0,\ or}$ | |
| | $T_{1-4}$ $N_{2-3}$ $M_{0,\ or}$ | |
| | $T_{1-4}$ $N_{0-3}$ $M_1$ | |

was staged as a T1N0 invasive squamous cell carcinoma of the glottis. The patient was treated with radiation therapy (6600 cGy). Six months following treatment he exhibited significant improvement in the appearance and functioning of the vocal folds, as shown in Figure 3–28. His voice progressed from moderately hoarse-harsh in quality, prior to radiation therapy, to mildly hoarse following treatment. Most important, he was judged to be disease-free at his most recent follow-up examination. Note that the tissue of the entire laryngeal inlet appears healthier in this figure as compared to the pretherapeutic illustration. The gross lesion abnormalities have been essentially resolved, and the vocal folds have re-mucosalized with relatively smooth free edges and glistening covers.

Carcinoma in situ is considered a proliferative disorder of the epithelium, with the essential cytologic manifestations of malignancy except for invasive qualities and the ability to metastasize. When the disease involves the larynx it is most commonly found in the anterior commissure region of the vocal folds. Mobility is usually unimpaired, and there is no distinctive clinical appearance of this form of cancer. It may appear as circumscribed or diffuse, with a grayish or reddish thickening of the involved vocal fold(s).

The following chapter delves into alternative surgical methods of management for laryngeal pathologies. Chapter 5 addresses voice therapy strategies.

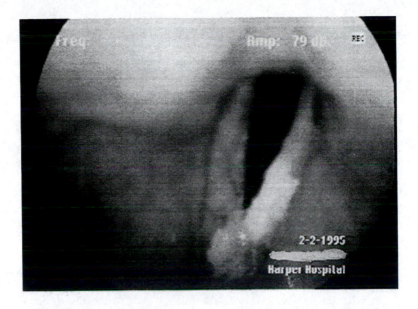

**FIGURE 3–24.** This patient is a 74-year-old female with a T2 glottic lesion involving the left true vocal fold. Note the extension of this squamous cell malignancy into the region of the anterior commissure. The associated voice is moderately hoarse-breathy, with low pitch dimensions.

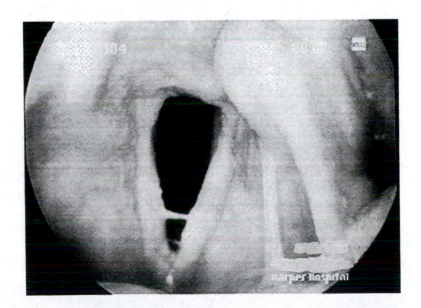

**FIGURE 3–25.** This photograph illustrates the responses of the patient in Figure 3–24 to radiation therapy. Note the marked improvement in the appearance of the left true vocal fold. Although there is evidence of bilateral anatomical irregularity along the covers and free edges of the vocal folds, the patient was considered to be free of disease at the time of this evaluation. Her voice, however, remained mildly hoarse in quality.

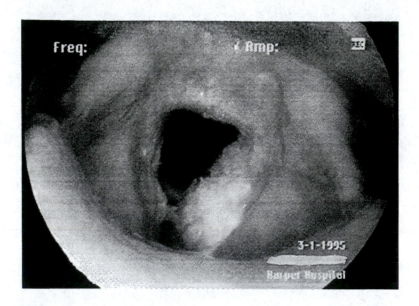

**FIGURE 3–26.** Verrucous cell carcinoma of the vocal folds bilaterally, more pronounced on the left side. Note the gross destruction of both true vocal folds and the patchy irregular texture and coloration of the tumor.

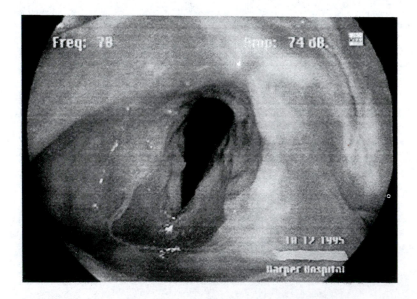

**FIGURE 3–27.** The appearance of the laryngeal inlet in a patient with a T1 N0 glottic squamous cell carcinoma. Note the widespread erythema and anatomical irregularity of the true and false vocal fold regions. Also note the white patchy leukoplakic changes along the left aryepiglottic fold, with extension into the apex of the arytenoid cartilage and postcricoid region.

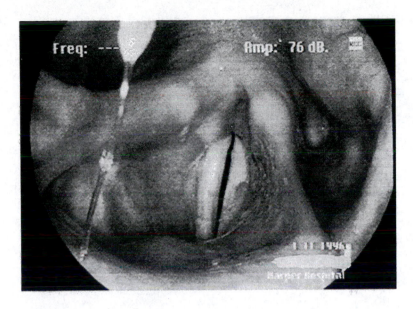

**FIGURE 3–28.** This photograph was obtained from the same patient in Figure 3.27 following full course radiation therapy. Note the significant improvements in the appearance of the entire larynx as a consequence of this treatment. This figure was obtained roughly 6 months following such therapy.

## SUGGESTED READINGS

Aronson, A. E. (1990). *Clinical voice disorders: An interdisciplinary approach* (3rd ed.). New York: Thieme-Stratton, Inc.

Aronson, A. E., & Hartman, D. E. (1981). Abductor spasmodic dysphonia as a sign of essential voice tremor. *Journal of Speech and Hearing Disorders, 46,* 52–58

Baer, H., Sasaki, C., & Harris K. S. (1985). *Laryngeal function in phonation and respiration.* San Diego: College Hill Press.

Boone, D. R., & McFarlane, S. C. (1994). *The voice and its disorders,* (3rd, ed.). Englewood Cliffs, NJ: Prentice-Hall.

Colton, R. H., & Casper, J. K. (1990). *Understanding voice problems: A physiologic perspective for diagnosis and treatment.* Baltimore, MD: Williams & Wilkins.

Davis, C. N., & Harris, T. (1992). Teachers' ability to accurately identify disordered voices. *Language, Speech, and Hearing Services in Schools, 23,* 136–140.

Davis, S. (1979). Acoustic characteristics of normal and pathologic voices. *Speech and Language: Advances in Basic Research and Practice, 1,* 271–314.

Fitz-Hugh, G. S., Smith, D. E., & Chiong, A. T. (1958). Pathology of 300 clinically benign lesions of the vocal cords. *Laryngoscope, 68,* 855–875.

Ford, C. M., & Bless, D. M. (1992). *Phonosurgery: Assessment and surgical management.* New York: Raven Press.

Greene, M. C., & Mathison, L. (1991). *The voice and its disorders* (5th, ed.). San Diego: Singular Publishing Group, Inc.

Greene, M. C. (1972). *The voice and its disorders* (2nd, ed.). Philadelphia, PA: J. B. Lippincott Co.

Fujimura, O. (1988). *Vocal physiology: Voice production, mechanisms and functions.* New York: Raven Press.

Hirano, M., Kirchner, J. A., & Bless, D. M. (1991). *Neurolaryngology.* San Diego: Singular Publishing Group, Inc.

Hirano, M., & Sato, K. (1993). *Histological color atlas of the human larynx.* San Diego: Singular Publishing Group, Inc.

Hirano, M. (1981). *Clinical examination of voice.* New York: Springer.

Kitzing, P. (1985). Stroboscopy: A pertinent laryngological examination. *Journal of Otolaryngology 14,* 151–157.

Klingholz, F. (1990). Acoustic recognition of voice disorders: A comparative study of running speech versus sustained vowels. *Journal of the Acoustical Society of America, 87,* 2218–2224.

Ludlow, C. L. (1981). Research needs for the assessment of phonatory function. Proceedings of the Conference on Assessment of Vocal Pathology, *ASHA Reports 11,* 3–10.

Moore, P. (1991) *Organic voice disorders.* Edgewood Cliffs, NJ Prentice-Hall.

Morrison, M. D., Nichol, H., & Rammage, A. (1986). Diagnostic criteria and functional dysphonia. *Laryngoscope, 96,* 1–8.

Murry, T. (1978). Speaking fundamental frequency characteristics associated with voice pathology. *Journal of Speech and Hearing Disorders, 43,* 374–379.

Murry, T. & Doherty, E. T. (1980). Selected acoustic characteristics of pathologic and normal speakers. *Journal of Speech and Hearing Research, 23,* 361–369.

Murry, T., Singh, S., & Sargent, M. (1977). Multidimensional classification of abnormal voice qualities. *Journal of the Acoustical Society of America, 61,* 1630–1635.

Najata, K., Kurita, S., Yassimoto, S., Maeda, T., Kawasaki, H., & Hirano, M. (1983). Vocal fold polyps and nodules, a ten year review of 1,156 patients. *Aurus Nasus Larynx Suppl. 10,* 27–35.

Netsell, R., Lotz, W., & Shaughnessy, A. L. (1984). Laryngeal aerodynamics associated with selective voice disorders. *American Journal of Otolaryngology, 5,* 397–403.

Olson, N. R. (1991).Laryngopharyngeal manifestations of gastroesophageal reflux disease. Otolaryngologic *Clinics of North America, 24,* 1201–1213.

Parnell, F. W., & Brandenburg, J. H. (1970). Vocal cord paralysis: A review of 100 cases. *Laryngoscope,* 1036–1045.

Rammage, L. A., Nichol, H., & Morrison, M. D. (1987). The psychopathology of voice disorders. *Human Communication, 11,* 21–25

Sataloff, R. T. (1992). The human voice. *Scientific American, 267,* 108–115.

Stasney, C. R. (1996). *Static and dynamic laryngeal pathology.* San Diego: Singular Publishing Group, Inc.

Stemple, J. C. (1984). *Clinical voice pathology: Theory and management.* Columbus, OH: Charles E. Merrill.

Stemple, J. C., Glaze, L., & Gerdman, B. K. (1994). *Clinical voice pathology: Theory and management* (2nd, ed.).San Diego: Singular Publishing Group, Inc.

Titze, I. R. (1973). The human vocal cords: A mathematical model: Part I *Phonetica, 28,* 129–170.

Titze, I. R. (1974). The human vocal cords: A mathematical model: Part II *Phonetica, 29,* 1–21.

Tucker, H. M. (1987). *The larynx.* New York: Thieme Medical.

Tucker, H. M. (1993). *The larynx: Neurologic disorders* (2nd ed.). New York: Thieme Medical.

Wilson, F. D. (1977). *Voice Disorders.* Austin, TX: Learning Concepts.

Wolfe, V. I., Cornell, R., & Palmer, C. (1991). Acoustic correlates of pathologic voice types. *The Journal of Speech and Hearing Research, 34,* 509–516.

Wolfe, V. I., Fitch, J., & Cornell, R. (1995). Acoustic correlates of dysphonia in commonly occurring voice problems. *Journal of Speech and Hearing Research, 38,* 273–279.

Yanagasawa, E., & Yanagasawa, R. (1991). Laryngeal photography. *Otolaryngology Clinics of North America, 24,* 999–1022.

# CHAPTER
# 4

# Surgical Alternatives for Nonmalignant and Malignant Laryngeal Pathologies

## INTRODUCTION

This chapter provides an overview of surgical alternatives for both nonmalignant and malignant laryngeal pathologies. Within this framework, some of the procedures discussed might be considered to be elective, phonosurgery techniques designed specifically to facilitate voice production. Others may be construed as mandatory, focused on improving phonation, but more importantly, providing airway protection during swallowing. Surgical options for advanced stage laryngeal carcinoma will also be addressed. For more detailed discussions on these topics a list of suggested readings has been included at the end of the chapter.

## HISTORY BEHIND PHONOSURGERY

The many sophisticated phonosurgical procedures of today can be largely ascribed to the early work of Kirstein (1895), who first introduced the technique of direct laryngoscopy, thus establishing the surgical specialty of laryngology. During this time period most direct laryngoscopic procedures were performed to diagnose and treat laryngeal cancers. Little emphasis was placed on voice restoration after ablative cancer operations, or voice improvement after treatment of benign laryngeal pathologies. However, in 1911 surgery to improve or restore voice gained wider acceptance when Brunings introduced the concept of paraffin injection into the vocal fold of patients suffering from unilateral vocal fold paralysis and associated breathy dysphonia. In 1915, Payr performed the first documented laryngeal framework operation, a medialization thyroplasty. It was designed to improve breathy dysphonia in a patient suffering from unilateral recurrent nerve paralysis by medializing the affected vocal fold, thus reducing glottal incompetency. Although the procedure was successful, it did not generate significant interest by other laryngologists until many years later.

Despite these early landmark contributions to the field of laryngology, the modern era of laryngeal surgery was truly born in 1954 when Albrecht coupled the operating microscope with direct laryngoscopy, thus establishing the technique of microlaryngoscopy. In 1974 Isshiki published his classic article describing four laryngeal framework operations designed to alter voice. These techniques remain the cornerstone for the many laryngeal framework procedures that are commonly performed today. One year later, Hirano (1975) described the cover-body theory of vocal fold vibration. His investigations of vocal fold vibration laid the groundwork for many of the current microlaryngeal vocal fold surgical procedures discussed in this chapter.

## ANATOMY OF THE VOCAL FOLD

The anatomy of the human vocal fold is unique because all other mammals lack a vocal ligament. In fact, humans are born without a vocal ligament and only after age 1 does this structure begin development.

As described in Chapter 1, the anatomy of the vocal fold consists of an outer mucosa layer that covers a more deeply located thyroarytenoid muscle complex. The mucosa includes an outer nonkeratinizing, stratified squamous epithelium, and a deeper lamina propria that can be subdi-

vided into superficial, intermediate, and deep layers, as illustrated in Figure 4–1. The superficial layer of the lamina propria is known as Reinke's space, and the intermediate and deep layers combine to form the vocal ligament.

The epithelium and superficial layer of the lamina propria form the "cover," the intermediate and deep layers of the lamina propria constitute a "transition zone," and the thyroarytenoid muscle complex represents the "body." The gelatinous consistency of the superficial layer of the lamina propria permits fluency of motion of the epithelial cover over deeper structures in the vocal fold body during normal vocal fold vibration. This rolling or gliding movement of the cover over the body is referred to as the mucosal wave, and is readily visualized using stroboscopic techniques. Most benign laryngeal pathologies, and even early laryngeal carcinomas, develop in the epithelium or superficial layer of the lamina propria, thus inhibiting fluency of movement of the mucosal wave. Because these lesions develop superficial to the vocal ligament, laryngologists are now careful to limit the dissection plane for the removal of benign vocal fold lesions to the superficial layer of the lamina propria. Preservation of the vocal ligament is thought to ultimately result in healing with significantly decreased scarring and, therefore, better voice results postoperatively. Indeed, this philosophy is the foundation of microlaryngeal surgery of the vocal fold as we know it today.

## LESIONS OF THE COVER AND BODY

During normal phonation, the vocal folds vibrate with relative symmetry, which limits the amount of unwanted noise in the voice signal. This symmetry of movement is referred to as entrainment of the vocal folds. Asynchrony of vocal fold vibration causes loss of entrainment, and usually,

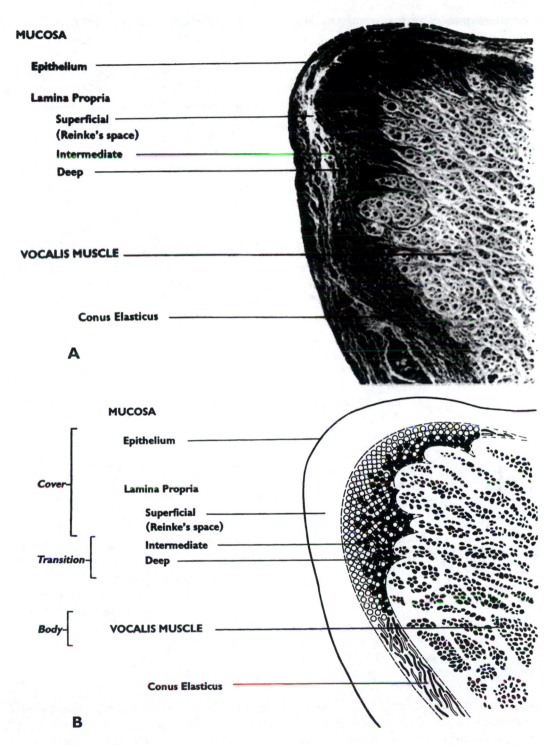

**MUCOSA**

    **Epithelium**

    **Lamina Propria**

        **Superficial**
        **(Reinke's space)**

        **Intermediate**
        **Deep**

**VOCALIS MUSCLE**

    **Conus Elasticus**

**A**

**MUCOSA**

    **Epithelium**

*Cover*

    **Lamina Propria**

        **Superficial**
        **(Reinke's space)**

        **Intermediate**
*Transition*        **Deep**

*Body*    **VOCALIS MUSCLE**

    **Conus Elasticus**

**B**

**FIGURE 4–1.** Photograph (**A**) and schematic (**B**) of the layered anatomy of the vocal fold. (From *Videostroboscopic Examination of the Larynx* by M. Hirano and D. M. Bless, 1993, p. 24. San Diego: Singular Publishing Group. Copyright 1993 Singular Publishing Group, Inc. Reprinted by permission.)

poor vocal quality. Such vibratory disruptions may be caused by cover lesions affecting the epithelium, superficial lamina propria, or both. These pathologies may include vocal fold polyps, diffuse polypoid changes or Reinke's edema, nodules, cysts, sulcus vocalis, squamous cell carcinoma, and scar formation. Likewise, loss of entrainment may result when the thyroarytenoid muscle complex, or body of the vocal fold, is flaccid due to unilateral vocal fold paralysis.

Mass lesions involving the cover of the vocal fold may disrupt the mucosal wave, thus altering the normal symmetric vibratory pattern of the folds. This disturbance occurs as a result of the load effect induced by increased vocal fold tissue density. When this occurs, abnormal airflow through the glottis produces sound energy at nonharmonic frequencies, perceived by the listener as hoarseness. Because most lesions produce irregular changes in the anatomy of the vocal fold cover, or free edge, abnormal and excessive transglottal airflow may occur, resulting in voice breathiness. If a mass lesion is located at the mid portion of a vocal fold, the anterior and posterior regions of the fold around the mass may simultaneously vibrate at different fundamental frequencies, causing features of diplophonia.

Vocal fold body flaccidity, secondary to paresis or paralysis of the thyroarytenoid muscle complex, results in asynchronous vibratory activity. Excessive escape of unphonated air through an incompetent glottal valve will distort vocal quality. Stroboscopic examination of the larynx may reveal irregular mucosal wave characteristics, which resemble the wave of a flag on a windy day. Mucosal wave amplitude may be increased, but velocity is diminished. Voice output is usually perceived as abnormally soft and breathy-hoarse in quality. Chapter 3 describes and illustrates these types of laryngeal pathologies.

# PHONOSURGERY FOR COVER LESIONS

In the last 20 years, with the aid of sophisticated diagnostic equipment and improved surgical instrumentation, the ability to diagnose and treat benign and malignant laryngeal abnormalities has greatly improved. Based on knowledge of the layered anatomy of the vocal fold, combined with a large number of patients suffering poor voice results postoperatively, the once universally accepted "vocal cord stripping" operation for benign lesions and selected superficial cancers has been replaced by mucosal sparing techniques. Because the vocal ligament is unique to humans, no animal model exists for study and comparison of different surgical techniques for removal of vocal fold lesions. Therefore, modern mucosal sparing procedures have been designed based on a combination of knowledge of the physiology and layered anatomy of the vocal fold, unsatisfactory phonosurgical results in the past, and common sense. With respect to generally predictable poor voice results following vocal cord stripping techniques, such outcomes are believed to be attributable to (1) uncontrolled, nonprecise tearing of mucosa off of the vibratory margin, which damages the vocal ligament and induces scar formation during healing, and (2) excessive removal of mucosa from the entire vocal fold, which results in a large raw surface area that the opposite fold contacts during phonation. These effects result in continual irritation of the exposed vocal ligament and increases the likelihood of scarring.

## Microflap Technique

In 1986 Sataloff described a mucosal sparing technique requiring (1) elevation of a "microflap" of epithelium by dissection in the superficial lamina propria, (2) excision of a subepithelial lesion, and (3) replacement of the flap with approximation of the raw epithelial edges to allow for primary healing. This procedure is designed to spare the underlying vocal ligament from injury during vibratory contact with the opposite vocal fold. Figure 4–2 illustrates this surgical approach, which has been generally accepted by laryngologists. It is currently the procedure of choice for removal of benign and selected superficial malignant vocal fold abnormalities. Figure 4–3 demonstrates a pretreatment photograph of a vocal fold cyst. This lesion was approached surgically using a mucosal sparing (microflap) technique. Even without postoperative voice therapy, the voice of this patient was converted from profoundly hoarse-breathy to near normal.

As our knowledge of vocal fold anatomy and physiology matures, surgical techniques will be modified to improve voice results. The availability of sophisticated laboratory instrumentation, as described in Chapter 2, has enabled voice scientists and laryngologists to discretely measure acoustic, aerodynamic, anatomic, and physiolog-

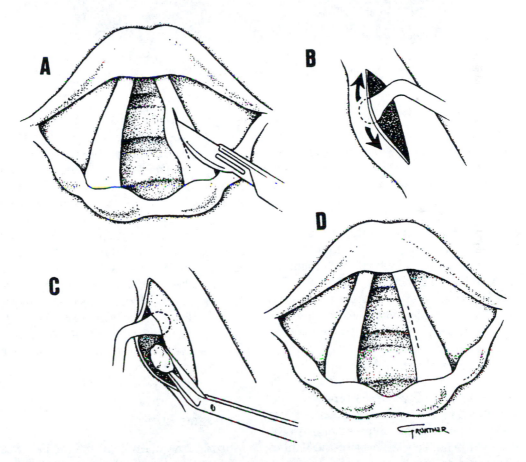

**FIGURE 4–2.** In the microflap technique an incision is made over the superior surface of the vocal fold (**A**). Blunt dissection is used to elevate a microflap of tissue over the lesion (**B**). The lesion is removed (**C**). The mucosal flap is replaced (**D**). (From *Professional Voice: The Science and Art of Clinical Care* (2nd ed.) by R. T. Sataloff, 1997, p. 620. San Diego: Singular Publishing Group, Inc. Copyright 1996 San Diego Publishing Group, Inc. Reprinted with permission.)

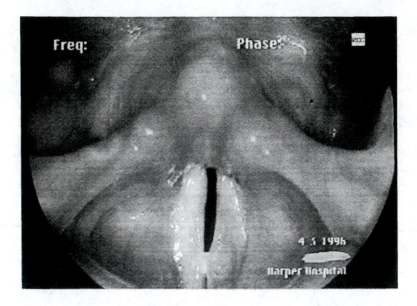

**FIGURE 4–3.** Preoperative view of a left-sided vocal fold cyst.

ic gains obtained following phonosurgery. Although subjective evaluation of voice quality remains the most important pre- and postoperative assessment tool, objective analyses have helped to reduce debate about treatment outcomes.

A report by Gray (1991) on electron microscopy of the mucosal surface of the vocal fold has enriched our knowledge of this delicate structure, which in turn has initiated changes in phonosurgery technique. He revealed a complex basement membrane zone structure located between the epithelium and superficial layer of the lamina propria, illustrated in Figure 4–4. The epithelium and basement membrane are attached to the superficial layer of the lamina propria by an elaborate array of type III and VII collagen fibers. Based on these findings, Sataloff (1995) proposed that unnecessary dissection in the superficial layer of the lamina propria may result in disruption of this basement membrane structure and scar formation during healing. He proposed a mini-microflap technique, whereby only the subepithelial lesion and its overlying epithelium are excised. The inferiorly based

epithelial flap is redraped over the mucosal defect to provide coverage of the vocal ligament, as shown in Figure 4–5.

Objective data supporting the use of mucosal sparing techniques are lacking. However, it makes intuitive sense that a less traumatic surgical technique will promote healing of the vocal fold with decreased scarring. Our experiences, and those of many others, suggest that conservative dissection strategies usually yield the best postoperative voice outcomes. Mucosal sparing techniques can be utilized for treatment of Reinke's edema, and for removal of vocal fold polyps, nodules, cysts, and selected superficial vocal fold cancers.

## Collagen Injection

Mucosal irregularities of the medial (free) edge of the vocal fold caused by scarring, senile bowing, sulcus vocalis, or atrophy secondary to vocal fold paralysis can result in severe dysphonia. These abnormal changes, examples of which have been reviewed in Chapter 3, may be treated with

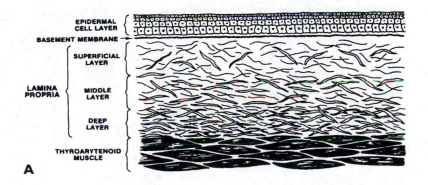

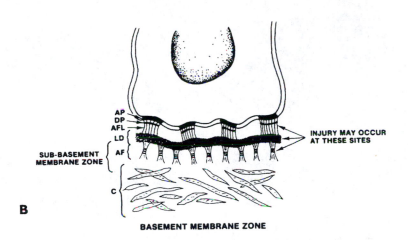

**FIGURE 4–4.** The basement membrane zone lies between the epithelium and the superficial layer of the lamina propria (**A**). Schematic illustrating epithelium and basement membrane attachments to the superficial layer of the lamina propria by an elaborate array of type III and VII collagen fibers (**B**). (From *Vocal Fold Physiology* by J. Gauffin and B. Hammarberg, 1991, p. 22. San Diego: Singular Publishing Group. Copyright 1991 by Singular Publishing Group, Inc. Reprinted by permission.)

glutaraldehyde-cross-linked bovine collagen (GAX-collagen, Zyplast®) injections. Collagen is a liquid material that is injected into the superficial layer of the lamina propria using a 27-gauge laryngeal needle, as shown in Figure 4–6. Injection of 0.3–3.0 mls, depending on the glottal defect, in the posterior aspect of the membranous vocal fold, just superficial to the vocal ligament, will allow infiltration of the liquid in a posteroanterior direction along the free edge of the vocal fold. Studies have shown an approximate 20–30% resorption rate after a mean follow-up of 4.5 years. Therefore, overcorrection of the glottal defect by 20–30% is recommended to allow for this anticipated effect. Skin testing with a 0.1 ml subcutaneous injection of GAX-collagen in the patient's forearm is recommended with a 10–30 day observation period for any signs of intolerance, such as localized redness or induration around the injection site.

A, B

C, D

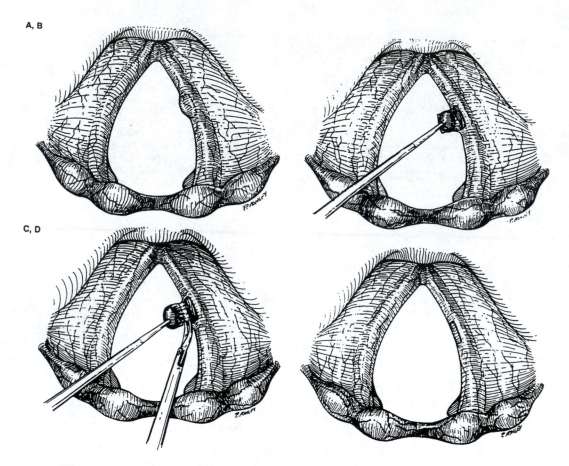

**FIGURE 4–5.** In the minimicroflap technique, only the subepithelial lesion and its overlying epithelium are excised. The minimicroflap is redraped over the mucosal defect to provide coverage of the vocal ligament. (From

*Professional Voice: The Science and Art of Clinical Care* (2nd ed.) by R. T. Sataloff, 1997, p. 621. San Diego: Singular Publishing Group, Inc. Copyright 1996 San Diego Publishing Group, Inc. Reprinted with permission.)

## $CO_2$ Laser

Coupling the operating microscope with the $CO_2$ laser launched a new era in the field of microlaryngeal surgery. With the development of microsurgical instrumentation and a micromanipulator attachment, which produces a reduced spot size diameter of 0.25 mm at a 400 mm working distance, the $CO_2$ laser combines surgical microprecision with capillary size hemostatic capability. This has become a useful instrument for a number of laryngeal pathologies. The glottis is an ideal structure for use

of a $CO_2$ laser because of its high tissue water content, especially in Reinke's space. Thermal energy created by the laser diffuses away from the impact site of the beam, resulting in less surrounding tissue injury. The benefits of minimal thermal damage from $CO_2$ laser surgery are realized with less postoperative tissue edema, limited scarring, and rapid wound healing. This surgical modality is ideally suited for vaporization of recurrent laryngeal papillomas, vocal fold ectasias or superficial vessels, hemangiomas, hemorrhagic polyps, and early glottic carcinomas.

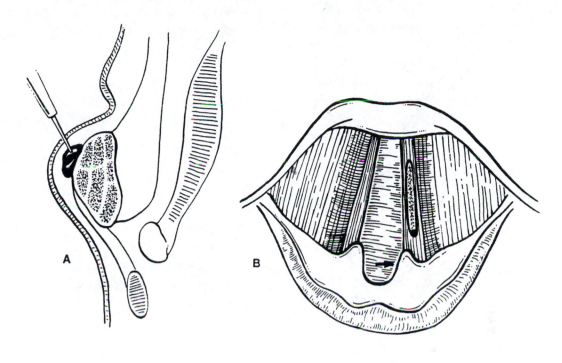

**FIGURE 4–6.** Proper placement of collagen is in the lamina propria **(A).** Additional collagen may be inject-ed (arrow) superficially over the cartilaginous portion of the vocal fold to provide better posterior glottic clo-sure **(B).** (From *Voice Surgery* by W. J. Gould, R. T. Sataloff, & J. R. Spiegel, 1993, p. 255. St. Louis, MO: Mosby. Copyright 1993 by Mosby Year-Book. Reprinted by permission.)

# PHONOSURGERY ALTERNATIVES FOR GLOTTAL INCOMPETENCY SECONDARY TO ADDUCTOR VOCAL FOLD PARALYSIS

Unilateral vocal fold paralysis, resulting in inadequate glottic closure, typically mani-fests with symptoms and signs of hoarse-ness, breathiness, a weak and ineffective cough, and episodic aspiration, especially with liquids. A number of phonosurgical procedures have been described to move the paralyzed vocal fold(s) to the midline of the glottis, thus enabling compensatory vibrato-ry activity and compression forces for better phonation, an effective cough, and airway protection when swallowing. A brief review of these surgical options is provided next.

## Teflon Injection

Teflon[R] (polytetrafluoroethylene) injection into the thyroarytenoid muscle was once the treatment of choice for permanent vocal fold paralysis. However, this technique is now being used less frequently because of the development of newer, potentially re-versible procedures that yield comparable, or even better, voice results. A Teflon injec-tion procedure is indicated for patients suf-fering from glottic incompetency secondary to irreversible vocal fold paralysis. Teflon, once injected into the vocal fold, cannot be easily removed. Therefore, accurate place-ment into the thyroarytenoid muscle com-plex, as far laterally as the thyroid cartilage, is of critical importance. This technique is il-lustrated in Figure 4–7. Injection just lateral

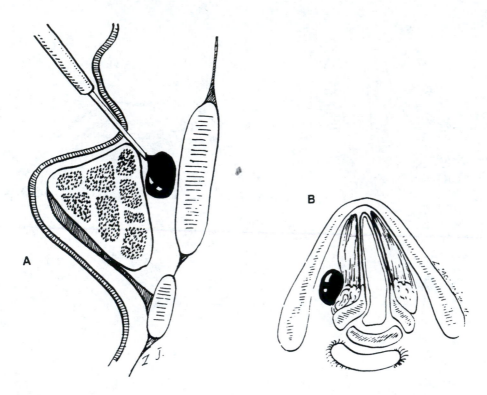

**FIGURE 4–7.** Proper placement of Teflon is lateral to the vocalis muscle, at the level of the vocal process. (From *Voice Surgery* by W. J. Gould, R. T. Sataloff, & J. R. Spiegel, 1993, p. 260. St. Louis, MO: Mosby. Copyright 1993 by Mosby Year-Book. Reprinted by permission.)

to the tip of vocal process of the arytenoid will provide medialization of the membranous vocal fold. A second injection can be placed in the mid membranous region if the vocal folds remain bowed. This technique is not indicated for closure of a large posterior commissure gap, vocal folds resting at unequal levels, or folds that are hypomobile or paretic. Complications associated with Teflon injection include airway compromise because of overinjection of the vocal fold, poor voice quality secondary to increased vocal fold stiffness, migration of material from the original injection site, and granuloma formation when the substance is injected too superficially.

## Gelfoam^R Injection

For those patients who suffer from suspected temporary vocal fold paralysis or paresis (neurapraxia), yet are symptomatic because of poor voice or aspiration, Gelfoam^R injection may prove very useful. This substance is biodegradable, and therefore it is reabsorbed by the vocal fold within 2 to 10 weeks following injection. For patients whose symptoms persist beyond this time period, multiple injections may be performed until recovery of function is evident. Gelfoam may also be used initially, with few risks, to predict the results of Teflon injection for patients who will require long-term or permanent augmentation. Voice results with gelfoam are comparable to those achieved with Teflon. Gelfoam powder is mixed with 3.5 ml of saline and injected in a similar fashion as Teflon. However, 30% overcorrection of the glottal defect is suggested to compensate for absorption of the saline, which occurs during the first few days postinjection. Complications associated with Gelfoam injection include airway compromise as a result of overinjection, and granuloma formation when the material is injected too superficially.

## Autologous Fat Injection

In 1992 Brandenburg introduced the technique of autologous fat injection into paralyzed vocal folds to achieve the same objectives as those described for Teflon, but with greater surgical flexibility and safety. Fat can be injected into vocal folds that are temporarily or permanently paralyzed, hypomobile, or bowed secondary to senile induced atrophy of the thyroarytenoid muscle complex. Multiple injections can be performed, if needed, and vocal fold inflammatory reactions to the fat have not been reported. The technique is particularly effective for compensating "elliptical" shaped glottal defects, which are readily visualized when the patient is asked to phonate. Such glottic incompetency is characterized by complete closure of the posterior commissure, and an elliptical shaped defect restricted only to the membranous vocal fold, as illustrated in Figure 4–8. The fat is usually harvested from the abdomen by utilizing an open technique, or by performing liposuction with a blunt tipped 14 gauge microextraction needle. If an open technique is used, the fat is minced into tiny pieces, washed with a saline solution and loaded into a Bruning syringe. The injection technique is similar to that used with Teflon, except that 50% overcorrection is attempted to compensate for expected resorption, which occurs within 6 months after injection. Unfortunately, because of overcorrection of the glottal defect initially, voice improvement is a gradual process that may be prolonged for as long as 6 months postsurgery. Complications associated with autologous fat injection include hematoma at the donor site and airway compromise from overcorrection.

## Laryngeal Framework Surgery

In 1974 Isshiki published a landmark article describing four laryngeal framework operations, each designed to alter voice in a specific way. Figure 4–9 illustrates these four techniques. Type I thyroplasty is a vocal fold medialization procedure utilized for treatment of membranous vocal fold incompetency. Type II creates lateral widening of the glottis to compensate for a compromised airway. Type III thyroplasty produces shortening and decreases tension of the vocal folds bilaterally, and was originally used to either lower the pitch of the voice or to treat adductor spasmodic dysphonia. The Type IV technique increases length and tension of the vocal folds bilaterally, which may raise pitch of the voice. Alternatively, the Type IV procedure can be

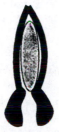

## A. Elliptical glottic defect

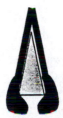

## B. Triangular glottic defect

**FIGURE 4–8.** An elliptical glottic defect occurs when there is anterior glottal incompetency, but closure of the posterior glottis during phonation **(A).** A triangular shaped defect results when an anterior and posterior glottic gap persist during phonatory efforts **(B).**

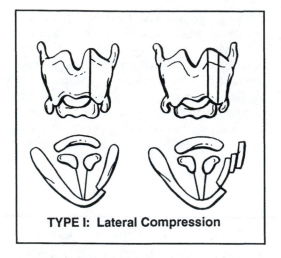

**TYPE I: Lateral Compression**

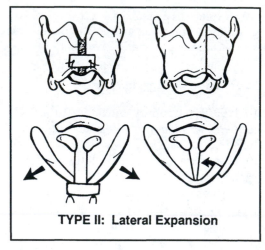

**TYPE II: Lateral Expansion**

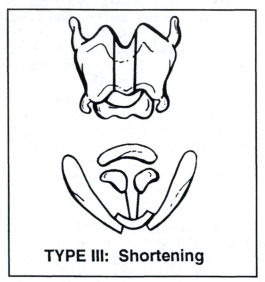

**TYPE III: Shortening**

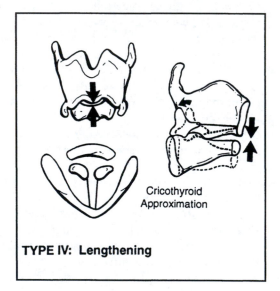

Cricothyroid
Approximation

**TYPE IV: Lengthening**

**FIGURE 4–9.** Four laryngeal framework procedures (types I-IV) first described by Isshiki. (From *Professional Voice: The Science and Art of Clinical Care* (2nd ed.) by R. T. Sataloff, 1997, p. 634. San Diego: Singular Publishing Group, Inc. Copyright 1996 San Diego Publishing Group, Inc. Reprinted with permission.)

performed in conjunction with a Type I thyroplasty if glottal incompetency persists after performing the latter technique.

Of the thyroplasty techniques described by Isshiki, the one most commonly performed today is the vocal fold medialization procedure. It is utilized for treatment of patients suffering from dysphonia or aspiration secondary to glottal incompetence. Because it is a potentially reversible proce-

dure, medialization thyroplasty is considered an effective method of treatment for temporary/permanent vocal fold paralysis/paresis that results in an elliptical shaped glottic defect, and for senile vocal fold bowing, where unilateral or bilateral implants may be used to straighten the leading edge(s) of the involved vocal fold(s). It should be noted, however, that this procedure will not provide closure of the posterior commissure. The medialization thyroplasty technique is performed using local anesthesia with sedation so that the patient is able to phonate while the surgeon adjusts the size and shape of the implant intraoperatively, thus allowing for fine tuning of the voice. The technique is illustrated in Figures 4–10 and 4–11. A small window is created in the thyroid lamina at the level of the affected vocal fold. A custom designed silastic implant is then inserted and secured within the cartilage window to provide a constant pushing force against the vocal fold toward the midline of the glottis. Complications associated with me-

dialization thyroplasty include hematoma formation, wound infection, implant extrusion or dislodgement, polypoid or inflammatory changes of the vocal fold, laryngocutaneous fistula, and airway compromise.

## Arytenoid Adduction

An injury to the vagus nerve high in the neck may result in paralysis of the superior and recurrent laryngeal nerves. This type of injury commonly causes glottic incompetence because of poor closure of the posterior commissure. Loss of both motor innervation to the cricothyroid muscle and

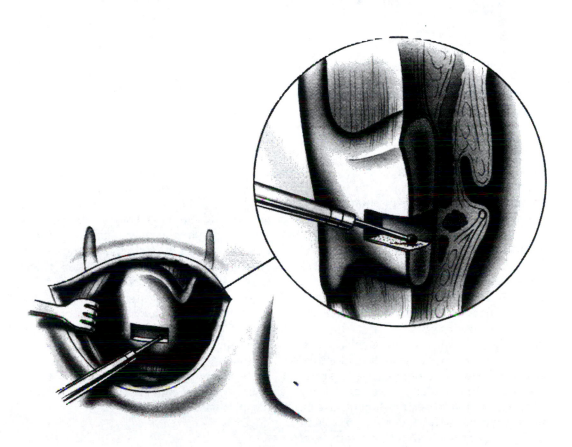

**FIGURE 4–10.** Medialization thyroplasty technique. A window is created in the thyroid lamina for placement of a silastic wedge. (From Phonosurgery: Silastic medialization for unilateral vocal fold paralysis by J. R. Wanamaker. In: *Operative Techniques in Otolaryngology—Head and Neck Surgery.* 1993;4(3): p. 210. Reprinted with permission.)

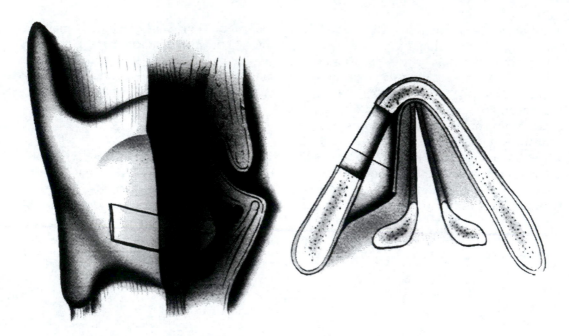

**FIGURE 4–11.** Medialization thyroplasty technique. The vocal fold is shown in a Medialized position after placement of the silastic wedge. (From Phonosurgery: Silastic medialization for unilateral vocal fold paralysis by J. R. Wanamaker. In: *Operative Techniques in Otolaryngology—Head and Neck Surgery.* 1993;4(3): p. 215. Reprinted with permission.)

sensation from the supraglottic larynx, because of superior laryngeal nerve injury, compounds problems of dysphonia and increases the risk for aspiration. Such glottic defects have been described as "triangular" in shape, in contrast to an "elliptical" shaped glottis that results when posterior commissure closure does occur, as shown in Figure 4–8. Triangular shaped glottal defects can be managed primarily with an arytenoid adduction procedure. Introduced by Isshiki in 1978, this technique provides rotation and rocking of the arytenoid into an adducted position by placing a suture around the muscular process of the arytenoid and strategically positioning and fixing the suture to the anterior thyroid lamina. This approach is shown in Figure 4–12. Arytenoid adduction can also be used to provide alignment of vocal folds that rest at different levels. Glottal defects that are only partially compensated by medialization

thyroplasty may be further corrected at the time of the initial operation by the addition of an arytenoid adduction procedure. Arytenoid adduction is contraindicated for those patients who may regain vocal fold motion because the technique is thought to be relatively irreversible. In addition, elderly patients who have poor pulmonary reserve and loss of elasticity of the thyroid cartilage may not tolerate sudden reduction of the glottal inlet area after such a procedure. Complications associated with arytenoid adduction include hematoma, wound infection, slipped arytenoid sutures, pharyngocutaneous fistula, and airway compromise.

## Reinnervation

Although vocal fold medialization techniques may improve the voice, they usually

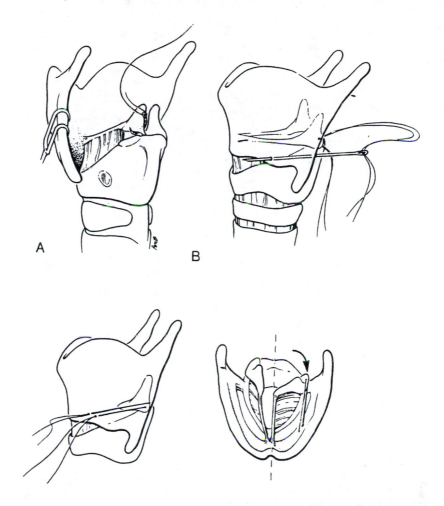

**FIGURE 4–12.** Arytenoid adduction procedure. A suture is placed around the muscular process of the arytenoid **(A)**. The muscular process is rotated anteriorly, resulting in medialization of the vocal fold **(B)**. (From "Laryngoplastic Phonosurgery," by J. A. Koufman, 1991, pp. 1163–1164. *The Otolaryngologic Clinics of North America*, 24(5). Copyright 1991 by W. B. Saunders. Reprinted with permission.)

do not produce completely normal voice quality, especially in patients whose etiology is recurrent laryngeal nerve paralysis. Denervation of the musculature causes atrophic changes of the vocal folds and inherently limits the potential phonation improvements that can be obtained with these forms of phonosurgery. To overcome such limitations, reinnervation of the intrinsic muscles has evolved as an alternative or complimentary surgical procedure. The primary objectives include improving underlying muscle tone and increasing muscle tensing capability, often improving the voice quality to near normal. Reinnervation does not, however, result in restoration of "normal" vocal fold movement. The literature suggests that the ansa cervicalis to recurrent laryngeal nerve anastomosis, illustrated in Figure 4–13, produces consistently good results. The procedure is often performed at the time of the vocal fold medialization procedure because recovery of muscle function usually takes from 3 to 6 months.

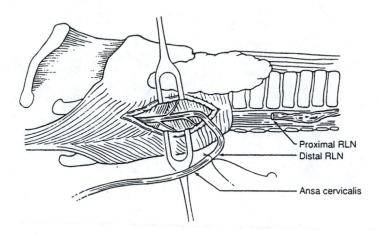

Proximal RLN
Distal RLN

Ansa cervicalis

**FIGURE 4–13.** Ansa cervicalis to recurrent laryngeal nerve anastomosis. (From "Laryngeal Reinnervation Techniques by R. L. Crumley, 1991, p. 209. In: *Phonosurgery: Assessment and Surgical Management of Voice Disorders*, edited by C. N. Ford & D. M. Bless. New York: Raven Press. Reprinted with permission.)

## BOTULINUM TOXIN INJECTIONS FOR VOICE DISORDERS

Botulinum toxin (Botox) is produced by the bacterium *Clostridia botulinum*. It creates its effects at the nerve-muscle junction by inhibiting the release of acetylcholine, a neurotransmitter, thus producing a flaccid muscle paralysis. The initial clinical use of Botox was for the treatment of strabismus, a disorder characterized by uncontrolled deviation of the eye secondary to hypertonicity of extraocular musculature. Since its introduction, Botox has been used successfully to treat a number of voice disorders. These include spasmodic dysphonia, vocal process ulceration secondary to a hyperfunctional speech disorder, and pharyngoesophageal segment muscle spasm in total laryngectomy patients suffering from failed tracheoesophageal speech.

### Spasmodic Dysphonia

Spasmodic dysphonia (SD) is most often a sequela of focal laryngeal dystonia. The cause is unknown and the disorder is characterized by abnormal involuntary movements of the vocal folds, resulting in breaks in speech fluency. In some patients there may be a strong psychogenic contribution to these disabling symptoms. This disorder has been subdivided into adductor, abductor, and mixed (adductor/abductor) types. The most common form is the adductor type, distinguished by tight closure of the true vocal folds during phonation, causing episodic phonatory breaks and a strangled sound to the voice. A less common form is the abductor type, characterized by periodic involuntary abduction of the vocal folds, with sudden interruption of speech by low intensity and breathy voice segments. Voice interruptions are especially evident with voice onset. The mixed form is more difficult to diagnose and is a combination of voice characteristics representative of both adductor and abductor forms.

Treatment options described for SD include voice therapy, recurrent laryngeal nerve transection, electrical stimulation of the recurrent laryngeal nerve, anterior laryngoplasty, and botulinum toxin injection. Presently, most experts consider botulinum toxin injection to be the therapy of choice for patients with SD, especially the adductor form, with recovery of voice to an average of 90% of normal function in response to each injection. However, botulinum toxin therapy for the abductor and mixed forms of this disorder has been less encouraging, with average improvement to 70% of normal voice function. Less impressive results may be partially attributable to the technical difficulty in accurately localizing and injecting botulinum toxin into the posterior cricoarytenoid muscle (PCA).

Botulinum toxin injections for treatment of adductor SD are usually given using an anterior percutaneous laryngeal approach, as illustrated in Figure 4–14. The injection can be performed either through the cricothyroid membrane and into the undersurface of the true vocal fold (thyroarytenoid muscle), or directly through the thyroid cartilage at the level of the true vocal fold, with submucosal injection into the thyroarytenoid muscle. These techniques can be performed using both electromyography (EMG) guidance for accurate localization of the thyroarytenoid muscle and flexible transnasal laryngoscopy to help visualize needle tip placement. The injections are relatively painless, quick, and easily given in the office, and voice improvement lasts an average of 3 months. Most patients will experience breathiness and minor swallowing difficulties within the first 24 to 48 hours postinjection. They may remain symptomatic for the following 1 to 2 weeks, with return to a more normal voice, without swallowing difficulties, during the remaining 3 months. If the spasmodic voice quality redevelops, a repeat injection can be performed, sometimes with longer lasting effects.

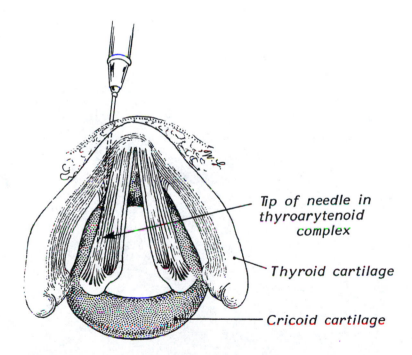

Tip of needle in
thyroarytenoid
complex

Thyroid cartilage

Cricoid cartilage

**FIGURE 4–14.** Anterior percutaneous botulinum toxin injection technique for treatment of adductor spasmodic dysphonia. The injection can be performed either through the cricothyroid membrane and into the undersurface of the true vocal fold, or directly through the thyroid cartilage and submucosally into the vocal fold.

Botulinum toxin injection approaches to the PCA for treatment of abductor SD include either lateral or anterior percutaneous laryngeal routes as illustrated in Figures 4–15, 4–16, and 4–17. Brin, Blitzer, Stewart, and Fahn (1990) originally described a lateral percutaneous approach. It involves rotation of the larynx away from the injection site and percutaneous placement of an EMG needle lateral to the larynx, along the posterior and inferior border of the thyroid cartilage, and finally into the PCA. This technique is currently the most popular method for botulinum toxin injection of the PCA. However, accurate localization of the muscle is often difficult. In addition, patients sometimes experience considerable discomfort from both laryngeal manipulation and needle placement.

Because of difficulties experienced with the lateral cervical injection technique, a new approach to the PCA was developed by Bastian (Meleca, Hogikyan, & Bastian, 1996) for the treatment of abductor SD. The technique includes directing a needle, with EMG guidance, through the cricothyroid membrane. After entering the laryngeal lumen the needle is directed 30 degrees laterally, and 15 to 20 degrees superiorly toward the posterior cricoid lamina. The needle is then directed through the cricoid cartilage and into the PCA. EMG documentation of increased activity when the patient is asked to sniff assures that the needle is accurately placed into the PCA. Botulinum toxin is injected into the muscle, the needle tip is then withdrawn into the laryngeal lumen, and injection of the opposite PCA is performed using the same technique. This procedure can be performed using transnasal flexible endoscopy to visualize needle placement. Complications associated with Botox injections to the PCAs are uncommon, but may include exertional stridor and dysphagia.

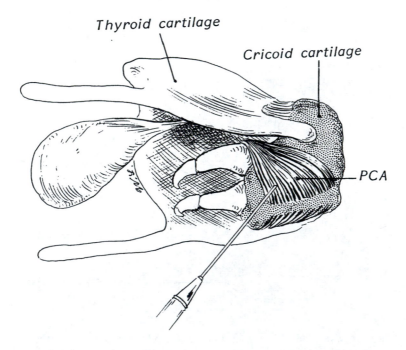

**FIGURE 4–15.** Lateral percutaneous botulinum toxin injection approach for treatment of abductor spasmodic dysphonia.

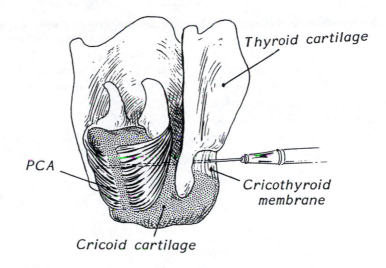

FIGURE 4–16. Lateral oblique view of the transcricoid botulinum toxin injection technique to the posterior cricoarytenoid muscle(s) for treatment of abductor spasmodic dysphonia.

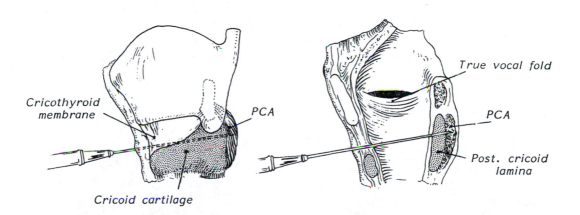

**FIGURE 4–17.** Lateral (left) and midsagittal (right) view of the transcricoid botulinum toxin injection technique to the posterior cricoarytenoid muscle(s) for treatment of abductor spasmodic dysphonia.

These effects are usually transient, lasting 1 to 2 weeks postinjection.

## Vocal Process Ulcerations

Patients with vocal process ulcerations or granulomas from a hyperfunctional voice disorder, characterized by forceful and traumatic vocal fold closure, can usually be effectively treated with conservative man-

agement, including speech therapy and the use of H2 blockers. When patients fail conservative treatment they may benefit from unilateral or bilateral Botox injection(s) to the thyroarytenoid muscle complex, as described by Berke (Nasri, Sercarz, McAlpin, & Berke, 1995). The injection technique is similar to that used for treatment of adductor SD. The aim of therapy is to weaken the vocal fold closing forces by inducing a paresis of the thyroarytenoid muscle(s). This reduces contact trauma to the vocal processes during phonation. Because the effects of Botox last approximately 3 months, healing of vocal process ulcerations will likely occur during this time period. Continuation of speech therapy after resolution of these lesions is of vital importance to prevent recurrence.

## Pharyngoesophageal Segment Spasm

Total laryngectomy patients, after undergoing a tracheoesophageal (TE) puncture, may develop abnormal TE speech because of pharyngoesophageal (PE) segment spasm. This disorder is characterized by phonatory breaks and a strangled sound to the voice, or an inability to produce any sound. It is caused by interruption of airflow through an abnormally hypertonic or spasmodic PE segment muscle complex. Vibration of the PE segment mucosa is disrupted and the aforementioned voice characteristics occur. The treatment of choice for this disorder is cricopharyngeal myotomy. However, there is a subset of patients who fail to develop fluent TE speech, despite undergoing a myotomy procedure. Blitzer, Komisar, Baredes, Brin, and Stewart (1995) reported that these patients may benefit from Botox injection of the PE segment to provide relaxation of this muscle complex and therefore allow fluency of vibration of the PE segment mucosa. This technique is shown in Figure 4–18. Three vertically aligned injections are performed in the anterior lateral neck region, just above the stoma. The first injection is performed approximately 1 cm above the lateral margin of the stoma. The needle is directed perpendicular to the plane of the neck and inserted until the tip of the needle abuts the vertebral body. The tip of the needle is then retracted 3 mm and an injection of approximately 15 units of Botox is given. The needle is then withdrawn and two other injec-

tions are similarly given, each approximately 2 cm above the previous injection site. Complications associated with this technique include hematoma formation and localized infection at the injection site.

## TREATMENT OF LARYNGEAL CARCINOMA

The diagnostic work-up and treatment for laryngeal carcinoma is performed by a team of multidisciplinary specialists, including an otolaryngologist, medical and radiation oncologists, speech and swallowing pathologists, a dentist, an oral surgeon, a pathologist, a radiologist, and multiple other ancillary personnel. A detailed staging work-up for such lesions was described in Chapter 2. Therapeutic options for laryngeal carcinoma include surgery, radiation therapy, chemotherapy, or a combination of these modalities. If surgical treatment is chosen, the particular technique utilized re-

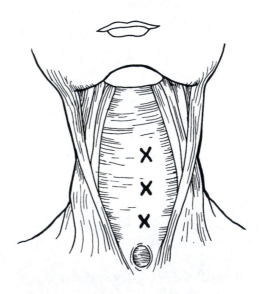

**FIGURE 4–18.** Botulinum toxin injection sites (X) marking the pharyngoesophageal (PE) segment. These injections are performed to ease PE segment muscle spasm and to improve tracheoesophageal speech.

lies upon a number of factors, including tumor location and staging, patient health, and surgeon preference. A number of surgical techniques are available, including excision of vocal fold cover lesions using microflap, vocal fold stripping, or laser techniques, cordectomy via either a thyrotomy or endoscopic laser approach, partial laryngectomy, or total laryngectomy. The principles behind such operations center on performing the most conservative, organ-sparing procedure that will provide voice quality and swallowing ability, combined with an oncologically sound technique that offers the best chance for cure. A detailed description of these operations is beyond the scope of this text, thus, a list of suggested readings is given at the end of this chapter, and only a general overview of surgical alternatives is provided here.

Excision of selected T1 vocal fold cover lesions is an oncologically sound treatment option, with local control and survival rates comparable to similar lesions treated with radiation therapy. These techniques were discussed earlier in the chapter.

Although radiation therapy is the treatment of choice for T1 glottic carcinomas, a cordectomy procedure can also be utilized for such lesions. The technique is performed either endoscopically using the knife or laser, or by making an incision in the neck and splitting the thyroid cartilage (thyrotomy) with excision of the involved vocal fold. The procedure is illustrated in Figure 4–19.

Partial laryngectomy refers to a variety of procedures designed to maintain function of the laryngopharynx by preserving voice quality and swallowing ability. Many of these procedures allow for tracheotomy removal after recovery from surgery. The most commonly used laryngeal conservation procedures include supraglottic, vertical hemi-, vertical partial, and supracricoid laryngectomies. Tumor location and stage are the primary features determining which surgical technique is utilized.

Supraglottic laryngectomy involves removal of supraglottic structures above the true vocal folds for selected carcinomas involving the epiglottis, aryepiglottic folds, false folds, or anterior or lateral piriform sinus. This laryngeal conservation approach, depicted in Figure 4–20, preserves the true vocal folds, thus allowing for more normal phonatory function postoperatively. The tracheotomy tube can usually be removed

**CORDECTOMY**

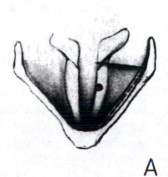
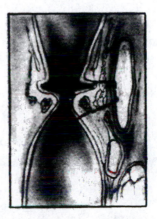
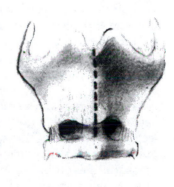

A

**FIGURE 4–19.** Cordectomy procedure using a midline thyrotomy approach. The margins of resection are outlined by the dashed line. (From *Surgery of the Larynx*, edited by B. J. Bailey & H. F. Biller, 1985, p. 264.

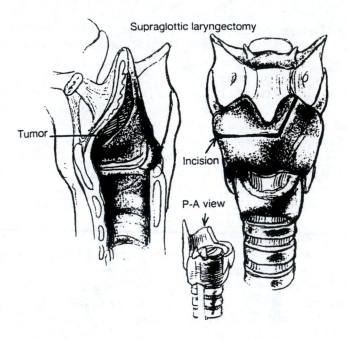

**FIGURE 4–20.** Supraglottic laryngectomy. Excision usually includes the supraglottic ipsilateral thyroid cartilage, the aryepiglottic folds, false vocal folds, and epiglottis. The excision can be extended to include the hyoid bone and arytenoid cartilages. (From "Advanced Cancer of the Larynx" by M. P. Fried & H. V. Girdhar-Gopal, 1993, p. 1355. In: *Head and Neck Surgery—Otolaryngology* (Vol. 2), edited by B. J. Bailey. Philadelphia: J. B. Lippincott. Copyright 1993 J. B. Lippincott. Reprinted with permission.)

once swelling subsides. Unfortunately, those patients receiving postoperative radiation therapy often suffer from severe dysphagia. This problem has been somewhat alleviated using an endoscopic laser supraglottic laryngectomy technique, thus preserving normal strap muscle attachments to the hyoid bone and sensory innervation of the supraglottic larynx.

Vertical hemi- and vertical partial laryngectomies are primarily performed for selected T1, T2, and T3 laryngeal carcinomas involving a unilateral true vocal fold or arytenoid, as shown in Figure 4–21. The technique may also be utilized for anterior commissure lesions, or cancers involving the anterior one third of the contralateral vocal fold. Reconstruction of the resected glottis

can be performed using mucosal advancement flaps, bipedicled muscle flaps, or an epiglottoplasty technique. Postoperatively, the patient may suffer from dysphonia, but swallowing function is usually maintained and the tracheotomy tube can normally be removed once swelling subsides.

The supracricoid laryngectomy was first introduced by Majer and Rieder (1959), and later modified by Laccourreye. It can be utilized for selected T2 and T3 carcinomas involving the supraglottis and glottis. The technique includes removal of laryngeal structures located between the hyoid bone and cricoid cartilage, as illustrated in Figure 4–22. The tissues not excised include the arytenoids, hyoid bone, and cricoid cartilage. The defect is closed by approximat-

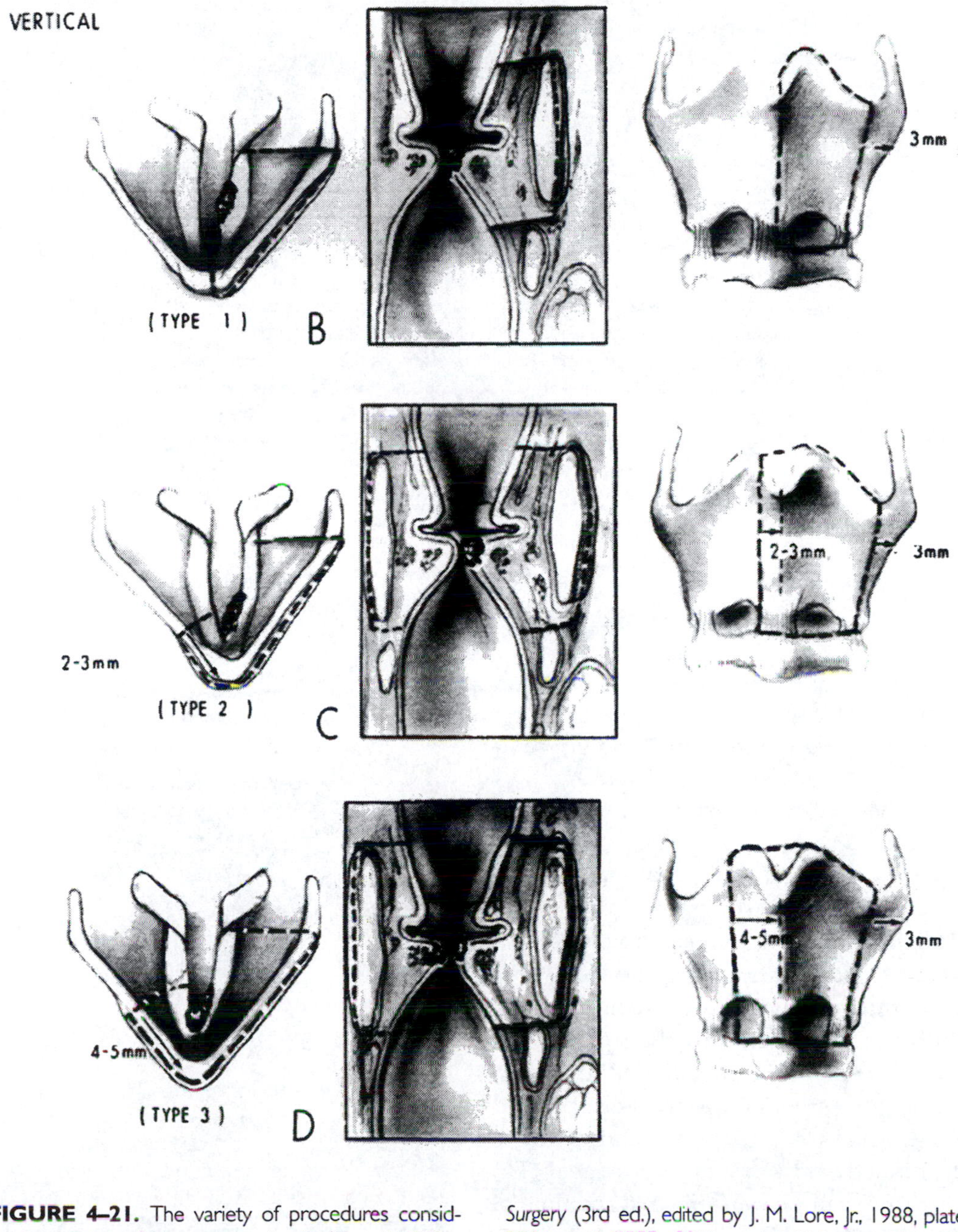

VERTICAL

( TYPE 1 )   B

3 mm

( TYPE 2 )   C

2-3 mm

2-3 mm   3mm

( TYPE 3 )   D

4-5 mm

4-5mm   3mm

**FIGURE 4–21.** The variety of procedures considered vertical partial laryngectomies (**B, C,** and **D**). The technique employed depends on the location and extent of the tumor. (From *An Atlas of Head and Neck Surgery* (3rd ed.), edited by J. M. Lore, Jr., 1988, plates 380A and 380B, 381B and 381C, pp. 895, 897. Philadelphia: W. B. Saunders. Copyright 1988 W. B. Saunders. Reprinted with permission.)

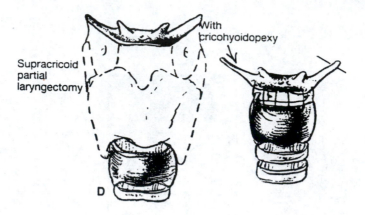

**FIGURE 4–22.** Supracricoid laryngectomy. Excision usually includes the entire thyroid cartilage, true and false vocal folds, aryepiglottic folds, and epiglottis. Leaving one or both arytenoids will allow for phonation. The defect is reconstructed by suturing the hyoid bone to the cricoid cartilage (cricohyoidopexy). (From "Advanced Cancer of the Larynx" by M. P. Fried & H. V. Girdhar-Gopal, 1993, p. 1355. In: *Head and Neck Surgery—Otolaryngology* (Vol. 2), edited by B. J. Bailey. Philadelphia: J. B. Lippincott. Copyright 1993 J. B. Lippincott. Reprinted with permission.)

ing the hyoid bone to the cricoid cartilage (cricohyoidopexy). The large majority of patients achieve "physiologic" phonation and are decannulated within the first postoperative month. However, approximately 50% of patients suffer from swallowing impairment lasting between 6 and 12 months.

For advanced laryngeal carcinomas demonstrating cartilage invasion (stage T4), the treatment of choice is a total laryngectomy, illustrated in Figure 4–23. This procedure involves en-bloc removal of the entire larynx, including the hyoid bone, thyroid, epiglottic, cricoid, and arytenoid cartilages, proximal trachea, and true and false vocal folds. A permanent stoma is fashioned and a tracheoesophageal (TE) puncture can be performed at the time of the original resection or at a second operation to provide TE speech. Most patients develop good quality speech and are able to swallow without difficulty.

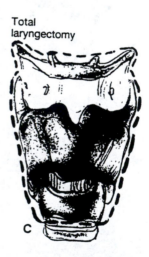

**FIGURE 4–23.** Total laryngectomy includes removal of the entire larynx, including the hyoid bone, thyroid and cricoid cartilages, arytenoids, true and false vocal folds, aryepiglottic folds, and epiglottis (excision outlined by dashed line). (From "Advanced Cancer of the Larynx" by M. P. Fried & H. V. Girdhar-Gopal, 1993, p. 1355. In: *Head and Neck Surgery—Otolaryngology* (Vol. 2), edited by B. J. Bailey. Philadelphia: J. B. Lippincott. Copyright 1993 J. B. Lippincott. Reprinted with permission.)

## CONCLUSION

In summary, laryngeal surgery is routinely performed not only to improve or restore voice, but also to treat problems with aspiration. Laryngeal pathology, either benign or malignant, may involve the cover or body of the vocal fold; modern surgical procedures have been developed to treat such lesions. Neurological disorders may lead to dystonic movements of the intrinsic and extrinsic laryngeal musculature. Botulinum toxin has proven to be beneficial for the treatment of such disorders, as well as other conditions of muscle spasticity or hypertonicity. The principles behind modern laryngeal techniques rely on the application of sound rationale, combined with a thorough understanding of the complex anatomy and physiology of the vocal folds. Certainly, pre- and postoperative treatment programs designed by the speech pathologist play an indispensable role in providing the patient with continuity-of-care and long-lasting therapeutic success.

## SUGGESTED READINGS

Albrecht, R. (1954). Uber den wert koloskopischer untersuchungsmethoden bei leukoplakien und carcinomen des mundes und kehlkopes. *Arch fur Ohren Nasen und Kehlkopfheilkunde, 165,* 459–463.

Arnold, G. E. (1962). Vocal rehabilitation of paralytic dysphonia. *Archives of Otolaryngology, 76,* 358–368.

Aronson, A. E., & Hartman, D. E. (1981). Adductor spastic dysphonia as a sign of essential tremor. *Journal of Speech and Hearing Disorders, 46,* 52–58.

Aronson, A. E. (1985). *Clinical voice disorders* (2nd ed.). New York: Thieme Medical Publishing.

Bailey, B. J., & Biller, H. F. (Eds.). (1985). *Surgery of the larynx.* Philadelphia: W. B. Saunders, Inc.

Benninger, M. S., Jacobson, B. H., & Johnson, A. F. (1994). *Vocal arts medicine: The care and prevention of professional voice disorders.* New York: Thieme Medical Publishing.

Berke, G. S. (1993). Voice disorders and phonosurgery. In B. J. Bailey (Ed.), *Head and neck surgery—Otolaryngology* (pp. 644–657). Philadelphia: J. B. Lippincott.

Blitzer, A., & Brin, M. F. (1993). Botulinum toxin in the management of adductor and abductor spasmodic dysphonia. *Operative Techniques in Otolaryngology—Head and Neck Surgery, 4(3),* 199–206.

Blitzer, A., Brin, M. F., Fahn, S., & Lovelace, R. E. (1988). Localized injections of botulinum toxin for the treatment of focal laryngeal dystonia (spastic dysphonia). *Laryngoscope, 98,* 193–197.

Blitzer, A., Brin, M. F., Sasaki, C. T., Fahn, S., & Haris, K. S. (1992). *Neurologic disorders of the larynx.* New York: Thieme Medical Publishing.

Blitzer, A., Brin, M. F., Stewart C., Aviv, J. E., & Fahn, S. (1992). Abductor laryngeal dystonia: A series treated with botulinum toxin. *Laryngoscope, 102,* 163–167.

Blitzer, A., Komisar, A., Baredes, S., Brin, M. F., & Stewart, C. (1995). Voice failure after tracheoesophageal puncture: Management with botulinum toxin. *Otolaryngology—Head and Neck Surgery, 113(6),* 668–670.

Bouchayer, M., Cornut, G., Witzig, E., Loire, R., Roch, J. B., & Bastian, R. W. (1985). Epidermoid cysts, sulci and mucosal bridges of the true vocal cord: A report of 157 cases. *Laryngoscope, 95,* 1087–1094.

Brandenburg, J. H., Kirkham, & W., Koschkee, D. (1992). Vocal cord augmentation with autogenous fat. *Laryngoscope, 102,* 495–500.

Brin, M. F., Blitzer, A., Stewart, C., & Fahn, S. (1990). Botulinum toxin: Now for abductor laryngeal dystonia. *Neurology, 40(Suppl. 1),* 381. (Abstract)

Brunings, W. (1911). Eber eine neue Behandlungsmethode der Rekurrenslahmung. *Verh Deutsch Laryngol, 19,* 93–151.

Clayman, D. A., Booth, R. P., Isaacs, J., & Russo, L. S. (1994). Percutaneous electromyography of the posterior cricoarytenoid muscles: Electromyographic needle placement with computed tomographic guidance. *Laryngoscope, 11,* 1393–1396.

Fawett, D. W. (1986). *A textbook of histology* (11th ed.). Philadelphia: W. B. Saunders, Inc.

Ford, C. N., & Bless, D. M. (1991). *Phonosurgery assessment and surgical management of voice disorders.* New York: Raven Press, Inc.

Ford, C. N. Bless, D. M. & Loftus, J. M. (1992). Role of injectable collagen in the treatment of glottal insufficiency: A study of 119 patients. *Annals of Otology, Rhinology, and Laryngology, 101*, 237–247.

Ford, C. N., Martin, D. W., & Warner, T. F. (1984). Injectable collagen in laryngeal rehabilitation. *Laryngoscope, 94*, 513–518.

Gay, T., Hirose, H., Strome, M., & Sasashima, M. (1972). Electromyography of the intrinsic laryngeal muscles during phonation. *Annals of Otology, 81*, 401–409.

Gould, W. J., Sataloff, R. T., & Spiegel, J. R. (1993). *Voice surgery.* St. Louis: Mosby.

Gray, S. (1991). Basement membrane zone injury in vocal nodules. In J. GauffinNN & B. Hammar-berg (Eds.). *Vocal fold physiology: Acoustic, perceptual and physiologic aspects of voice                    mechanics* (pp 21–27). San Diego: Singular Publishing Group, Inc.

Hirano, M. (1975). Phonosurgery. Basic and clinical investigations. *Otologia (Fukuoka), 21*, 239–442.

Hirano, M. (1981). *Clinical examination of voice.* New York: Springer-Verlag, Inc.

Hoffman, H. T., McCulloch, T. M., Peterson, L., & Van Demark, D. (1992). Botulinum neurotoxin injection after total laryngectomy. *National Center for Voice and Speech Status and Progress Report*, pp. 167–172.

Isshiki, N., Morita, H., & Okamura, H. (1974). thyroplasty as a new phonosurgical technique. *Acta Otolaryngology, 78*, 451–457.

Isshiki, N., Tanabe, M., & Sawada, M. (1978). Arytenoid adduction for unilateral vocal cord paralysis. *Archives of Otolaryngology, 104*(10), 555–558.

Isshiki, N. (1989). *Phonosurgery theory and practice.* Tokyo: Springer-Verlag.

Jankovic, J., & Orman, J. (1987). Botulinum A. toxin for cranial–cervical dystonia: A double-blind, placebo-controlled study. *Neurology, 37*, 616–623.

Johns, M. E., & Rood, S. R. (1987). *Vocal cord paralysis: Diagnosis and management. A self-instructional package* (2nd ed.). Washington, DC: American Academy of Otolaryngology—Head and Neck Surgery.

Kirstein, A. (1895). Autoskopie des larynx und der trachea (laryngoscopia directa, euthyskopie, bisichtigung ohne spiegel). *Archiv fur Laryngologie und Rhinologie, 3*, 156–164.

Koufman, J. A., & Isaacson, G. (Eds.). (1991). Voice disorders. *The Otolaryngologic Clinics of North America, 24*(5).

Laccourreye, H., Brasnu, D., Lacau St. Guily, J., & Fabre, A. (1988). New concepts in conservation surgery of the larynx. In M. P. Fried (Ed.). *The larynx: A multidisciplinary approach* (pp. 503–513). Boston: Little Brown.

Laccourreye, H., Lacau St Guily, J., Brasnu, D., Fabre, A., & Menard, M. (1987). Supracricoid hemilaryngopharyngectomy. Analysis of 240 cases. *Annals of Otology, Rhinology, and Laryngology, 96*, 217–221.

Laccourreye, O., Merite-Drancy, A., Brasnu, D., Chabardes, E., Cauchois, R., Menard, M., & Laccourreye, H. (1993). Supracricoid hemilaryngopharyngectomy in selected pyriform sinus carcinoma staged as T2. *Laryngoscope, 103*, 1373–1379.

Majer, H., & Rieder. W. (1959). Technique de laryngectomie permettant de conserver la permeabilite respiratoire la cricohyoidopexie. *Ann Otolaryngol Chir Cervicofac, 75*, 677–683.

Meleca, R. J., Hogikyan, N. D., & Bastian, R. W. (1996). A comparison of methods of botulinum toxin injection for abductory spasmodic dysphonia. Manuscript submitted for publication.

Miller, R. H., & Woodsn, G. E. (1991). Treatment options in spasmodic dysphonia. *The Otolaryngologic Clinics of North America, 24*, 1227–1237.

Morrison, M. D., & Rammag, L. A. (1993). Muscle misuse voice disorders: Description and classification. *Acta Otolaryngology (Stockh), 113*, 428–434.

Mu, L., & Yang, S. (1990). A new method of needle-electrode placement in the posterior cricoarytenoid muscle for electromyography. *Laryngoscope, 100*, 1127–1131.

Nasri, S., Sercarz, J. A., McAlpin, T., & Berke, G. S. (1995). Treatment of vocal fold granuloma using botulinum toxin type A. *Laryngoscope, 105*(6), 585–588.

Payr. (1915). *Belenkverletzungen, Gelenkeiterungen und ibre Behandlung.* Wehnschr: Munchen med.

Ramacle, M., Dujardin, J. M., & Lawson, G. (1995). Treatment of vocal fold immobility by glutaraldehyde-cross-linked collagen injection: Long-term results. *Annals of Otology, Rhinology, and Laryngology, 104*(6), 437–441.

Robbins, K. T., Medina, J. E., Wolfe, G. T., Levine, P. A. Sessions, R. B., & Pruet, C. W. (1991). Standardizing neck dissection terminology. *Archives of Otolaryngology, 117*(6), 601–605.

Rontal, M., Rontal, E., Rolnick, M., Merson, R., Silverman, R., & Truong, D. D. (1991). A method for the treatment of abductor spasmodic dysphonia with botulinum toxin injections: A preliminary report. *Laryngoscope, 101,* 911–914.

Sataloff, R. T. (1992). Office evaluation of dysphonia. *The Otolaryngologic Clinics of North America, 25,* 843–855.

Sataloff, R. T. (1995). Rational thought: The impact of voice science upon voice care. *Journal of Voice, 9*(3), 215–234.

Sataloff, R. T. (1986). The professional voice. In C. W. Cummings, J. M. Frederickson, L. A. Harker, C. J. Krause, D. E. Schuller (Eds.), *Otolaryngology—Head and Neck Surgery, vol. 3* (pp. 2029–2056). St. Louis: Mosby.

Sataloff, R. T., Spiegel, J. R., Carroll, L. M., Scheibel, B. R., Darby, K. S., & Rulnick, R. (1987). Strobovideolaryngoscopy in professional voice users: Results and clinical value. *Journal of Voice, 1,* 359–364.

Sataloff, R. T., Spiegel, J. R., Heuer, R. J., Baroody, M. M., Emerich, D. A., Hawkshaw, M. J., &

Rosen, D. C. (1995). Laryngeal mini-microflap saga. *Journal of Voice, 9*(2), 198–204.

Singh, W., & Soutar, D. S. (1993). *Functional surgery of the larynx and pharynx.* London: Butterworth-Heinemann.

Wanamaker, J. R., Netterville, J. L., & Ossoff, R. H. (1993). Phonosurgery: Silastic medialization for unilateral vocal fold paralysis. *Operative Techniques in Otolaryngology—Head and Neck Surgery, 4*(3), 207–217.

Woo, P., Colton, R., Casper, J., & Brewer, D. (1991). Diagnostic value of stroboscopic examination in hoarse patients. *Journal of Voice, 5,* 231–238.

Zeitels, S. M. (1993). Microflap vocal fold cover excisional biopsy for atypia and microinvasive glottic cancer. *Operative Techniques in Otolaryngology—Head and Neck Surgery, 4*(3), 218–222.

Zeitels, S. M. (1995). Premalignant epithelium and microinvasive cancer of the vocal fold: The evolution of phonomicrosurgical management. *Laryngoscope, 105*(3), 1–51.

# CHAPTER
# 5

# *Nonsurgical Voice Improvement Strategies*

This chapter is devoted to a brief overview of nonsurgical voice improvement strategies for both malignant and benign laryngeal pathologies. The information provided is not intended to represent an exhaustive account of voice improvement treatment alternatives. Rather, the suggestions are cursory in design, and they are based largely on the successful clinical experiences of the authors. It is beyond the scope of this text to delve too deeply into this subject matter. For more detailed information the reader is referred to the suggested readings at the end of the chapter, from which some of the material reviewed originates.

## VOICE THERAPY AS THE PRIMARY TREATMENT MODALITY: CURATIVE AND PALLIATIVE APPROACHES

### Patients with Small Growths or Lesions

Small or relatively immature vocal fold growths or lesions, which are caused by chronic vocal abuse or misuse, often respond completely to voice therapy as the primary mode of treatment. This includes conditions such as generalized edema, dysplasia, nodules, polyps, granulomas, contact ulcers, and cysts. When compliant patients learn to modify behaviors that are known to traumatize the vocal folds, these types of pathologies may resolve without medicosurgical intervention.

### Patients with Nonorganic (Functional) Dysphonia

Many patients exhibit clinically significant dysphonia without evidence of associated laryngeal pathology. Voice difficulties may range from mild to severe, and the symptoms may be intermittent or persistent. In some patients, there may be a psychogenic explanation for the dysphonia. Those patients with conversion disorders often exhibit either protracted or frequently recurring episodes of aphonia. For virtually all of these individuals, behavioral management is instrumental in restoring voice to within normal limits. Adjunctive psychotherapy is often indicated to facilitate this process.

Other patients demonstrate faulty vocal habits, which may be sequelae to professional or social stress factors, personality traits, health problems, or general muscle tension syndromes. The laryngeal examination often reveals glottal incompetency, owing either to underlying true vocal fold weakness and hypotonicity or stiffness and hypertonicity. Co-occurring hyperactivity of the ventricular folds is not uncommon in this population. At times, this perverse condition can be so severe as to obscure views of the true cords during phonation efforts. The dysphonia may range from mild to severe. All of these types of patients are potential candidates for voice therapy as the primary and sole treatment modality. In many cases, voice is restored to within normal limits. Success in therapy is usually fostered when patients adopt coordinated efforts to modify stress factors and adjust their lifestyles. It should be noted, however, that patients with chronic poor health do not always enjoy the same levels of voice improvement; their general level of ill health tends to interfere with the physiologic and concentration demands of the voice therapy program.

## Patients with Neurogenic Dysphonia

Many patients with voice difficulties caused by neurologic disease, illness, or injury do not have the benefit of surgical or pharmacologic treatment options, and voice therapy may be the only alternative. This is typically the case for those whose dysphonias are sequelae to cerebral palsy, cerebral vascular accidents, Parkinson's disease, multiple sclerosis, amyotrophic lateral sclerosis, organic voice tremor, Huntington's disease, or tic syndromes. It should be noted that, in most cases, voice exercises are not capable of restoring phonatory skills to normal lev-

els. At best, those who respond to treatment may learn to acquire compensatory "functionally" useful voices.

## VOICE THERAPY FOLLOWING SURGICAL INTERVENTION: FACILITATIVE AND PREVENTIVE APPROACHES

### Patients with Large Growths and Lesions

Treatment applications, alternatives, and sequences usually vary in accordance with the underlying etiology of the vocal fold lesion or growth. Voice disorders that are due to severe, generalized, or focal swelling of the vocal folds (e.g., Reinke's edema or hemorrhagic polyps) usually do not respond to behavioral therapy alone. Large, fibrotic vocal fold nodules and various types of cysts are equally difficult, if not impossible, to treat effectively with voice therapy only. Similarly, large ulcerative lesions (contact ulcers and granulomas), webs, papillomas, and advanced leukoplakias or hyperplasias are not ordinarily candidates for voice therapy as the initial treatment modality. For all of these types of abnormal growths or lesions, surgical removal is almost always necessary prior to the institution of a therapy program. Antacid, nasal steroid, antibiotic, antihistamine, decongestant, and mucolytic medications are often prescribed for many of these conditions in advance of and to facilitate voice therapy. In cases such as these, behavioral therapy is usually indicated to begin within 2 weeks postoperatively.

Patients are usually instructed to remain silent for a minimum of 10 days following surgery. Those patients whose conditions are causally linked to abusive vocal fold behaviors are advised that the planned therapy programs may be indispensable to voice rehabilitation. Warnings are issued about recurrence of the pathology, if the underlying voice abuse patterns are not formally addressed and extinguished in therapy. It is made clear that surgery and prescription drugs cannot treat the root of the voice problem prior to proceeding with these forms of management. It has been our experience that the patient who realizes good to excellent medicosurgical voice results, and is motivated to do whatever it takes to avoid recurrence of the problem, usually does not require extensive therapy. At most, a few exercise sessions are prescribed that address basic issues of vocal fold functioning, voice hygiene, and optimal pitch and loudness contours appropriate to different speaking situations.

In contrast, we have discovered that the patient whose voice difficulty persists or worsens following medicosurgical treatment requires comprehensive therapy. When voice improvement occurs, it usually does so gradually. When the end result of treatment is disappointing, the prognosis for further gains, even in the highly motivated patient, is ordinarily guarded and influenced by the surgical outcome. Occasionally, neither surgery, medicine, nor therapy, either singly or in various combinations, makes a difference. Many different idiosyncratic factors may account for such failures.

Patients who seem cavalier about their voice difficulties frequently prove to be non-compliant with postoperative follow-up appointments and therapeutic recommendations. These individuals usually do not do well in the long run. They may demonstrate significant improvements initially, owing to good surgical results, but these gains are often short-lived. Laryngologists and voice therapists should be wary of individuals whose attitudes are virtually certain to interfere with rehabilitation.

## Patients with Neurogenic Dysphonia

In virtually all cases of neurogenic dysphonia, voice therapy is necessary, either in lieu of, concurrent with, or immediately following medicosurgical treatments. For most patients, neither single nor multimodality treatments are capable of restoring voice to within normal limits.

Surgical treatments of neurogenic voice disorders are most often indicated for patients with flaccid paralysis secondary to recurrent laryngeal nerve damage. Phonosurgical options have been described in Chapter 4. Generally speaking, implant materials such as Teflon, Gelfoam, collagen, and autologous fat have all been used successfully to plump and medialize atrophic vocal folds for compensatory glottal closure and improved phonation. Thyroplasty and arytenoid adduction procedures are also commonly performed to augment glottal competency in patients with adductor vocal fold paralysis.

# VOICE THERAPY CONCURRENT WITH MEDICAL-PHARMACOLOGIC TREATMENT: A FACILITATIVE APPROACH

## Patients with Spasmodic Dysphonia: Focal Laryngeal Dystonia

With the exception of botulinum toxin A (Botox), there are no known drugs that are prescribed specifically to treat voice disorders. However, patients with neurogenic dysphonias may experience secondary voice motor control benefits from medications that are used to relieve their overall pathophysiologic symptoms. These types of treatments are not usually prescribed in lieu of, but rather in conjunction with, voice therapy.

The most common current treatment for focal laryngeal dystonia (spasmodic dysphonia) is the injection of Botox into the vocal fold musculature to induce paralysis.

For predominantly adductor spasms, the vocalis and/or lateral cricoarytenoid muscles are injected either unilaterally or bilaterally. Abductor spasms require injections into the posterior cricoarytenoid muscles, usually unilaterally, to ensure an adequate airway for respiratory purposes. Occasionally, the cricothyroid muscle must also be injected in the patient with abductor spasmodic dysphonia.

## Patients with Dysarthria

Various combinations of levodopa and carbidopa (Sinemet), and bromocriptine (Parlodel) pharmacologic therapy often provide some degree of relief from the hypokinetic movement disorder of Parkinson's disease. At the very least, these drugs usually facilitate voice therapy with such patients. The following drugs modify the effects of dopamine, and therefore may provide some relief for patients with quick hyperkinetic movement disorders, such as Huntington's disease and Tourette syndrome: lithium (Lithobid) and tetrabenozine (Nitoman) inhibit the neuronal uptake and storage of dopamine, haloperidol (Haldol) and chlorpromazine (Thorazine) are phenothiazine neuroleptic agents that interfere with the activity of dopamine receptors, and diazepam (Valium) and clonazepam (Klonopin) are sedating agents that may suppress choreiform movement patterns. Slow hyperkinesias, observed in patients with generalized dystonia, dyskinesia, and athetosis, may be treated systemically for symptomatic relief with high doses of the following anticholinergic agents: trihexyphenidyl (Artane), ethopropazine (Parsidol), and benzotropine (Cogentin). Baclofen (Lioresal), an antispasticity agent, Sinemet, and Valium may be used as supplemental agents with these populations. The beta-adrenergic (blocker) agents propranolol (Inderal) and Klonopin are often prescribed to relieve or decrease the limb symptoms of essential tremor syndrome, and intention tremors in patients with ataxia. Those patients who, in general, respond favorably to these drugs may realize further voice motor control improvements with secondary behavioral exercises.

## Patients with Systemic Disease

Corticosteroids are typically successful in restoring voice to near normal levels in patients with systemic vocal fold erythematosus, secondary to lupus. The anticholinesterase drug Mestinon often provides effective relief from the bulbar muscle weakness and vocal fatigue symptoms associated with myasthenia gravis, a lower motor neuron disorder. Voice therapy is often indicated to facilitate the effects of medication.

## Patients with Gastro-Esophageal-Reflux Disease

Laryngitis and granulomatous lesions classified as pachydermia laryngis may result from gastric reflux into the hypopharynx and laryngeal inlet. A 4- to 6-week regimen of prescription drugs, such as Zantac, Prilosec, or Propulsid, is frequently used as the first line treatment defense to thwart the production of stomach acids and enhance esophageal motility and food digestion. Concurrent voice therapy often boosts the recovery period and helps prevent recurrence of the problem. A modified diet is also recommended that includes avoidance of late night meals, unusually hot and spicy foods, and excessive amounts of caffeinated beverages or chocolate candy.

## Patients with Ventricular Dysphonia

Figure 5–1 illustrates the larynx of a young man who demonstrated a voice quality that sounded very much like Mickey Mouse. He suggested that this difficulty was induced by a very frightening experience during an amusement park ride. At the time of presentation, the patient had

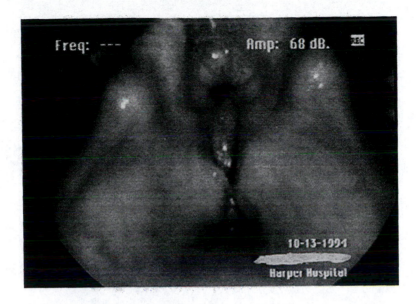

**Figure 5–1.** Appearance of the laryngeal inlet of a 29-year-old male with profound degrees of hyperventricular activity during phonation efforts. This was considered to be of psychogenic origin. Note that the true vocal folds are virtually obliterated from view.

been struggling with this profound dysphonia profile for more than 3 months. His medical and voice histories were both relatively unremarkable. The status of the true vocal folds could not be examined, neither at rest nor during phonation, because of pronounced hypertrophy, tonic hypertension, and hyperfunctional activity of the overlying ventricular folds. The patient subsequently underwent six 1-hour sessions of voice therapy, which included various types of relaxation and biofeedback exercises. Unfortunately, no discernable improvements in voice were obtained.

In an effort to stifle ventricular vocal fold activity, which appeared largely responsible for the dysphonia, the laryngeal inlet was bathed with 4% topical lidocaine. This was accomplished by piercing the cricothyroid membrane with a 25 gauge hypodermic needle and releasing 3 cc of this anesthetic agent. Vigorous coughing activity, induced by the lidocaine, ensured a widespread anesthetic effect. Three minutes later the patient was requested to prolong the vowel

/a/. Although his voice was somewhat tremorous at the outset, the strained, high pitched dysphonia had virtually resolved. Within a few additional minutes, as the patient practiced prolonging vowels and articulating simple words, his vocal quality, pitch, and loudness controls began to approximate normal levels. Figure 5–2 was obtained roughly 10 minutes postinjection. Note the generally healthy-appearing true vocal folds, both at rest and during phonation efforts. Neither tonic contractions nor hyperactivity of the ventricular folds were evident. The patient left the office elated. He returned, however, 2 days later with partial recurrence of the original voice difficulty. A repeat injection was performed with excellent results. This time the effect was long lasting, as the patient returned 2 weeks later with normal voice features.

We have experienced similar success with other patients who did not respond to voice therapy for intractable ventricular dysphonia. In each case, the true vocal folds were uninvolved, and psychogenic distur-

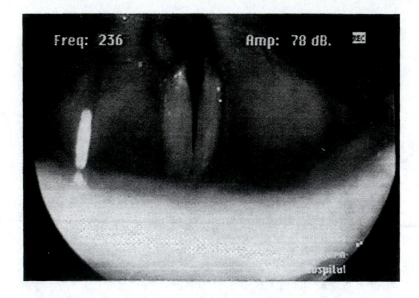

Freq: 236                    Amp: 78 dB.

**Figure 5–2.** This laryngeal photograph illustrates the patient shown in Figure 5–1 following lidocaine injection into the laryngeal inlet to stifle false vocal cord; activities. Note that this objective was accomplished as the true vocal folds are now readily visible for examination. During phonation the patient exhibited mild glottal incompetency, likely as a result of disuse weakness. No gross lesions were evident on the covers or free edges of the true vocal cords. Abductory and adductory biomechanical functions of the cords were adequate for both phonation and respiratory events.

bances were judged responsible for the problem. Those patients who recruit the ventricular folds during phonation because of underlying true vocal fold pathologies generally are not good candidates for this experimental approach to management. In fact, attempting to suppress contributions of this supraglottal compensatory mechanism may prove counterproductive to both phonation and swallowing capabilities. In these types of patients, attention should be focused on treating the (primary) vocal fold abnormalities. Success at this level, with subsequent voice therapy to reduce any residual laryngeal hyperfunctioning, often results in significant overall voice improvements.

## TENETS OF VOICE THERAPY

Whether therapy is rendered initially, with hopes of bypassing surgery, or secondarily,

it is designed with common objectives. These include: (1) educating patients about their disorders and the suspected etiologies, (2) vocal exercises with biofeedback to help train improvements in voice output, and (3) ensuring maintenance (i.e., prevention of recurrence) of the effects achieved with all forms of intervention.

Patients with histories of excessive use of tobacco products, consumption of alcoholic beverages, or both undergo an additional educational therapeutic component. The ill-effects of these habits on the health of the larynx are explored in detail. Photographs and videotapes of nonmalignant, precancerous, and malignant neoplasms are reviewed. Throughout the treatment program we do not hesitate to reiterate the importance of terminating the smoking and drinking behaviors. Homework assignments are given, which include various types of voice exercises and schedules of gradual weaning from the addictive substances that the patient may be using daily.

## SPECIFIC VOICE THERAPY TECHNIQUES

The overall objective in voice therapy for patients with benign laryngeal pathologies is to achieve the best voice possible, given the constraints of the underlying cause, and any other treatment rendered such as laryngeal surgery. A functionally satisfying voice, one that permits the patient to continue professional goals and to get along effectively in virtually all speaking situations, is the general target of therapy. This goal applies regardless of whether therapy is administered as the primary treatment modality, in lieu of surgical intervention, or postoperatively to augment the outcome of surgery and prevent recurrence. Aiming for a perfect or "normal" voice is much too subjective and hardly ever an appropriate goal, regardless of the underlying laryngeal pathology. Although patients occasionally experience remarkable gains following surgery, therapy, or both—gains that by any definition would constitute normal outcomes—we have discovered that predicting such results can lead to very disappointing posttreatment discussions.

## Indirect Methods of Therapy

### Short course on the patient's specific voice problem

In this form of therapy patients are counseled about the underlying causes of their voice disorders. Techniques and the importance of behavioral modification are also addressed. A short course on normal anatomy and physiology of phonation is provided at the outset of the therapy program for comparison with the patient's disorder. Schematic illustrations and anatomical models of all speech subsystems are included in the discussion. Patients learn about the normal coordinated interaction of these systems for voice and speech production. Scaled down descriptions are offered of various abnormal laryngeal growths and lesions that may result from chronic vocal fold abuse or misuse, so that patients understand fully the potential gravity of their own clinical conditions and faulty habits. In this vein, a comprehensive clinical review of the specific laryngeal pathology exhibited by the patient is held following this short course. Explanations of the acoustic, speech aerodynamic, and perceptual disturbances are provided, as are discussions of the therapeutic objectives. Promises of normal voice outcomes are never rendered, for obvious reasons.

### Logging patient's responses to therapy

Charts, similar to the one shown in Figure 5–3, are used routinely to record and track patient responses to different therapeutic exercises. These graphic tools also enable the patient to appreciate both the gains made as well as the areas of dysfunctioning that still need improvement.

### Involvement of family members

Where appropriate, family members are familiarized with the overall goals of the treatment program. This component is especially necessary when working with children. Parents and older siblings are usually instrumental home program facilitators. They may serve as clinical assistants, ensuring that the rules of vocal hygiene are followed and the homework exercises are practiced daily.

### Importance of homework assignments

Adult patients are advised that they must set aside at least 20 minutes a day for voice exercises that are prescribed during therapy sessions. Adults with quiet lifestyles and free time to spend as they wish usually do not have difficulty with this requirement. However, most adults with busy work and

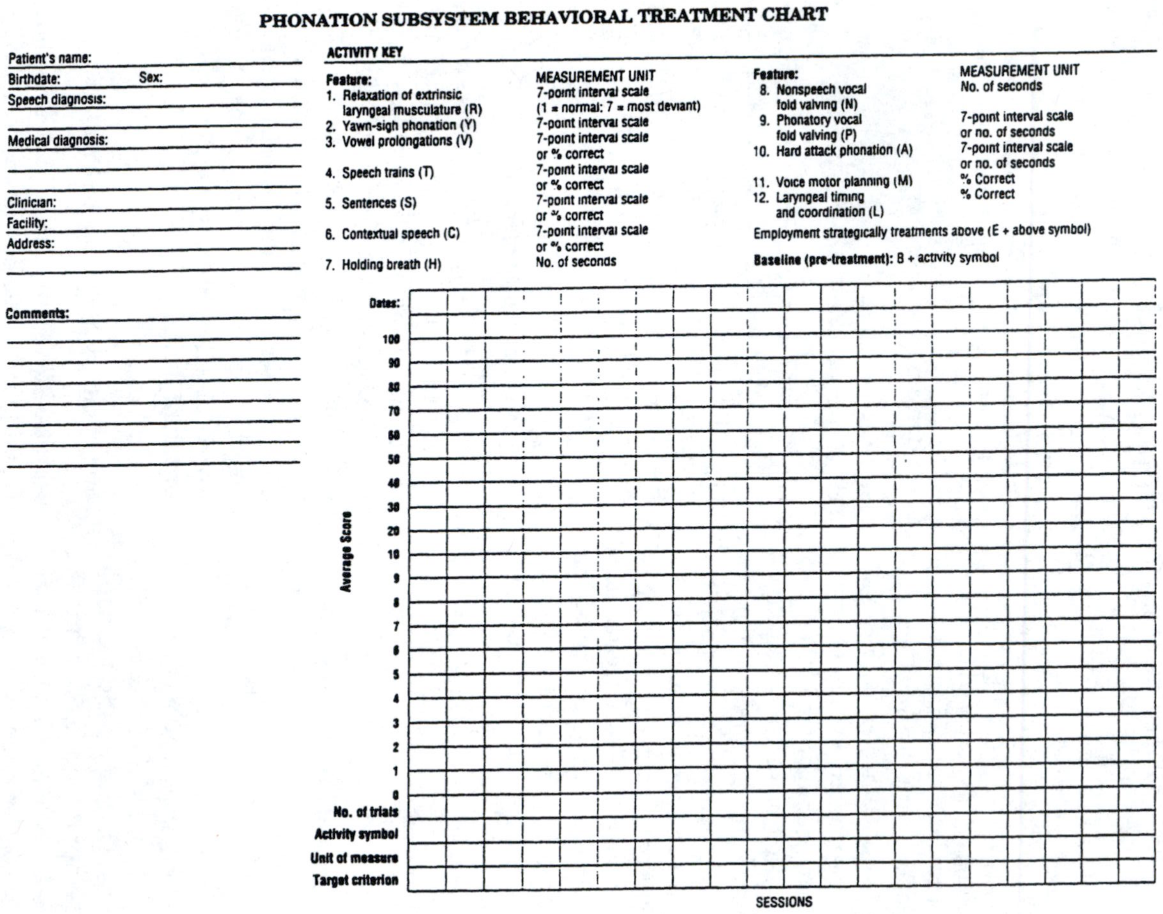

**PHONATION SUBSYSTEM BEHAVIORAL TREATMENT CHART**

Patient's name:
Birthdate: Sex:
Speech diagnosis:
Medical diagnosis:
Clinician:
Facility:
Address:

Comments:

**ACTIVITY KEY**

| Feature: | MEASUREMENT UNIT |
|---|---|
| 1. Relaxation of extrinsic laryngeal musculature (R) | 7-point interval scale (1 = normal: 7 = most deviant) |
| 2. Yawn-sigh phonation (Y) | 7-point interval scale |
| 3. Vowel prolongations (V) | 7-point interval scale or % correct |
| 4. Speech trains (T) | 7-point interval scale or % correct |
| 5. Sentences (S) | 7-point interval scale or % correct |
| 6. Contextual speech (C) | 7-point interval scale or % correct |
| 7. Holding breath (H) | No. of seconds |
| 8. Nonspeech vocal fold valving (N) | No. of seconds |
| 9. Phonatory vocal fold valving (P) | 7-point interval scale or no. of seconds |
| 10. Hard attack phonation (A) | 7-point interval scale or no. of seconds |
| 11. Voice motor planning (M) | % Correct |
| 12. Laryngeal timing and coordination (L) | % Correct |

Employment strategically treatments above (E + above symbol)

**Baseline (pre-treatment):** B + activity symbol

Dates:

Average Score: 100, 90, 80, 70, 60, 50, 40, 30, 20, 10, 9, 8, 7, 6, 5, 4, 3, 2, 1, 0

No. of trials

Activity symbol

Unit of measure

Target criterion

SESSIONS

**Figure 5–3.** Phonation subsystem behavioral treatment chart, which can be used for tracking the patient's responses to specific voice exercise. (From, J. P. Dworkin, *Motor Speech Disorders: A Treatment Guide* (p. 146), 1991. Mosby Year Book. Reprinted with permission.)

home schedules often argue that they simply do not have the time to squeeze this assignment into their daily routines, despite their desire for improved phonation skills. For these patients a compromise approach is suggested that is usually acceptable, even to the busiest of individuals. We request patients to capitalize on time spent in their cars to and from work. Most voice exercises can be easily practiced in this setting, without sacrificing valuable time needed for work and family responsibilities.

## Direct Methods of Voice Therapy for Patients with Strained-Strangled, Harsh, or Tremorous Dysphonia

Behavioral modification of so-called hyperfunctional vocal fold vibratory patterns, as observed in patients with strained-strangled, harsh, or tremorous voice disorders, can be a challenging clinical objective. This is especially evident when the problem is caused by neurologic disease or injury. In this vein, patients with spasmodic dysphonia, spastic dysarthria, or organic voice tremor may only experience minimal therapeutic gains. However, greater levels of improvement may be achieved by those patients who have developed such difficulties because of faulty vocal habits secondary to emotional or psychological disturbances. The assistance of a psychiatrist or clinical psychologist in the treatment of some of these individuals may prove necessary and helpful.

The following types of exercises can be attempted with a modicum of enthusiasm. Setting strict discontinuation criteria will prevent untoward exhaustion of the patient who is not responding to the therapy.

### Muscle relaxation

Patients with the strained-harsh vocal quality characteristic of spasmodic dysphonia, spastic dysarthria, and certain psychogenic conditions often suffer from hypertensive/hyperfunctional vocal fold activity. Therapy for the resulting dysphonia may consist of several different techniques. Head, neck, and jaw musculature relaxation exercises, including the popular "rag doll" and "chewing" techniques, may help patients who complain of unusual tension and stiffness in these regions, regardless of etiology. Any relief of these symptoms may pay voice improvement dividends. Gentle massage of the larynx and interconnecting strap musculature has been shown to induce relaxation of both the extrinsic and intrinsic laryngeal musculature. This result may facilitate voice improvement exercises.

### Breath support exercises

Use of the Kay Elemetrics Visi-Pitch device is very helpful in providing biofeedback of nonvocal airflow control and various sound production parameters. This is accomplished by setting the instrument to collect data for 7.5 seconds using the *Intensity* mode display. The patient can be requested to speak into the microphone for detailed graphics and acoustic analyses of loudness features. With a mouth-to-microphone distance of 2 inches, the patient can display airflow control characteristics by blowing a stream of air into the unit. Creating a horizontal cursor at 35 dB on the monitor affords a target for the patient to demonstrate and practice steady and uninterrupted transglottal airflow. The minimal objective is to prolong the air stream for the entire 7.5 seconds (left to right across the screen) without the microphone signal deviating significantly off of the target line.

Many patients with hyperfunctional vocal fold activity cannot perform this task without either running out of breath prematurely, struggling to maintain steady and controlled airflow dynamics, or both. With practice, improvements are usually realized. Gains made may translate into reduced glottal airflow resistance and enhanced respiratory support during voice activities.

For homework, patients who struggle with this behavior are requested to hold a facial tissue in front of the lips while blowing a steady stream of air. The tissue will flutter in response to the degree and nature of the airflow source. Patients are requested to practice increasing the duration of flow, improving the steadiness of the emission, and developing the ability to vary the respiratory efforts utilized during the task from light to forceful. Any gains made can be measured against the Visi-Pitch apparatus at follow-up therapy sessions.

### Adjusting the pitch used in conversational speech

Sometimes adjusting the patient's (habitual) pitch level helps to relieve hyperfunctional vocal fold behavior. We have discovered that higher pitched, sing-song patterns of contextual speech may evoke periods of relatively fluent voice in patients with adductor spasmodic dysphonia. Although underlying spasmodic characteristics are not completely resolved using this approach, for some patients the improvements achieved have been rather remarkable. Perhaps for these types of responders there may be a strong psychogenic component to the disorder. Similarly, patients with organic voice tremor may moderately benefit from this technique.

### Easy initiation of voice

Regardless of the etiology and underlying dysphonic features, patients who exhibit hyperfunctional vocal fold behaviors often benefit from easy onset voice exercises. Transitions are made from breathy-easy voice initiation through gradual degrees of more natural sounding voice efforts. The popular "Yawn-Sigh" technique is used to foster this approach, wherein the patient begins the approach with a yawning, inspiratory gesture, and completes the task by

protracting an audible sigh. This procedure enforces practice of voice under conditions of mild to moderate glottal compression or resistance forces. If the patient demonstrates the ability to generate breathy-easy vocalizations, vowels are practiced in isolation and in various combinations with focus on progressively increasing phonatory power without causing harsh-strained vocal quality. Success with vowels is the precursor to practice material that includes individual words, phrases, complex sentences, and conversational speech.

### Airflow biofeedback techniques during speech

The speech aerodynamics instrument rack may be used to provide biofeedback of transglottal airflow rate during steady-state vowel prolongations. In the beginning of the therapy program, increased glottal resistance limits mean airflow rate to less than 100 cc/sec in most patients with hyperfunctional voice disorders. Visual biofeedback of the airflow signal during the aforementioned vowel exercises may prove helpful for some of these individuals, as they attempt to modify the interruptive glottal squeezing forces and improve voice output. Successful relaxation at the level of the glottis usually results in increased airflow rate and perceptually less strained or harsh vocal quality.

For those therapists who do not have airflow transducers for these types of measurements and feedback, the See Scape device (Pro-Ed) may serve as an acceptable alternative. Designed for detecting nasal airflow abnormalities, the styrofoam float mechanism will respond to any type of airflow stimulus through the connective tubing. The nasal olive is placed in the patient's most patent nostril, so that nasal airflow associated with humming activities can be visualized, as shown in Figures 5–4A and 5–4B. Once the olive is in position, the patient is requested to prolong a humming sound. Hyperfunctional vocal fold behav-

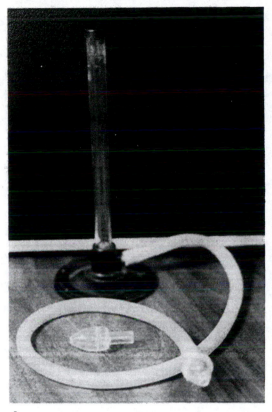

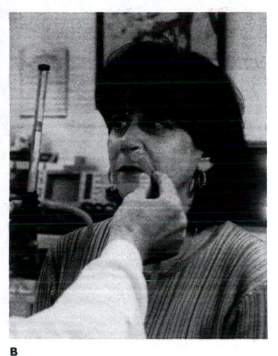

**A**

**B**

**Figure 5–4 A.** See Scape device (Pro Ed) showing the styrofoam float within a test tube and a plastic nasal olive connected to the rubber hose. **B.** Use of the See Scape device to provide visual feedback of nasal air emission that may be associated with the production of the consonant /m/. Note that the float rises toward the top of the tube as the patient generates sufficient nasal resonance and nasal airflow dynamics during production of this sound.

iors will disrupt the airflow through the vocal tract and limit styrofoam movements in the See Scape tube. Practicing easy voice initiation and control may improve the fluidity of vocal fold vibrations by reducing glottal resistance. Gains obtained will be appreciated by means of smooth, upward movement of the float in response to the humming sounds produced by the patient. Interrupted airflow, caused by hyperactivity of the vocal folds associated with strained vocal quality, will be evident as the float descends to or remains near the bottom of the tube. This biofeedback exercise can be very effective for some patients.

Those who demonstrate improvements with this approach may practice humming familiar tunes or pitch scales to induce fluent, controllable, upward float activity within the See Scape tube during all vocalizations.

A 2-inch piece of drinking straw can be substituted for the nasal olive furnished by the manufacturer. The straw is placed between the patient's lips, as shown in Figure 5–5, with the open end held in light contact with the central incisor teeth. After a normal inhalation the patient is requested to prolong the vowel /i/. If the sound generated is characterized by strained-harsh vocal quality, which is usually indicative of

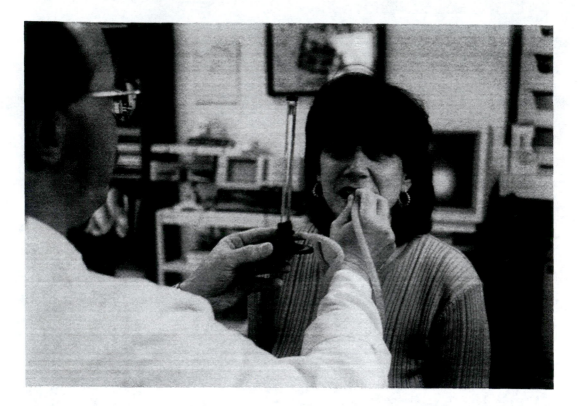

**Figure 5–5.** Use of the See Scape device to demonstrate airflow dynamic control associated with production of the vowel /i/. Note that a piece of drinking straw is connected to the rubber tubing, in lieu of the plastic nasal olive. Intraoral air pressure associated with the production of this vowel is generated through this straw and rubber tubing for movements of the styrofoam float mechanism, as can be seen in this illustration.

abnormally increased glottal resistance, the float will not move significantly from the bottom of the tube. The objective of this therapy technique is to provide the patient with visual biofeedback of the degree of transglottal airflow as easy voice initiation and control are practiced. As vocal fold hyperfunctioning is reduced, through easy voice production efforts, the float will move upward in the tube. Ultimately, the patient is requested to prolong the vowel for at least 10 seconds; the float must be elevated to within 1 inch of the top of the tube and remain at or near this position throughout the utterance. In the beginning, breathy vocal quality can be practiced for immediate success. Voice can be gradually superimposed, and float dynamics will provide

feedback regarding the status of glottal resistance and transglottal airflow.

The following list can be incorporated into the practice sessions for additional stimuli material: /u/, /o/, /hi/, /hu/, /shi/, /shu/, /pi/, /pu/, /po/, /si/, /su/, /so/, /ipi/, /upu/, /opo/, and so on. Sentences can also be practiced using the same See Scape technique with similar objectives. Select sentences that are loaded with the consonants and vowels [i, u, o, sh, s, p, m, h, ch]; for example, *stay put, pet the puppy,* and *may I go to the store.* Note that as the words in the sentence are produced with good vocal quality and speech aerodynamics, albeit at times with slight articulatory imprecision owing to the presence of the straw between the lips, the float moves toward or remains near the top of the tube, except during normal breaths and intersyllabic pauses. Simple sentences are best in the beginning, with progression to longer, more complex word combinations.

### Visual biofeedback of vocal fold vibrations

Use of videolaryngostroboscopy affords the patient and therapist the opportunity to visualize glottal and supraglottal activity during vowel exercises. Tremorous movements, prolonged closure time, recruitment of the ventricular folds, and reduced amplitudes of vibration are some of the most common difficulties exhibited by patients with strained, harsh, and/or tremorous voice disorders. Real time visual biofeedback of the larynx enables the patient to experiment with phonatory modifications to reduce or eliminate these interruptive vibratory behaviors.

### Manual compression and stabilization for patients with voice tremors

Patients with predominantly tremorous vocal quality usually do not respond to the aforementioned palliative therapeutic techniques. Before abandoning hopes for voice improvement with this population, therapists may wish to experiment with manual stabilization of the larynx and its extrinsic musculature. For this maneuver the therapist stands behind the patient and firmly grasps the neck and larynx region with both hands, analogous to a choke hold. We hypothesize that this technique may inhibit uncontrollable laryngeal and strap musculature tremors. Some patients have suggested that the compression grasp of these structures reduces the inherent shimmy and facilitates phonation efforts. Patients can be taught to use their own hand(s) to try to effect such relief. When indicated, this maneuver is coupled with the aforementioned biofeedback exercises, with hopes of stimulating even slight improvements in voice fluency and motor control. On occasion, patients make remarkable gains, and

they can be weaned from using the hands to stabilize the phonatory mechanism during conversation.

### Artificial larynx applications

Transcervical or intraoral electronic larynges may be used with the patient who cannot generate functionally useful voice for verbal communication. Provided that the individual possesses reasonably precise articulation capabilities, benefits may be derived from using one of these types of artificial larynx devices. Essentially, this type of instrument permits the user to communicate verbally without normal dependence upon contributions from the respiratory, phonatory, or resonatory subsystems. We have discovered that the patient who must use a nonverbal system of communication because of profound laryngeal dysfunctioning may readily accept these instruments as last-resort alternatives to nonvocal means of communication. It is important to note that in the beginning the patient may have difficulty when using the artificial instrument learning not to use the natural voice while articulating.

## Direct Methods of Voice Therapy for Patients with Hoarse-Breathy Dysphonia

Hypotensive/hypofunctional voice disorders are most commonly seen in patients with histories of paralyses, growths, and generalized swelling of the vocal folds. These conditions restrict or retard vibratory mobility and midline phase symmetry during phonation, resulting in unnatural glottal chinks and escape of unphonated air pulses. Associated vocal quality is usually hoarse-breathy, pitch is typically lower than normal with limited range, volume is generally soft, and voice production may be effortful. Vocal fatigue is not uncommon, as patients may tax and weaken the respiratory musculature as they compensate at that level for underlying glottal insufficiency, excessive transglottal airflow, and a reduced number of syllables per breath.

Patients with hypofunctional dysphonias may respond more favorably to voice therapy than those whose difficulties are caused by hyperadduction of the vocal folds. Contributing to these outcome differences are the potential augmentative effects of various phonosurgery alternatives for the former population. It should be noted that patients with progressive or degenerative neurogenic dysphonias, as observed in individuals with amyotrophic lateral sclerosis and Parkinson's disease, often make good gains early in the therapy program but experience setbacks as their conditions worsen. Also, patients who continue to abuse or misuse the vocal folds, despite warnings to the contrary, do not usually achieve long-lasting voice improvements, regardless of the initial treatment results.

The overall objectives of therapy are to improve underlying vocal abuse and misuse behaviors, voice quality, habitual pitch level, pitch range, loudness control, inflection patterns, respiratory support, the number of syllables produced per breath, and the degree of effort to vocalize. To meet these goals therapy may consist of the following techniques: (1) breath support activities, (2) various vocal fold valving maneuvers that incorporate the patient's hands and arms for pushing, pulling, and squeezing activities during phonation, (3) vocal quality, pitch, and loudness exercises, (4) artificial, external compression of the larynx, (5) hard glottal attack voice drills, (6) acoustic, speech aerodynamic, and videostroboscopic biofeedback exercises, (7) motor voice programming stimulation using a metronome to pace phonation, and (8) connected discourse practice. Each of these therapeutic components will be briefly discussed.

### Breath support activities

As previously described, the Visi-Pitch apparatus can be effectively used to train improvements in nonspeech airflow regulation. To transduce airflow input, the instrument is set in the *Intensity* data collection mode, and the microphone is held at a distance of 2 inches from the mouth. As the patient blows a steady stream of air into the microphone a signal display appears on the monitor. A horizontal cursor should be placed at between 35 and 40 dB as a biofeedback target. Patients with poor breath support and control usually are unable to sustain a steady airstream for more than a few seconds at any designated intensity level. At first, practice may focus on increasing the length and steadiness of airflow without varying the target. As the patient improves, variable intensity and time length targets can be incorporated into the therapy program to increase the complexity of the exercise.

Use of the See Scape device may also facilitate improvements in breath support. The patient can blow into the nasal olive or a piece of drinking straw fastened to the tubing of the instrument. A marking pen can be used to select segments along the length of the tube that will serve as targets during the blowing tasks. Patients can be instructed to blow into the olive or straw with sufficient control of the expiratory force so as to position the styrofoam float at specific target locations. Dropping three or four standard paper clips onto the float offers resistance to airflow input, which makes the blowing task more challenging and valuable. The therapist can create any number of tasks within this exercise paradigm that tax the patient to demonstrate both gross and fine breath support abilities. As a general rule of thumb, the patient should be able to prolong a silent airstream at the 35 dB target level for at least 7 seconds without significant signal variability from beginning to end. Additionally, the patient should be able to demonstrate expiratory force control by varying, upon command, the degree of airflow at any given moment in time within the exercise trial.

We have discovered that patients who make good gains in this area of rehabilitation generally succeed with subsequent voice exercises. Those who fail to establish or develop adequate control of expiratory airflow usually struggle when voice activities are introduced into the treatment plan. For homework, patients are asked to practice similar nonspeech blowing against a facial tissue, the long end of which is held approximately 1 inch from the mouth. As with the Visi-Pitch and See Scape devices, the tissue serves as a biofeedback tool. Abnormal airflow features cause the tissue to flutter aperiodically. Patients can recognize disturbed performance and modify and compare subsequent efforts.

### Phonatory vocal fold valving exercises

The primary aims of these types of exercises are to increase the contact forces of vocal folds during the closed phases of vibration associated with voice, and to convert these adductory forces into improved phonation during connected discourse. There are three alternative valving techniques that work equally well for most patients: (1) clasping the hands together at chest level, with arms bent 90° at the elbows, and squeezing the palms together as hard as possible, (2) sitting in a chair, grasping the bottom with both hands, and pulling up as hard as possible, as if to lift the chair off the ground, and (3) sitting in a chair and pushing down on the seat bottom with both hands, as if to cause the chair to collapse. Experimentation with all three maneuvers may prove necessary to determine if any one is superior to the others in facilitating vocal fold valving.

Initially, the patient is taught to employ the maneuver of choice while simultaneously producing prolonged vowels. The objective of this exercise is to increase maximum phonation time over the baseline level. A minimum of 10 seconds is the early therapeutic target, with 2-second increments as subsequent targets. Pushing the patient to prolong a vowel for more than 16 seconds on one breath is unnecessary. Focus is not placed on quality, pitch, or loudness features of the voice produced. Individual words, short phrases, and connected discourse can be practiced next using the same valving maneuvers. Fading employment of the technique as the patient demonstrates improved vocal fold valving capabilities should be an ultimate therapeutic objective. A stopwatch, See Scape device, tape recorder, or Visi-Pitch unit can provide important biofeedback regarding the time components and/or adequacy of the voice signals produced by the patient during this exercise program.

### Vocal quality, pitch, and loudness exercises

We regularly use the Visi-Pitch device with our patients as a tool for training pitch and loudness control, and for biofeedback of vocal quality during isolated sound productions and connected discourse. Vocal quality can be roughly analyzed by examining the degree of fundamental period perturbation in the voice signal. This measurement is generally analogous to the (pitch) jitter ratio. We have discovered that improvements in vocal quality can often be induced by altering the habitual pitch level, which in most cases is too low. The Visi-Pitch can facilitate this alteration. Once the unit is programmed to collect data in the *Pitch* mode, various pitch targets can be set with the horizontal cursors. By experimenting with these progressively higher level pitch targets during isolated vowel productions the patient can observe the effects of such adjustments on the voice signal line curves. Generally speaking, poor vocal quality is represented by a disjointed, unpatterned series of dots on the monitor. The associated perturbation factor is usually greater than 1.0%; patients with moderate to severe hypofunctional voice disorders commonly exceed 5.0% levels. Normal or near normal vocal quality is characterized by a cohesive series of dots or a uniform line curve that closely adheres to the horizontal target cursor. The perturbation score is predictably less than 1.0%. The Visi-Pitch permits statistical analyses of the differences in perturbation between one voice attempt and another. This measurement provides important objective data about underlying variations in the vocal quality of the sounds produced. Use of the computerized acoustic instrumentation rack also permits objective measures of perceived vocal quality improvements by comparing pretherapeutic jitter data with those obtained following this stimulation program.

Once the pitch level that stimulates the best voice output is discovered, practice material consists of various isolated vowels, two, three, and four vowel combinations, individual words, short phrases, and sentences. In the beginning of the program, the patient is requested to generate a monotone voice and to remain flat on the pitch level established. The Visi-Pitch device provides biofeedback regarding deviation from the target pitch cursor. Through this reinforcement technique the (new) fundamental frequency of phonation becomes habituated. Attention is then turned to running speech exercises so that more natural prosodic balance and inflection patterns can be rehearsed, while preserving optimum pitch, loudness, and quality of voice control.

Similar exercises are introduced with loudness control as the focus of therapy. The Visi-Pitch is set to record voice in the *Intensity* mode, and various loudness targets are set using the horizontal cursors. In most cases, the treatment objective is to train habitual loudness to not exceed 70 dB (SPL) during conversational speech. Patients who achieve this goal, and who realize gains with the preceding breath support, valving, and pitch modification exercises, usually experience clinically significant improvements in overall vocal quality.

### Artificial compression of the larynx

The primary purpose of external compression of the larynx is to achieve artificial medialization of the vocal fold on the side of stimulation. This may prove to be especially helpful for patients with glottal incompetency secondary to vocal fold paresis, paralysis, or bowing. The digital compression technique requires the therapist to use an open hand to push the larynx gently while the patient simultaneously generates voice. Variation in the degree of compression force can be attempted as the contralateral side of the larynx is supported with the opposite hand. Often the results of this experimental procedure lend support to the need for surgical vocal fold repositioning or medialization.

Another technique that may offer greater therapeutic advantage than digital compression involves the use of a neck band that contains a firm bulge. This device can be easily constructed using an elastic band (12 x 3/4 in.), velcro material, a piece of cotton fabric, a styrofoam wedge (1 x 1/2 x 1/2 in.), and common household thread. The styrofoam wedge is sewn into the cotton fabric and then connected to the middle of the elastic band to form a relatively firm bulge. The velcro is sewn onto the ends of the elastic band so that it can be fastened securely around the patient's neck. The bulge is positioned against the thyroid ala on the side of vocal fold weakness. The band tension is adjusted around the neck for relatively tight yet comfortable compression against the larynx. This device simulates the effects of digital and surgical medialization techniques. Patients can wear the band away from the therapy session for constant stimulation without difficulty. This approach is especially helpful for patients with neurapraxic (usually temporary) glottal incompetency, often occurring as a consequence of reversible trauma to the vagus nerve during head and neck surgery. A note of caution is warranted, however. Therapists should clear this anticipated treatment with the referring physician, as some patients may be placed at risk for cerebral blood flow difficulty or wound formation with protracted use of the compression neck band.

Objective measures of the potential beneficial effects of these compression techniques should be obtained using acoustic, speech aerodynamic, and videostroboscopic instrumentation. Coupled to perceptual impressions, these types of data may offer important information regarding whether or not vocal fold medialization surgery would be helpful if the dysphonia persists or worsens throughout the therapy period.

### Hard-attack phonation

The therapeutic use of hard-attack phonation should only be incorporated with patients who have failed to improve with the preceding vocal fold adduction exercises. Instructing the patient to drive the vocal folds together with forceful, abrupt phonatory efforts should be done with limitations in order to prevent the possibility of short-term abusive side effects. Additionally, patients should be reminded about the ill-effects of habitual hard glottal contact on the health of the vocal folds.

To induce this effect the therapist can place the palm of an open hand on the patient's abdomen. The patient is requested to take a deep breath and hold it, while the therapist firmly pumps the abdomen with the open palm to cause air to be exhaled. The patient is instructed to try to resist this external force by bearing down as hard as possible at the level of the glottis. Strong glottal resistance should trigger audible vocal straining, which can be shaped into more fluent, controlled vowel prolongations by the patient. As voice is produced under this condition, the therapist gradually fades the abdominal pumping technique. Use of the Visi-Pitch affords biofeedback regarding quality, pitch, and loudness features of the voice produced. With further practice, the patient can work to reduce laryngeal tension and stress associated with hard attack phonation, and to improve volitional glottal resistance abilities. A stethoscope is quite useful in providing biofeedback of glottal attack behav-

iors. The ear pieces are worn by the patient as the diaphragm of the scope is alternately placed against the larynx of the therapist, for demonstration purposes, and against the larynx of the patient for comparative analyses.

### Acoustic, aerodynamic, and stroboscopic feedback

As mentioned earlier, the voice laboratory equipment can be used both diagnostically and therapeutically. Virtually all patients are intrigued by the opportunity to visualize their vocal folds, voice signals, and underlying airflow dynamics on these instruments during various phonatory maneuvers. With instruction from the therapist, the images obtained on the monitor screens can serve as valuable feedback regarding vocal fold vibratory efficiency and phonatory control. The objective data obtained from these measures during therapy can be compared to similar data gathered prior to therapy. Results of such comparisons add important details to final treatment summaries, and they often strengthen treatment outcome conclusions.

### Voice motor programming exercises

There is a select group of patients who, as a result of focal brain damage often secondary to stroke, exhibit faulty programming of voice initiation and control during volitional speech efforts. The ensuing disorder is known as apraxia of phonation, and it is generally characterized by episodic and variable aphonia, whispered speech, arrests of voice, asynchronous articulatory and exhalatory movements, and strident, squeal-like vocalizations that may be camouflaged by periods of normal voice production. Profound involvement may render the patient mute. Coexisting articulatory apraxia is more the rule than the exception. The overall objective of this voice therapy paradigm is to train the patient to access the vocal folds with discrete control for all volitional speech events. The program is modeled after one that has been successfully employed for the treatment of speech apraxia. A pacing technique is utilized with the aid of a standard metronome. Therapy begins with the speed of the pendulum set at 30 beats per minute. The patient is requested to produce a vowel repeatedly to the beat, one production per beat, on the beat. After 30 seconds of continuous practice, a brief rest period is permitted. The vowel can be changed at any time during the practice session. Once the patient demonstrates competence on this task, the speed of the metronome is changed to 60 beats per minute, and the same practice regulations apply. Most patients who respond to this intervention program are able to work their way up to 120 beats per minute without significant difficulty. At this point, two, three, and four vowel combinations are introduced according to the same treatment protocol, beginning at 30 beats per minute and progressing to higher speeds as competency is demonstrated at slower levels. Ultimately, monosyllable, trisyllable, and multisyllable words are practiced in similar fashion, as the patient is required to produce one syllable per beat and to recycle the word until the stimulus is changed. Short phrases, sentences, and running speech exercises are introduced next, following the same rules of metronomic use.

It has been hypothesized by several prominent clinical researchers that there exists a central rhythm generator normally responsible for voice and speech motor control. Metronomic pacing may induce rhythmic stimulation of this center, which in turn may facilitate output commands to the phonation subsystem. In this vein, we are reminded of a recent 74-year-old patient who came to us 12 years after suffering a moderate CVA, which resulted in very mild aphasia, mild speech apraxia, and moderate phonatory apraxia. She was also paretic on the right side, necessitating use of a cane. Although virtually all aphasic and speech apraxic features resolved within the first year following the stroke, the phonatory difficulties persisted without abatement. Unfortunately, the patient never received voice or speech therapy prior to her visit to our laboratory. With the exception of the aforementioned common voice difficulties that are characteristic of apraxia of phonation, the patient evidenced no other remarkable examination findings. The described metronomic pacing program was initiated. Within five sessions, at 1 hour per visit, she had regained approximately 90% of volitional voice motor control. Three sessions later, she had plateaued at a level of 95% error-free phonatory expression. To date, roughly 9 months following discharge from therapy, no regression in these voice motor planning or production skills is evident.

### Connected discourse practice

These exercises are designed to assist in the transition from routine, robotic-like therapeutic voice activities to more natural phonatory expression during conversational speech. Essentially, the patient engages in oral reading tasks, responds extemporaneously to simple questions, and evokes unsolicited conversation with the therapist. The Visi-Pitch is used throughout these sessions for biofeedback of prosody (inflection patterns, loudness features, degree of pausing, rate of speech, etc.), and overall voice characteristics. Placed in the *Walking* display mode, the instrument permits forward and backward scrolling of the patient's speech productions for comprehensive review and discussion. Improvements can be prompted, rehearsed, and reviewed for comparative purposes. When indicated, the monitor can be split into an upper and lower portion so that the therapist's voice and speech patterns can be stored on one half of the screen and the patient's on the other half. The patient can attempt to match the therapist's model during subsequent conversational voice attempts. Videotape and audiotape recorders are routinely used for this segment of intervention, the results of which are compared with pretherapy recordings.

Figure 5–6 is a composite recapitulation of voice therapy strategies that may be employed with different dysphonic populations.

## LARYNGECTOMEE REHABILITATION

### Esophageal Speech

Years ago, total laryngectomees either learned how to produce esophageal speech through intensive therapeutic exercises, or they were remanded to mastering use of an artificial larynx to communicate verbally. Acquisition of functional esophageal speech ability was not an easy task then, and it remains an equally difficult objective for current patients interested in this form of rehabilitation To meet this challenge, a variety of air charging methods must be utilized in therapy to teach these individuals how to insufflate the esophagus. This source of energy is necessary to generate vibrations of the pharyngo-esophageal (P-E) segment for voice production. The resultant sounds are converted into verbal speech by the usual types of vocal tract adjustments. Perhaps there are as many patients who fail to develop functional esophageal speech as there are who succeed in this therapeutic endeavor. Generally speaking, among those who eventually do acquire this skill, the total amount of time spent in therapy and the competency outcomes vary significantly both within and between patients. Even excellent esophageal speakers suffer from variably hoarse-harsh quality, periodic wet-gurgly overtones, soft volume, very low pitch, limited phonation time, abnormally few syllables per air charge, distracting clunking sounds associated with the injection technique of esophageal insufflation, occasional noise from stoma blast, and episodic dysfluency. These acoustic, aerodynamic, and perceptual disturbances occur because the P-E segment is, at best, a quasielastic sphincter mechanism. It is not supported by an abductor-adductor system of muscles like that of the vocal folds within the larynx. Rather, it functions as an unpaired, comparatively thick, and inelastic fibromuscular mechanism.

The fundamental frequency of good esophageal speakers averages around 80 Hz, whereas poor speakers usually do not exceed 60 Hz. The conversational voices of good esophageal speakers average 10 to 20 dB softer than individuals with normal laryngeal phonation. The good esophageal speaker may only generate an average of 10 to 12 syllables per air charge, and as few as 100 words per minute; intervals of silence (prosodic insufficiency) may be as high as 50% of the total speaking time.

### Methods to induce esophageal vibration

Figure 5–7 is an illustration of the anatomy of the neoglottis (P-E segment) and adjacent structures used for esophageal phonation. Note that at rest, air pressure in the pharynx is neither above nor below (0) that of the atmosphere, the P-E segment is closed, creating positive (+) pressure, the collapsed esophagus registers negative (−) pressure, and the lower esophageal sphincter registers positive (+) pressure. Insufflation for esophageal voice production can occur in at least three possible ways. First, pharyngeal air pressure can be increased beyond the level of resistance of the P-E segment so that air can be forced into the esophagus. The majority of esophageal speakers use an *injection method* for insufflation purposes, wherein pumping, sweeping, or pressing movements of the tongue against the palate and pharynx compress air molecules in the pharynx into the esophagus. These actions may be produced prior to attempts at speech, or they may be coupled to the act of articulating specific voiceless consonants, such as /s, sh, p, t, k/.

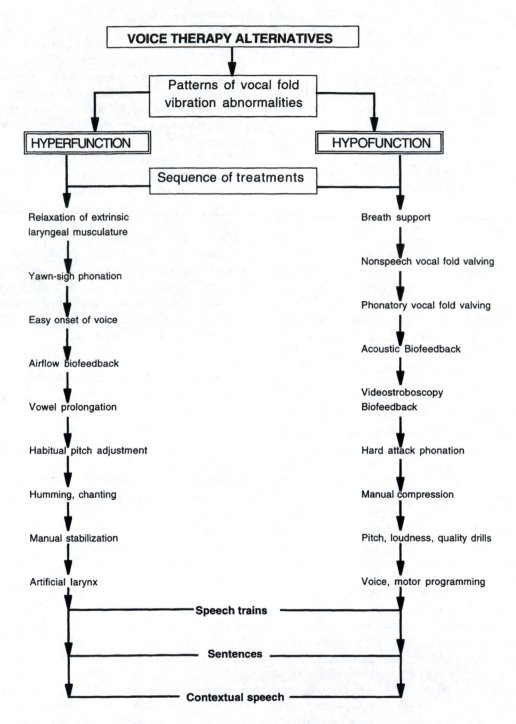

**Figure 5–6.** Phonation subsystem voice therapy hierarchy that is segregated by type of vocal fold vibration abnormality.

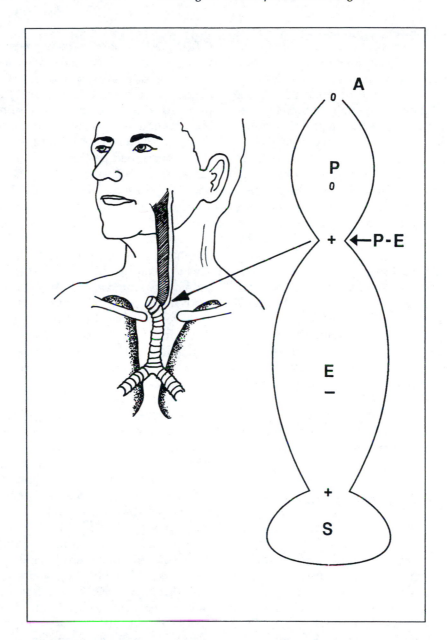

**Figure 5–7.** Schematic illustration of the anatomical changes following total laryngectomy. Note that the arrow points to the pharyngo-esophageal segment (neoglottis). Also note the pressure differentials between the atmosphere (A), pharynx (P), P–E segment, esophagus (E), and stomach (S). These pressure differentials must be altered for insufflation of the esophagus to occur, which is necessary for esophageal voice production.

Second, if esophageal air pressure can be reduced further, air may be sucked through the P-E segment with a vacuum effect. This is accomplished by some esophageal speakers using the *inhalation method* of insufflation, which involves little or no tongue movement during air intake. This is accomplished in synchrony with the biomechanics of pulmonary breathing. As the volume of the lung-thorax unit increases, prior to inhalation, the volume of the esophagus increases slightly. These volume increases reduce air pressure in the lungs and esophagus below atmospheric and pharyngeal levels, which creates a vacuum for airflow into the lungs and esophagus. Learning to coordinate pulmonary and esophageal speech breathing is very difficult, perhaps accounting for the small percentage of laryngectomees who use this method of insufflation.

Third, if a *deliberate puncture tract* is surgically created between the posterior tracheal and anterior esophageal walls, slightly below the level of the P-E segment, a prosthesis can be fitted within this tunnel that permits pulmonary air to be shunted into the esophagus. The segment is therefore charged with air pressure from the lungs. Vibrations of this neoglottis are powered by this source of energy, not unlike the aerodynamic contributions that normally underlie true vocal fold vibratory activity.

## Tracheo-Esophageal Puncture

In 1958 Conley and his associates first discussed the tracheo-esophageal shunt method of surgical voice restoration for the total laryngectomee. At first, Conley's shunt consisted of a tunnel of mucosal tissue from the esophagus to the trachea, just above the level of the stoma. A year later, this same researcher modified this technique by using a great saphenous vein graft for the shunt. Due to the propensity for spontaneous stenosis of the shunt and tracheal leakage during swallowing, this procedure was not widely accepted as a viable alternative to traditional esophageal speech rehabilitation. Many other surgical voice reconstruction techniques came and went over the years following Conley's initial pioneering efforts. However, it was not until

20 years later that Blom and Singer published their work on a tracheo-esophageal puncture (TEP) technique that employed a medical grade silicone prosthesis for the shunt. Since then, this relatively simple procedure and design has become the gold standard alternative to traditional esophageal speech rehabilitation.

As mentioned earlier, the P-E segment serves as the vibrator for both esophageal and TEP speech activities. For the latter, voice is produced by occluding the stoma during exhalation, which shunts airflow through the valved prosthesis into the esophagus for responsive P-E vibration. This is illustrated in Figure 5–8. Driven by pulmonary support, the vibrations are generally more periodic, continuous, forceful, and controllable than those produced through the aforementioned injection and inhalation insufflation methods used by esophageal speakers. Good to excellent speech and voice results are usually achieved by most patients within 1 month following placement of the prosthesis. In therapy, most patients develop moderate loudness and pitch variation abilities, which enhance the prosodic balance of speech. Maximum phonation time often approximates that achieved by normal speakers, as does the mean number of syllables that can be produced per breath. The quality of voice, however, varies considerably from patient to patient. Some have resounding, only mildly hoarse-breathy voices. Others have strained-harsh voices, with intermittent dysfluency. Still others may struggle with chronic wet-gurgly vocal quality. A small percentage do not acquire functional TEP speech, despite hard clinical work and motivation to succeed. Such outcome variations depend on different factors: (1) the anatomy and physiology of the neoglottis; (2) the architecture of the T-E tract and tracheostoma; (3) pulmonary functioning; (4) the extent of postirradiation fibrosis and mucositis; (5) skin and mucosal sloughing, susceptibility to fistula formation, and overall tactile sensitivity level; (6)

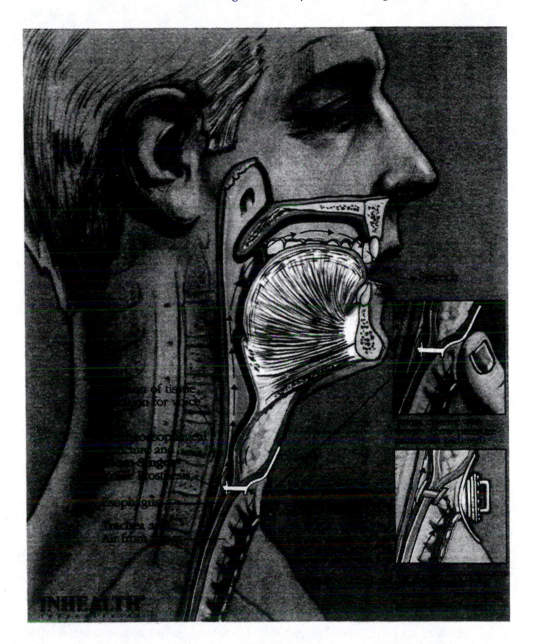

**Figure 5–8.** Illustration of the tracheo-esophageal puncture surgical reconstruction technique following total laryngectomy. Note the position of the silicone prosthesis in the surgically created tunnel between the trachea and esophagus. Collars on both the esophageal and tracheal sides of the prosthesis ensure stable fit of the appliance within this tract. Reprinted from *InHealth Technology* publication.

articulatory skills, and (7) the ability to place, remove, evaluate, and care for the prosthesis.

Because chronic salivary leakage through the prosthesis rarely occurs, and most patients acquire relatively quick and functional verbal communication skills, the TEP technique has become the most popular rehabilitation alternative. For those patients who do not desire to use or cannot learn successful finger-to-stoma valving skills, breathing valves may be coupled to the tracheostoma to overcome this problem. Perhaps as many as 30% of patients require a cricopharyngeal myotomy to reduce spasms of the P-E segment that interfere with fluent airflow and successful voice and speech outcomes. An air insufflation test is often performed prior to the TEP procedure to estimate the tonal status of the segment. Patients who fail this examination usually benefit from a myotomy in concert with the puncture. In some facilities, the TEP, with and without myotomy, is performed at the same time as the primary laryngectomy. In other centers, laryngologists prefer to delay this procedure for as many as 3 to 6 months following the primary operation. The rationale for this secondary approach rests on the value of more time to allow for additional healing and all adjuvant therapy to be completed. Neither philosophy has proved more efficacious or harmful than the other.

## Artificial Instrument Speech

There is an assortment of different types of artificial larynges that virtually all laryngectomees can be taught to use for vocal expression. These devices offer an immediate means of communication, and they are much more helpful than gesturing or a piece of paper and a pencil. Every laryngectomee should own and learn to use an artificial larynx. It is a tool that facilitates communication during the early stages of esophageal or TEP speech training and development. Also, it may prove invaluable during emergencies or when other forms of alaryngeal speech fail. A critical prerequisite to successful use is the possession of at least minimally efficient articulation abilities. Even manual dexterity difficulties can be overcome using special sensors and toggle

switches, which can activate most commercially available devices via contractions of forehead, facial, or articulatory musculature.

### Types of Instruments

There are two basic types of artificial instruments for alaryngeal communication: *transcervical* and *transoral*

### Transcervical Devices

These types of electronic instruments are most commonly used by laryngectomees. They are battery-operated tone generators designed to be hand held. Perhaps the most sophisticated model is the Servox, manufactured by Siemens Corporation. Patients are trained to locate a spot on the neck (or cheek) that permits good penetration of the sound emitted from the instrument into the vocal tract. This artificial sound source is then articulated in the usual manner, but speech is distinctly robotic (monopitched and monoloud). Patients must be taught how to find this so-called sweet spot consistently and with ease. Learning how to coordinate speech efforts with finger depression of the activation button is another challenge. In the beginning, many laryngectomees either prolong the sound generated by the device beyond the end of the last word spoken, cut the sound off prematurely, or both. Attempting to say too many words on a long, continuous (buzzing) sound is another early problem experienced by many patients. Rapid-fire, short bursts of sound generation are also common features that make speech choppy and threaten intelligibility.

There are three major contraindications to use of a transcervical instrument. These include (1) excessive scarring, post-op edema, or postradiation fibrosis on both sides of the neck, which may dampen or impede sound transmission; (2) anesthetic neck tissue, which may reduce kinesthetic feedback necessary for efficient and consistent positioning of the instrument against the desired neck region; and (3) fistulization in the neck or pharynx, which may also dampen or divert sound waves.

### Transoral Devices

These instruments are hand held electronic or pneumatic (reed driven) devices that direct sound to the oral cavity through a plastic or rubber tube. They are especially beneficial for laryngectomees who either temporarily or permanently cannot use a transcervical device, for reasons discussed earlier. The Cooper-Rand (Luminaud) unit is probably the most commonly used device designed exclusively for transoral application. It is composed of a transducer, which is hand held, a short piece of tubing, and a wire-connected sound oscillator with an on/off switch usually carried in the shirt pocket. There are two primary disadvantages to the use of a transoral device. The tube may interfere periodically with lingual and labial articulatory adjustments and proficiency, and saliva may clog the tube and disrupt sound penetration and transmission to the oral cavity.

Early in the post-op period, most patients experience significant edema and tenderness, which preclude placement of an instrument against the neck or cheek. For many laryngectomees these conditions are considered temporary side effects. Rather than purchasing transoral devices, many patients and clinicians opt to make modifications of the transcervical devices for transoral use. This is accomplished by coupling a rubber oral adapter with extended tubing to the diaphragm. Once neck placement is possible, the adapter and oral tubing can be discarded. However, acquisition of a transoral instrument is indicated from the beginning of the rehabilitation program for the patient who will probably never be able to use a transcervical device.

The Tokyo pneumatic transoral device is designed to couple the tracheostoma and oral cavity. This interconnection enables pulmonary airflow to stimulate vibration of the reed mechanism located within the main body of the instrument. Artificial sound generation is therefore regulated by respiratory subsystem forces, akin to the aerodynamics underlying normal voice and speech production. As a consequence, intensity variations, inflection patterns, speaking rate, and phrasing may be controlled in a relatively natural manner. The tension of the reed can be adjusted to raise or lower the fundamental frequency of the sound produced. Whereas voice and speech are often good to excellent in patients who use pneumatic artificial larynges, this method of alaryngeal speech rehabilitation is surprisingly unpopular.

The previously mentioned disadvantages of transoral instruments may also be experienced by patients who use pneumatic devices. Additionally, some patients find it necessary to use both hands to position and stabilize the instrument. This poses a problem for those who cannot learn to coordinate use of the device with one hand only. Further, odd stomal architecture may prohibit achieving a consistent air-tight seal when the instrument is being used. Still others struggle to learn to coordinate breathing with instrument placement over the stoma for speech purposes.

## SUBTOTAL LARYNGECTOMEE REHABILITATION

Whereas years ago the total laryngectomy procedure was generally performed for most Stage III and Stage IV malignancies, more recently, head and neck surgeons have stressed the importance of organ preservation treatment strategies, even for patients with advanced disease. National research protocols have encouraged oncology teams to elect radiation therapy as the primary treatment modality for most T1, T2, and T3 laryngeal disease. Surgery for salvage is considered when necessary, along with planned neck dissections. Many patients with Stage III and Stage IV disease are being treated with a variety of subtotal procedures, including the supraglottal laryngectomy, near total laryngectomy, supracricoid hyopexy, and vertical hemilaryngectomy. Adjunctive radiation therapy is often prescribed postoperatively. These alternatives are viewed as oncologically acceptable in most cases, and there are no data to support the premise that the percentage of postoperative disease persistence or recurrence is any greater than that following total laryngectomy.

From a functional, quality of life point of view, these subtotal surgical reconstruction methods usually provide patients with immediate verbal communication abilities that often equal or exceed the levels ultimately achieved by most total laryngectomees. Additionally, with the exception of the near total procedure, these conservative approaches do not usually require a permanent tracheotomy; voice is driven by pulmonary airflow, and respiratory exchange occurs in the usual way. Voice and speech outcomes generally range from fair in some cases to good to excellent in most others. There is rarely a need for an extensive vocal exercise program. On the downside, however, there is a fear of aspiration difficulty that threatens the feasibility of each of these subtotal laryngectomy options. Patients who are at risk for dysphagia, such as those with coexistent esophageal, base of tongue, and/or pharyngeal carcinoma, do not qualify as easily for these organ preservation protocols. If dysphagia occurs following surgery, swallowing therapy is indicated to try to reduce or eliminate the difficulty.

The supraglottal swallow maneuver is often employed in this program as a way to protect the airway during eating. Briefly, this technique requires the patient to hold the breath during each swallow. Immediately upon completion of the swallow effort, the patient must generate hard glottal attack phonation before taking another breath. If possible, a second, quick swallow is requested after the voice outburst, but before inhalation. These maneuvers accomplish two primary objectives: they train voluntary adduction of the vocal folds prior to swallowing, which helps to ensure airway protection and reduce the chances of aspiration, and they expel food particles away from the glottis that may have leaked into the laryngeal inlet during the swallow. Trace degrees of aspiration may persist even after therapy discharge, but most patients learn to tolerate the mild effects without clinically significant symptoms or signs.

In Chapter 6, numerous case studies are presented to coordinate, as realistically as possible, the information contained in the first five chapters of this text.

## SUGGESTED READINGS

Andrews, M. L. (1991). *Voice therapy for children.* San Diego: Singular Publishing Group, Inc.

Andrews, M. L., & Summers, A. (1988). *Voice therapy for adolescents.* Boston, MA: College-Hill Press.

Andrews, M. L. (1994). *Manual of voice treatment: Pediatrics to geriatrics.* San Diego, CA: Singular Publishing Group, Inc.

Andrews, M. L. (1991). *Voice therapy for children: The elementary school years.* San Diego, CA: Singular Publishing Group, Inc.

Arnold, G. E. (1962) Vocal rehabilitation of paralytic dysphonia. *Archives of Otarlyngology. 76,* 358–368.

Aronson, A. E. (1990). *Clinical voice disorders: An interdisciplinary approach* (3rd ed.). New York: Thieme Stratton, Inc.

Benninger, M. S., Gillan, J., Thieme, P., Jacobson, B., & Dragovich, J. (1994). Factors associated with recurrence in voice quality following radiation therapy for T1 and T2 glottic carcinomas. *Laryngoscope, 104,* 294–299.

Blom, E. D., & Singer, M. (1979). Surgical prosthetic approaches for post-laryngectomy voice restoration. In R. L. Keith & F. L. Darley (Eds.). *Laryngectomee rehabilitation,* Houston: College-Hill Press.

Boone, D. R. (1990). *The voice and voice therapy* (2nd ed.). Englewood Cliffs, NJ: Prentice-Hall, Inc.

Boone, D. R., & McFarlane, S. C. (1988). *The voice and voice therapy* (4th ed.). Englewood Cliffs, NJ: Prentice-Hall.

Brodnitz, F. (1958). Vocal rehabilitation and benign lesions of the vocal cords. *Journal of Speech and Hearing Disorders, 23*, 112–117.

Butcher, P., Elias, A., & Raven, R. (1993). *Psychogenic voice disorders in cognitive behavioral therapy.* San Diego, CA: Singular Publishing Group, Inc.

Casper, J. K., & Colton, R. H. (1992). *Clinical manual for laryngectomy and head and neck cancer rehabilitation.* San Diego, CA: Singular Publishing Group, Inc.

Conley, J. J., DeAmesti, F., & Pierce, J. K. (1958). A new surgical technique for the vocal rehabilitation of the laryngectomized patient. *Annals of Otology, Rhinology, and Laryngology, 67*, 655–664.

Crannell, K. C. (1987). *Voice and articulation.* Belmont, CA: Wadsworth Publishing Co.

Crumley, R. L. (1990). Teflon versus thryoplasty versus nerve transfer: A comparison. *Annals of Otology, Rhinology, and Larngology, 99*, 759–763.

Dedo, H. H. (1976). Recurrent laryngeal nerve section for spastic dysphonia. *Annals of Otology, Rhinology, and Laryngology, 85*, 451–459.

Dromey, C., Ramig, L. O., & Johnson, A. B. (1995). Phonatory and articulatory changes associated with increased vocal intensity in Parkinson disease: A case study. *Journal of Speech and Hearing Research, 38*, 751–764.

Fawcus, M. (1991). *Voice disorders and their management* (2nd ed.). San Diego, CA: Singular Publishing Group, Inc.

Froeschels, E. (1952). Chewing method as therapy. *Archives of Otolaryngology, 56*, 427–434.

Goldfarb, D., Keene, W. M., & Lowry, L. D. (1993). Laryngeal pacing as a treatment for vocal fold paralysis. *Journal of Medical Speech-Language Pathology, 1*, 179–185.

Greene, M. C. (1991). *The voice and its disorders* (5th ed.). San Diego, CA: Singular Publishing Group, Inc.

Hoit, J. D. (1995). Influence of body position on breathing and its implicatons for the evaluation and treatment of speech and voice disorders. *Journal of Voice, 9*, 341–347.

Kacse, J. L. (1991). *Clinical management of voice disorders* (2nd ed.). San Diego CA: Singular Publishing Group, Inc.

Kay Elemetrics Corp. *Acoustic, speech aerodynamic, and videostroboscopic instrument systems.* Lincoln Park, NJ: Kay.

Kotby, M. N. (1995). *The accent method of voice therapy.* San Diego, CA: Singular Publishing Group, Inc.

Lavorato, A., & McFarlane, S. (1983). Treatment of the professional voice. In W. Perkins (Ed.) *Current therapy of communication disorders: Voice disorder.* New York: Thieme Medical Publishers.

Morrison, M., & Rammage, L. (1994). *The management of voice disorders.* San Diego, CA: Singular Publishing Group, Inc.

Murry, T., & Woodson, G. E. (1995). Combined-modality treatment of adductor spasmodic dysphonia with botulinum toxin in voice therapy. *Journal of Voice, 9*, 460–465.

Ramig, L. O., Countryman, S., Thompson, L. L., & Horii, Y. (1995). Comparison of two forms of intensive speech treatment for Parkinson disease. *Journal of Speech and Hearing Research, 38*, 1232–1251.

Salmon, S. J., & Mount, K. H. (1991). *Alaryngeal speech rehabilitation: For clinicians by clinicians.* Austin, TX: ProEd.

Sapir, S. (1995). Psychogenic spasmodic dysphonia: A case study with expert opinions. *Journal of Voice, 9*, 270–281.

Saxon, K. G., & Schneider, C. M. (1995). *Vocal exercise physiology.* San Diego, CA: Singular Publishing Group, Inc.

Smith, M. E., Ramig, L. O., Dromey, C., Perez, K. S., & Samandari, R. (1995). Intensive voice treatment in Parkinson disease: Laryngostroboscopic findings. *Journal of Voice, 9*, 453–459.

Stemple, J. C. (1993). *Voice therapy: Clinical studies.* St. Louis, MO: Mosby Yearbook.

Stemple, J. C., Glaze, L., & Gerdman, B. K. (1994). *Clinical voice pathology: Theory and management* (2nd ed.). San Diego, CA: Singular Publishing Group, Inc.

Yamaguchi, H., Yotsukura, M., Sata, H., Watanabe, Y., Hirose, H., Kobayshi, N., & Bless, D. N. (1993). Pushing exercise program to correct glottal incompetency. *Journal of Voice, 7*, 250–258.

# CHAPTER

# 6

# *Case Studies*

This chapter contains 51 case studies of patients with different types of voice disorders. These cases are presented with focus on several pertinent factors, including the following: (1) the salient background history, (2) clinical and laboratory examination findings, including pretreatment laryngeal photographs, (3) the medical and speech diagnoses rendered, (4) treatment recommendations, (5) treatment results, including posttreatment laryngeal photographs, (6) comparisons with pretreatment status, and (7) theoretical discussion of the underlying disorder, and summary of the case.

References are made in the case studies to audiotape samples, which augment appreciation of the voice disorder exhibited by the patient. In some cases, two or more audiotape samples are provided to illustrate voice difficulties prior to and following intervention. The reader is advised to listen to the sample(s) provided on the companion audio CDs for each case presentation at the time the case is being read. The segments are correlated by number with case studies as they appear in this chapter. CD 1–33 on CD 1, Cases 34–74 appear as Tracks 1–41 on CD 2. This enables fast tracking to a specific voice sample for those who desire to review a case out of sequence.

The cases selected represent a cross-sec-tion of laryngeal pathologies, both benign and malignant. The evaluation procedures used to reach definitive diagnosis for each case study are not meant to be interpreted as an exhaustive account of the tests that could or should have been conducted. Similarly, the treatment recommended and that may have been provided for each patient presented highlights the methods that were employed, regardless of the outcome. Where applicable, alternative treatment approaches were discussed at the conclusion of the case study. Clinical and medicosurgical successes and failures have both been included in this chapter as a learning experience and for teaching purposes. It is hoped that the case studies that follow accomplish two primary objectives: first, that some stimulate new thoughts and discussions about potential evaluation and treatment strategies for patients with various types of voice disorders, and second, that others solidify well established and effective diagnostic and therapeutic techniques.

Please note that 23 cases have been added to the CDs. These patients (cases 52–74) were selected because they exhibit interesting voice disorders. Their medical backgrounds are briefly described in the appendix at the end of this chapter. Because of space limitations, photographs of the underlying laryngeal pathologies could not be included.

# CASE I
## T1N0M0 Laryngeal
## (Supraglottal) Carcinoma

## HISTORY

The patient is a 75-year-old female who presented with chief complaints of persistent hoarseness and mild dyspnea, which had persisted for 2 months. With the exception of these problems, she had enjoyed a relatively unremarkable medical history, despite smoking one pack of cigarettes per day for more than 50 years.

## EXAMINATION FINDINGS

Videostroboscopy of the larynx illustrated the following salient features: (1) an obstructive lesion emanating along, but confined to, the left ventricular vocal fold, which partially obscured views of both the right and left true folds; (2) difficulty visualizing true fold activity during phonation and respiratory efforts; however, bilateral arytenoid dynamics appeared unimpaired; and (3) aggressive contact between the edematous left ventricular fold with its right counterpart throughout all vocalizations. Although true vocal fold mobility could not be evaluated with confidence, actions of the arytenoid cartilages suggested that the lesion observed was confined to the supraglottal mechanism, as shown in Figure 6–1A.

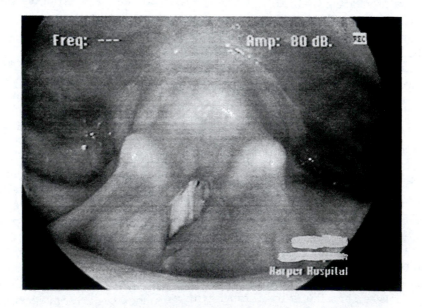

**FIGURE 6–1A.** This laryngeal photograph was obtained from a 75-year-old female with T1N0M0 supraglottal squamous cell carcinoma. Note the pronounced swelling of the left ventricular vocal fold, which partially obscures views of the underlying true vocal fold mechanism. This examination was conducted prior to the institution of full course radiation therapy.

Triple endoscopy and CT scan results supported this conclusion, as direct extension to or involvement of the true vocal folds was not evident. Biopsy confirmed the diagnosis of moderately well differentiated squamous cell carcinoma, which was staged T1N0M0 (supraglottis).

The **first voice sample** was obtained from this patient immediately prior to the institution of radiation therapy (6600 cGy/33 fractions planned), which was elected as the sole treatment modality. Note that her voice is moderately hoarse-harsh in quality. She also struggles with moderately low pitch and abnormal loudness variability. Notwithstanding these disturbances, maximum phonation time was within normal limits.

Acoustic analysis revealed the following: (1) fundamental frequency @ 210 Hz, (2) jitter @ 1.8%, (3) shimmer @ 0.80 dB, and (4) harmonic/noise ratio @ 1.2 dB. Overall, these data were interpreted as moderately abnormal.

Speech aerodynamic testing revealed (1) mean transglottal airflow rate @ 225 cc/sec, (2) subglottal pressure estimate @ 13 cmH$_2$O, and (3) glottal resistance @ 31.2 cmH$_2$O/lps. The flow findings represent roughly two times the normal degree of transglottal egress during phonatory efforts, suggestive of hypofunctional laryngeal valving. Higher than normal tracheal pressures are commonly exhibited by individuals with obstructive glottal lesions, as respiratory forces may be increased to compensate for underlying vocal fold vibratory inertia during phonation efforts. The resistance data are on the low end of normal, which points to reduced vocal fold compression forces. These findings are consistent with the theme of a hypofunctioning mechanism.

## POST-RT RESULTS

The **second voice sample** was obtained from the same patient after she completed one-third of the radiation therapy regimen. Perceptually, her voice remains moderately hoarse-breathy in quality with low pitch characteristcs. Maximum phonation time was within normal limits. Fundamental frequency dropped to 187 Hz, jitter improved to 0.83%, shimmer was normalized to 0.31 dB, and a slight improvement in the H/N ratio was evident @ 3.8 dB. Mean transglottal airflow rate during phonation was markedly lower and mildly restricted @ 20 cc/sec, subglottal pressure was virtually unchanged @ 12.5 cm H$_2$O, and glottal resistance increased to 90 cm H$_2$O/lps. Explanations for these findings were sought through videostroboscopy of the larynx. Note on Figure 6–1B the appearance of widespread erythema and mucositis of the laryngeal inlet. Hypertrophy of the left ventricular fold remains evident, and continues to obscure the anterior commissure and parts of the left and right true vocal folds. Also note the irregular appearances of the free margin of the left fold. Glimpses of the posterior one-third of the glottis were now evident during most phonatory efforts. These edematous changes help account for the mildly decreased airflow and moderately increased resistance results.

The **third voice sample** was obtained roughly 2 months following radiation therapy. She now exhibits only trace degrees of hoarse-breathy dysphonia. Habitual pitch remains lower than normal, as does her conversational loudness level. Overall, however, she is very pleased with the voice improvements she has made since the onset of treatment. Acoustic analyses revealed fundamental frequency @ 178 Hz, jitter @ 0.35%, shimmer @ 0.30 dB, and H/N ratio @ 4.1 dB. With the exception of the latter figure, which is indicative of a moderate amount of excess noise in the voice signal, these numbers are all within normal limits. Speech aerodynamic testing yielded data that were relatively unchanged from the previous examination findings, with one exception: glottal resistance measured 50 cm H$_2$O/lps, which is a clinically significant im-

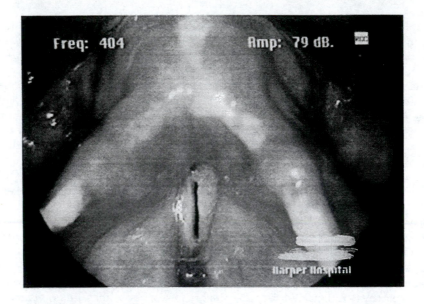

**FIGURE 6–1B.** This photograph was obtained roughly one-third of the way through radiation therapy. Note the marked improvement in the appearance of the ventricular vocal fold on the left. The true vocal folds can now be observed. Note the mildly irregular appearance of the covers and free edges, and the mild hemorrhagic abnormality at the level of the petiole of the epiglottis.

provement, and within normal limits. Figure 6–1C demonstrates the results of videostroboscopy, which illustrated (1) smooth free edges of both true vocal folds, with only a minimal chink in the posterior glottis during voice efforts, (2) a small anterior web with a white patchy appearance, (3) resolution of ventricular fold edema and the radiation-induced mucositis, and (4) adequate mucosal wave activity of both vocal folds during voice production.

## DISCUSSION

Radiation therapy cures approximately 85% of all patients who present initially with T1 glottic or supraglottic carcinoma. However, voice is rarely restored to normal quality, pitch, and loudness levels following successful treatment. Additionally, residual anatomical abnormalities are also quite common among this population, including lingering mucositis, diffuse laryngeal edema, glottal incompetency, and vocal fold atrophy. Our patient responded well to radiation therapy, and to date she remains disease free. However, like most others with similar histories, she struggles with some of these laryngeal anomalies, mild dysphonia, and chronic complaints of xerostomia and episodic sore throat symptoms. These results should signify that, although radiation therapy is not a benign treatment process, it is a relatively safe and effective organ preservation strategy for patients with T1 laryngeal carcinomas.

Our patient was not interested in voice therapy or medication for the dry mouth difficulties. Reasons for the web formation are unclear and perplexing. This side effect is not reported in the radiation oncology literature.

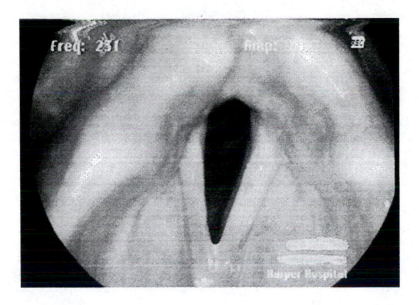

**FIGURE 6–1C.** This photograph was obtained 2 months following the completion of radiation therapy. Note marked improvement in the appearance of the laryngeal inlet. No gross lesions are evident. The patient was considered to be disease free at this point in time and doing well.

# CASE 2
## *Unilateral Adductor Vocal Fold Paralysis— Neurapraxia of Phonation*

### HISTORY

The patient is a 55-year-old male who presented with a 3-month history of dysphonia, characterized largely by breathy-hoarse quality and low volume features. He suggested that these voice difficulties began while he was in the hospital for severe pneumonia. During hospitalization, he received a tracheotomy and was placed on a respirator for 3 weeks. A PEG was performed for tube feeding purposes because of a moderate degree of aspiration symptoms. A diagnosis of left vocal fold neurapraxia (temporary paralysis) was rendered at that time, which was judged a sequela to intubation trauma. In addition to dysphonia and dysphagia the patient suffered from significant shortness of breath and vocal fatigue. Upon discharge, comprehensive voice and swallowing evaluations and therapy were recommended. His past medical history is positive for chronic use of tobacco and alcoholic products, untreated gastric reflux symptoms, and mild hearing loss in both ears. He denied voice misuse or other forms of potential vocal fold abuse.

### EXAMINATION FINDINGS

Perceptually, the patient's voice was moderately breathy-hoarse in quality and reduced in volume. Running speech was evidently labored and intermittently dysfluent, due to breaths that frequently occurred in the middle of words. He commented that there had been no discernable changes in voice functioning since the onset of the problem. Maximum phonation time was 4 seconds. The next **voice sample** illustrates these dysphonia features.

**CD1**
**Track 2**

Acoustic analysis revealed the following: (1) fundamental frequency @ 153 Hz, (2) jitter @ 2.17%, (3) amplitude shimmer @ 0.37 dB, and (4) harmonic/noise ratio @ 14 dB. The jitter findings suggest a substantial amount of instability and aperiodicity in the cycle to cycle vibratory characteristics of the vocal folds during phonation. The remaining acoustic data were all within normal limits.

Speech aerodynamic testing yielded the following: (1) mean airflow rate @ 2,196 cc/sec, (2) subglottal pressure @ 19 cm $H_2O$, and (3) glottal resistance @ 3.3 cm $H_2O$/lps. Transglottal egress was roughly 20 times the normal degree, indicative of a hypofunctional laryngeal valve and marked escape of unphonated air. Tracheal pressure was two times normal, suggestive of excess respiratory effort during phonation. The resistance data revealed less than one tenth the normal degree of vocal fold compression forces. All of these findings further substantiated the probable diagnosis of glottal incompetency and associated vocal fold hypofunctioning.

Videostroboscopy illustrated the following: (1) left paramedian vocal fold paralysis, (2) mild hyperactivity of the ventricular folds during voice efforts, (3) inconsistent compensatory action of the right true vocal fold across the midline of the glottis, (4) a persistent, full length glottal chink during all vocalizations, and (5) lack of mucosal wave activity, but aerodynamic fluttering of both vocal folds was evident. An adequate airway was demonstrated on various respiratory maneuvers. Figures 6–2A and 6–2B illustrate these laryngeal characteristics.

Intubation trauma was strongly considered the cause of the vocal fold paralysis. The diagnosis: neurapraxia of phonation. A 6-week stint of voice therapy was prescribed as a conservative method of management. The patient was not at great risk for aspiration pneumonia, as he remained NPO and on a tube feeding schedule only.

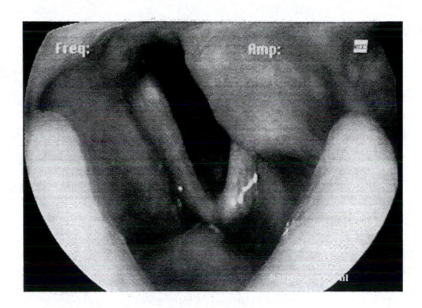

**FIGURE 6–2A.** Left vocal fold paralysis in a 55-year-old male. Note that the cord hangs in the paramedian position, and is essentially motionless during all phonation activities. Also note the overhanging flaccidity of the arytenoid soft tissue on the same side, which partially obscures the view of the underlying true vocal fold.

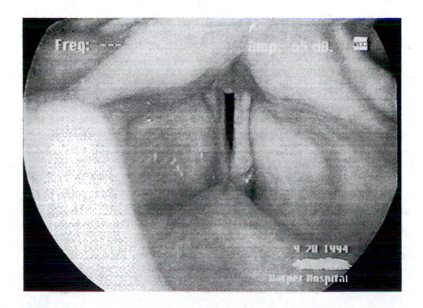

**FIGURE 6–2B.** This photograph illustrates the same patient during vigorous voice activity. Note the persistent glottal chink across the entire length of this mechanism. The right true vocal fold fails to make compensatory contact with the opposing side. The patient mildly recruits the ventricular vocal folds in an effort to compensate for the glottal incompetency.

## TREATMENT RESULTS

The patient attended twice weekly voice therapy sessions, 50 minutes per visit, for 6 weeks. Focus was placed on laryngeal valving techniques, including pushing, pulling, hard glottal attack, and manual compression exercises. The Visi-Pitch and videostroboscopy systems were woven into the sessions for biofeedback of voice and vocal fold dynamics. At the completion of this program, roughly 6 months following the onset of the dysphonia, no clinically significant voice improvements were obtained. Gelfoam injection was recommended at this time, but the patient was inclined to wait a few more months for potential spontaneous recovery of functioning before submitting to phonosurgery. He was thereafter lost to follow-up.

## DISCUSSION

Neurapraxia of phonation is a common sequela to intubation trauma. One or both vocal folds may become paretic or completely paralyzed, resulting in hoarse-breathy dysphonia. Depending on the extent of glottal incompetency, the patient may be at risk for aspration pneumonia. Knowledge of the medical history is of paramount importance in determining the probable etiology of the paralysis, diagnostic tests that should be administered, prognosis for spontaneous recovery, and most efficacious treatments that should be rendered at the outset. Definitive EMG studies of the intrinsic laryngeal musculature can be ordered at the outset to objectively measure underlying motor unit dysfunctioning and the potential for voice restoration. Regardless of the severity of dysphonia, if the patient also exhibits dysphagia, glottal augmentation surgery is indicated as soon as possible. Two primary alternatives include gelfoam injection to plump the paralyzed vocal fold or medialization thyroplasty. These techniques are preferable to more irreversible surgical options, such as Teflon, collagen, or autologous fat injections, because the gelfoam is typically fully resorbed within 2 months and can be reinjected if necessary, and the silastic implant can be removed if and when vocal fold functioning returns.

When the paralysis is mild to moderate in degree, the probability is usually high that the condition is temporary. If there are no co-occuring signs of aspiration, otolaryngologists may be inclined to resist surgical options in favor of stimulative voice exercises. We have discovered that therapy often provides a physiologic boost to the recovery process. In some cases, full recovery can be expected within a few short weeks following the onset of the problem. For others, improvements may occur over the course of several months. A small percentage of patients never demonstrate clinically significant gains, whether they receive intensive therapy or not. We operate under the assumption that, if after 12 months no improvements have occurred, phonosurgical intervention should be considered. The aforementioned longer lasting surgical alternatives have all been shown to be effective in the treatment of mild to moderate adductor vocal fold paralysis. Some otolaryngologists would elect the Isshiki I medialization thyroplasty procedure as the treatment of choice for patients with large glottal chinks and severe voice and deglutition difficulties.

# CASE 3
## *Adductor Spasmodic Dysphonia*

## HISTORY

The patient is a 70-year-old female who presented with a 1-year history of progressively worsening dysphonia. She complained of intermittent periods of voice arrest and a "squeezing sensation" in her throat during conversational speech. As an active participant in the family-owned business, she stopped interacting with customers because of these voice difficulties. She denied co-occuring limb or head tremors, blepharospasms, oral-buccolingual dyskinesia, torticollis, or any other type of dystonic behavior. She did not smoke, and she denied alcohol or illicit drug use. She had a positive medical history of hypertension, which was controlled with medication, and no hospitalization experiences within the past 65 years.

## EXAMINATION FINDINGS

The patient was alert and oriented to person, place, and time. No signs of language, cognitive, or perceptual disturbances were evident. Judgment and reasoning skills were also within normal limits. Cranial nerve examination was unremarkable. All other gross and fine motor and sensory examination results were within normal limits.

Perceptually, the patient's voice during connected discourse was profoundly breathy in quality. When she was urged to generate more voice, productions were marred by moderate to severe combinations of tremor and strained-strangled features. The next **voice sample** highlights this patient's speech and voice disturbances.

**CD1**
**Track 3**

Maximum (whispered) phonation time was less than 5 seconds. Acoustic analysis of forced phonation efforts revealed the following: (1) fundamental frequency @ 165 Hz, (2) jitter @ 1.3%, (3) shimmer @ 0.84 dB, and (4) harmonics-to-noise ratio @ 6.5 dB. These data were judged with caution because they were collected under unnatural phonation conditions for the patient. Notwithstanding this limitation, the jitter findings were roughly three times the normal degree of cycle-to-cycle vocal fold vibratory irregularity, shimmer was two times normal, and the harmonics data underscored the presence of excess noise in the voice signal.

Speech aerodynamic testing yielded the following results: (1) mean airflow rate @ 685 cc/sec during unstimulated, whispered phonation, (2) mean airflow rate @ 23 cc/sec when the patient was urged to try to generate voice, (3) subglottal pressure @ 16 cmH$_2$O during whispered voice, and 22 cmH$_2$O when phonation was attempted, and (4) glottal resistance @ 20 cmH$_2$O/lps during whispering, and 92 cmH$_2$O/lps when the patient was instructed to produce voice during the task. Collectively, these data suggest that the patient has developed laryngeal hypofunctioning as a compensatory strategy to combat an underlying hypertensive vocal fold valving disorder. When stressed to generate voice, the patient demonstrated severe, hyperfunctional difficulties on all of the aerodynamic measurements.

The results of videostroboscopy are illustrated in Figure 6–3. Note the presence of small nodules on the middle third free margin surfaces of both vocal folds. During voice efforts a persistent chink in the posterior glottis was evident. Prolonged closure time, vibratory stiffness, and voice induced tremors of the vocal folds, arytenoid cartilages, and aryepiglottic folds were prominent abnormalities.

The clinical diagnosis: adductor spasmodic dysphonia-essential voice tremor. Voice therapy was recommended as the initial method of management.

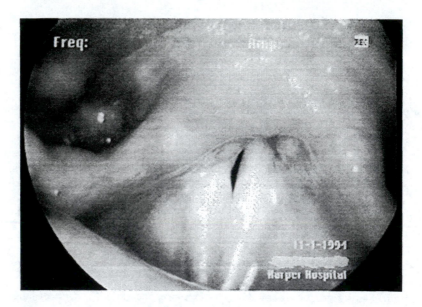

**FIGURE 6–3.** This patient exhibits predominantly strained-strangled voice quality, characteristic of adductor spasmodic dysphonia. She also exhibits a mild tremor overlay. Note on the middle one-third of both true vocal folds small, edematous nodules, likely sequelae to the tight adductory forces during phonation effort. There is a persistent chink in the posterior glottis during all voice activities.

## TREATMENT RESULTS

The patient underwent 10 sessions of voice therapy wherein the following stimulation techniques were employed: easy onset of voice production, increasing pitch, humming, sing-song voice activities, and manual stabilization of the larynx and strap musculature during all phonation efforts. Use of the Visi-Pitch apparatus provided visual biofeedback of the patient's voice and samples of the clinician's voice for modeling purposes. At the conclusion of this program the patient was able to generate significantly improved voice output; speech was more fluent, and whispering behaviors occupied less than 20% of all contextual utterances. However, carryover outside of the therapy environment was extremely poor. The next **voice sample** reveals this therapeutically induced improvement. Unilateral Botox injections were recommended because of this unsatisfactory outcome. The patient declined, and thereafter was lost to follow-up.

**CD1**
**Track 3**

## DISCUSSION

The pathogenesis of spasmodic dysphonia/essential voice tremor varies among patients. Although not histologically confirmed, the site of lesion for this condition has been postulated to be within the extrapyramidal system, possibly involving the dentato-rubro-olivary tract network. In cases like the present one, where the voice tremor component is largely camouflaged by more pronounced spasmodic vocal fold activities, focal laryngeal dystonia is usually rendered as the medical diagnosis. This hyperkinetic, laryngeal movement disorder is generally resistant to behavioral intervention and use of antispasmodic or beta-blocking drugs. However, we have had some clinical success with behaviorally stimulating speech fluency by using higher than normal pitch and sing-song voice patterns with several patients. Carryover has ranged from poor to good, with the chief complaint that it is very taxing mentally to employ this speaking strategy consistently.

Deliberate resection of one recurrent laryngeal nerve to induce vocal fold paralysis and reduce glottal hypertension has been reported in the literature with mixed, long term voice results. At present, the most common method of management involves botulinum toxin (Botox) injections into the vocal fold musculature. This technique was described in the phonosurgery chapter. Essentially, this pharmacologic agent causes paralysis of the recipient muscle tissue. Numerous research reports have unequivocally demonstrated that such injections may dramatically reduce adductor (and abductor) laryngospasms and improve overall voice and speech fluency. Because the peripheral nerve endings undergo a natural sprouting and regeneration process, repeat injections are necessary every 3 or 4 months to overcome recurrence of spasmodic symptoms.

# CASE 4
## *Hemorrhagic Vocal Fold Polyps*

## HISTORY

The patient is a 41-year-old attorney who presented with a 4-month history of persistent dysphonia. He suggested that the voice difficulty began following a severe upper respiratory infection, during which he suffered from chronic coughing and throat clearing for 5 days. He admitted to a long history of cigarette smoking, at one pack per day, as well as a moderate amount of alcohol consumption on a daily basis. He also conceded that he has been a voice abuser at work, home, and social events for many years. He denied gastric reflux symptoms, swallowing problems, or any other clinically relevant past medical history.

## EXAMINATION FINDINGS

Perceptually, the patient's voice was mildly to moderately hoarse-breathy in quality. He suggested that his pitch had dropped dramatically over the past 2 months. Indeed, his conversational voice was characterized by low-pitched, resonant overtones. No signs of voice fatigue were evident, and the number of syllables uttered per breath was within normal limits. Maximum phonation time was 16 seconds.

**CDI**
**Track 4**

The next **voice sample** illustrates this patient's voice features.

Acoustic analysis revealed the following: (1) fundamental frequency @ 105 Hz, (2) jitter @ 1.4%, (3) shimmer @ 0.33 dB, and (4) harmonic/noise ratio @ 12.7 dB. The jitter findings are abnormal, suggestive of a moderate degree of instability in the cycle-to-cycle vibratory activities of the true vocal folds. The remaining data were within normal limits.

Speech aerodynamic testing yielded the following: (1) mean airflow rate @ 798 cc/sec, (2) subglottal pressure @ 20 cm $H_2O$, and (3) glottal resistance @ 20 cm $H_2O$/lps. The transglottal egress is roughly four times the normal amount during sustained vowel production, which is usually indicative of glottal incompetency and vocal fold hypofunctioning. The tracheal pressure finding is approximately twice the normal degree, suggestive of a significant amount of respiratory effort during vocalization. Glottal resistance, which essentially measures the compression forces between the vocal folds during the closed phases of vibration, was one-half the normal level. This result substantiated preliminary impressions of a hypofunctional laryngeal valve. Figure 6–4A illustrates the results of videostroboscopy. Note the presence of a large hemorrhagic polyp on the left true vocal fold. There is a smaller hemorrhagic polyp on the anterior third of the opposing cord as well. During the closed phases of vibration associated with voice efforts these growths intermittently approximate one another at the midline of the glottis. As a consequence, they contribute to visual perceptions of complete glottal closure; views of the subglottal region during phonation and respiration activities are obscured. Observations of true vocal fold mucosal wave dynamics, vibratory phase symmetry, and amplitude excursions were virtually impossible. During deep inhalation-exhalatory maneuvers the left polyp was seen to flop in and out of the glottal lumen.

The diagnosis: bilateral true vocal fold hemorrhagic polyps, likely secondary to voice abuse and misuse. Because of the severity of this condition, phonosurgery was recommended followed by a stint of voice therapy.

## TREATMENT RESULTS

A microflap approach was used for both cords, and the patient was placed on total voice rest for 10 days. Voice laboratory reevaluation took place at 3 weeks post-op.

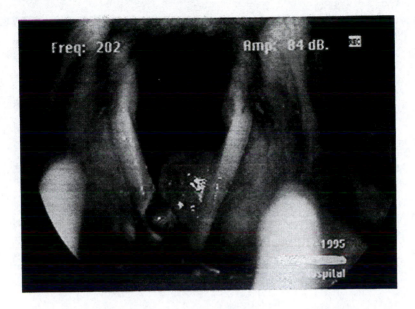

**FIGURE 6–4A.** Bilateral hemorrhagic polyps emanating off of the true vocal folds. During phonation these masses tended to flop in and out of the glottis.

Figure 6–4B illustrates the marked improvement in the appearances of the vocal folds. Note, however, that during the closed phase of vibration there is a slight asymmetry in the anatomy of the vocal folds. Notwithstanding this postsurgical side effect, vibratory actions and glottal competency were within normal limits. Both vocal folds exhibited adequate mucosal waves. The following lab results were obtained: (1) perceptually, voice was within normal limits, as can be appreciated by listening to the next **voice sample**, (2) maximum phonation time was within normal limits, (3) fundamental frequency @ 140 Hz, (4) jitter @ 0.50%, (5) shimmer @ 0.53 dB, (6) H/N ratio @ 15 dB, (7) mean airflow rate @ 93 cc/sec, (8) subglottal pressure @ 10 cm $H_2O$, and (9) glottal resistance @ 60 cm $H_2O$/lps. All of these data represent clinically significant improvements over the preoperative testing results. Two sessions of voice therapy followed, with focus on vocal hygiene issues. The ill effects of voice abuse and misuse were addressed in detail, and assorted reading material was provided to familiarize the patient with the relationship between polyp formation and these abnormal behaviors.

**CD1
Track 4**

## DISCUSSION

The patient's preoperative voice was not indicative of the severity of the underlying laryngeal pathology. In fact, most of his co-workers and family members were surprised when they learned of the initial evaluation results and recommendations. This situation is not uncommon in patients with very large vocal fold lesions that occupy and fill the glottis during phonation. These growths may give rise to mild or moderate quality disturbances, which may be partially camouflaged by the low pitched, resonant overtones that they generate. Female patients are usually more concerned about these voice changes than their male counterparts, primarily because of the low pitch features.

   The current patient helped substantiate that full-scale voice laboratory evaluations are indispensable to differential diagnosis and treatment. Had we relied on perceptu-

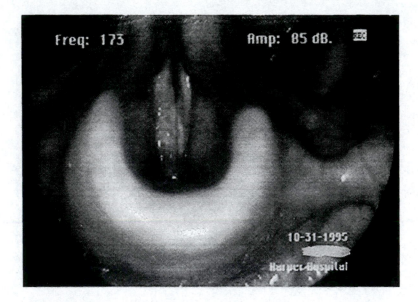

**FIGURE 6–4B.** Postoperative appearance of the laryngeal inlet. Note that the hemorrhagic polyps have been removed successfully and the patient achieves full glottal competency at the midline during phonation. These results were excellent not only with regard to laryngeal anatomy; the patient exhibited near normal phonatory skills as well.

al impressions alone, the patient might have been enrolled in a voice therapy program at the outset. We have discovered that hemorrhagic polyps, especially large ones, do not resolve with therapy. There is no doubt that the patient benefited most by undergoing surgery first, followed by a stint of therapy. In his case, the surgical results were excellent, limiting the need for direct voice exercises. For cases with less successful surgical outcomes, more extensive voice therapy is usually indicated. One final note: This case also reminds us that what we hear in the voice of the patient is not always reflective of the overall anatomic and physiologic status of the larynx.

# CASE 5
## *Subglottal Lymphoma*

## HISTORY

The patient is a 41-year-old female who was brought to the emergency room by her husband because of progressive dyspnea. She was admitted to the hospital for a tracheotomy, owing to a large obstructive airway lesion. A biopsy was also performed, and the diagnosis of low grade, non-Hodgkins lymphoma was rendered by the pathologist. She was referred as an inpatient to the voice lab for detailed laryngeal function studies. With the exception of seasonal hay fever symptoms, she did not present a remarkable medical background.

## EXAMINATION FINDINGS

Perceptually, with the exception of moderately low pitch features, the patient's voice was unimpaired. However, during conversation she suffered from moderately inefficient and irregular speech breathing patterns. As a consequence, the number of syllables per breath was moderately lower than normal, causing mild phonation dysfluency. Maximum phonation time was 10 seconds, which is roughly half the normal length.

The next **voice sample** highlights these dysphonic features.

**CD1**
**Track 5**

Acoustic analysis revealed the following: (1) fundamental frequency @ 171 Hz, (2) jitter @ 0.51%, (3) shimmer @ 0.40 dB, and (4) harmonic to noise ratio @ 11.6 dB. These data were all within normal limits, with the exception of moderately low habitual pitch. Speeh aerodynamic testing yielded the following results: (1) mean airflow rate @ 600 cc/sec, (2) subglottal pressure @ 7.5 cm $H_2O$, and (3) glottal resistance @ 18 cm $H_2O/lps$. The transglottal egress finding reveals roughly six times the normal amount of airflow during sustained vowel production, suggestive of vocal fold hypofunctioning and glottal incompetency. The resistance data point to approximately half of the normal degree of compression force between the vocal folds during the closed phases of vibration, which also indicates the presence of a weak glottal valve.

The results of videostroboscopy are illustrated in Figures 6–5A and 6–5B. Note the presence of an irregularly shaped, soft appearing, pink, relatively smooth subglottal mass on the left side. This lesion attaches to the lower lip of the ipsilateral vocal fold, and it extends inferiorly to the region of the upper tracheal ring, posteriorly to the interarytenoid zone, and medially to occupy approximately 30% of the airway. Mild inflammation of the posterior third of the left vocal fold is evident. Vibratory abnormalities include a mild degree of glottal incompetency, mildly irregular phase symmetry, and mildly retarded mucosal wave activity on the involved side. Note that during the closed phase of vibration the lesion is not visible.

The diagnosis: biopsies were taken for frozen and permanent sections. Histopathologically, the lesion was composed of small lymphocytes and condensed chromatin. A diagnosis of non-Hodgkin's lymphoma, small cell type, was reached. Chemotherapy (cyclophosphamide, vindesine, and prednisone) was prescribed as the primary treatment of choice, with locoregional radiation therapy and/or surgery for salvage.

## TREATMENT RESULTS

The patient returned 6 weeks later for videostroboscopy reevaluation to determine the degree of tumor response. She had received two courses of treatments to date.

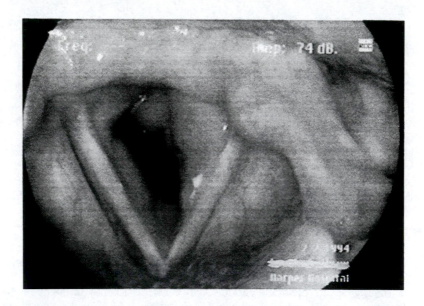

**FIGURE 6–5A.** This laryngeal photograph was obtained from a 41-year-old female who was diagnosed as having subglottal non-Hodgkins lymphoma. Note the bulky irregularity of this mass in the subglottic region. The true vocal folds are free of growths, as this tumor is confined entirely to the subglottal space.

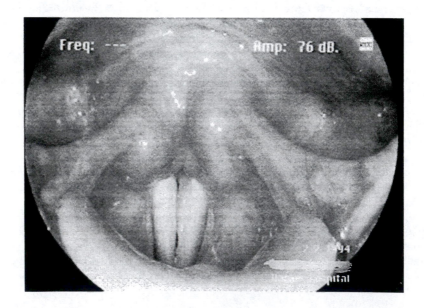

**FIGURE 6–5B.** This view demonstrates the appearance of the true vocal folds during voice efforts. Note that the subglottal lymphoma is hidden from view. There are no gross lesions on the surface or free margins of the vocal folds themselves.

**CD1**
**Track 5**

Perceptually, her voice and speech breathing patterns were within normal limits, and she was not dyspneic. This can be appreciated in the next **voice sample**. She was decannulated approximately 2 weeks ago. Figure 6–5C illustrates notable improvements in overall tumor size. A small degree of swelling is still evident subglottally, immediately inferior to the posterior third of the left true vocal fold. The remaining region is adequately patent with no evidence of disease. Both cords are white and glistening, normally characteristic of healthy mucosa. Physiologically, phase symmetry is very mildly depressed. In general, however, the vocal folds move fluently to and from the midline of the glottis during phonation. A small but persistent chink exists in the posterior glottis during phonation, due to residual left side abnormality. There is a very mild depression of the mucosal wave on the left, perhaps due to slight tethering subglottally.

The patient was scheduled to continue with chemotherapy treatments, but 2 weeks later she developed signs and symptoms of lymphoma involving the mediastinum. Reexamination in the voice laboratory revealed enlargement of the subglottal mass, as can be seen in Figure 6–5D. The patient was scheduled for 4 weeks of daily low dose radiation therapy, to be followed by home infusion therapy over the course of 5 months.

She returned for reevaluation roughly 3 months postirradiation and halfway through the home chemotherapy program. She complained only of episodic coughing spells. Perceptually, her voice remained within normal limits on all parameters. Examination was confined to videostroboscopy, the results of which are illustrated in Figure 6–5E. Note that full and complete glottal closure was evident. Adequate mucosal wave dynamics were observed on both vocal folds during various phonatory maneuvers. The subglottal area shows resolution of the previously described tumor recurrence. There remains, however, mild asymmetry in the anatomical appearance of the larynx from left to right. The left vocal fold is somewhat thinner than its counterpart. Additionally, both respiratory and phonatory activities demonstrate mild asym-

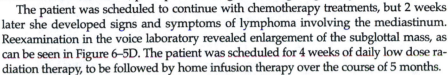
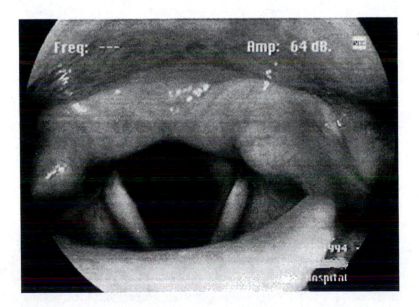

**FIGURE 6–5C.** This view was obtained from the patient following roughly two courses of chemotherapy. Note that the tumor has resolved to a large extent. There is still a remnant mass in the subglottis on the left side, but this is a significant improvement over the prechemotherapy observation.

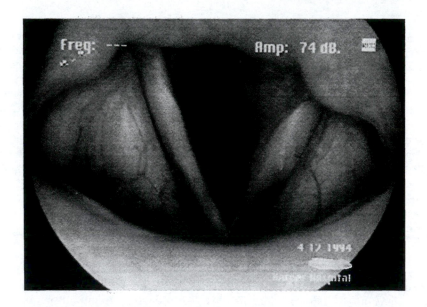

**FIGURE 6–5D.** Note that roughly 1 month later the patient now demonstrates recurrence of the lymphoma in the subglottal space on the left side. Note the mild swelling of the ipsilateral vocal fold as well.

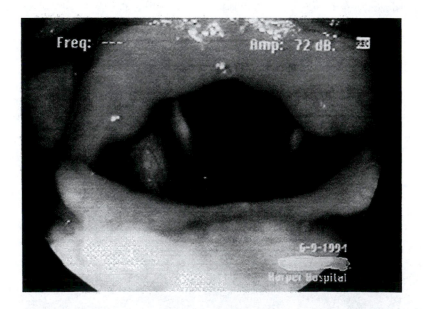

**FIGURE 6–5E.** Note that the patient has now undergone radiation therapy and continues on a home infusion chemotherapy program. This photograph was obtained roughly 2 months after Figure 6–5D. Observe that the subglottal mass has completely resolved, but that there is some mild asymmetry anatomically between the left and right true vocal folds, both at rest and during phonation efforts.

metry in the extent of vocal fold excursions; the left side lags and is responsible for this phasic disturbance. These mild abnormalities do not, however, adversely affect overall vibratory behaviors during voice production. These findings were viewed as evidence of a complete response to the treatments rendered.

## DISCUSSION

Primary non-Hodgkin's lymphoma limited to the subglottic larynx is extremely rare. Less than 10 cases have been reported in the literature to date. It is a potentially curable disease that can lead to profound airway distress if left untreated. Because of the high probability that the condition is not confined to the larynx, a thorough workup requires investigation of other possible sites of involvement. Careful physical examination, CT and basic radiographic studies, and bone marrow biopsies may prove helpful.

In the current patient, the initial biopsy results were somewhat surprising to us. Debate ensued regarding the best method of treatment for this condition, which included a discussion about surgical excision as the primary modality followed by radiation and chemotherapy. There are very few reports in the literature that favor only surgery. Most of the existing literature on laryngeal lymphomas recommends either chemotherapy, radiation therapy, or a combination of both as the best treatment approach, with surgery for salvage, if necessary. This was the track ultimately prescribed for the current patient. She began with chemotherapy and experienced a partial response. The tumor had shrunk roughly 75% in overall size. At this point, the possibility of surgery was remote. However, radiation therapy was considered necessary to boost the effects of chemotherapy and to shrink the remaining tumor. Home infusion chemotherapy was prescribed next as a maintenance program.

The patient did very well, and to date exhibits no evidence of disease. In this case, phonation was only minimally disturbed. Voice therapy was not indicated but ongoing voice laboratory studies have been prescribed according to a 6-month interval schedule. It is important to note that a complete response to treatment, like that obtained with the current patient, does not necessarily mean that the disease has been cured. Lymphomas have a tendency to occur at distant sites many years following succesful treatment. That is why regular follow-up evaluations are critical.

# CASE 6
## *Left Vocal Fold Paralysis*

## HISTORY

The patient is a 58-year-old male who presented with a 3-month history of persistent dysphonia, shortness of breath, and vocal fatigue. He suggested that these difficulties began following a severe bout of viral influenza, which lasted 10 days. He denied voice abuse behaviors, but admitted to a long history of cigarette smoking at one pack per day. Historically, he underwent radiation therapy for prostate cancer 3 years ago. He did not report any other significant medical background, prior difficulties with voice, or symptoms of dysphagia.

## EXAMINATION FINDINGS

**CD1**
**Track 6**

Perceptually, the patient's voice was severely breathy-hoarse in quality, with associated reductions in volume control and pitch range. Maximum phonation time was 3 seconds, and running speech was dysfluent because of abnormal pausing to breathe between words spoken. The next **voice sample** is an example of these dysphonic features.

Acoustic analysis revealed the following: (1) fundamental frequency @ 97 Hz, (2) jitter @ 2.9%, (3) shimmer @ 1.26 dB, and 4) harmonic to noise ratio @ 1.8 dB. These results are significantly abnormal. The jitter and shimmer findings are representative of substantial instability in the cycle-to-cycle vibratory dynamics of the true vocal folds. The harmonics data suggest a profound amount of noise in the voice signal, which correlates with his perceptual voice disturbances.

Speech aerodynamic testing yielded the following: (1) mean airflow rate @ 2,694 cc/sec, (2) subglottal pressure @ 9 cm $H_2O$, and (3) glottal resistance @ 3.9 cm $H_2O$/lps. Transglottal flow is roughly 26 times normal, and laryngeal resistance is about one-fifteenth the normal degree during phonation. These data suggest the presence of a hypofunctional laryngeal valve and coincident glottal incompetency.

Figures 6–6A and 6–6B illustrate the appearance of the laryngeal inlet captured during videostroboscopy. Note that the following salient features were observed: (1) midline paralysis of the left vocal fold, with no discernable movement during various phonation and breathing tasks, (2) faulty attempts by the right vocal fold to compensate for the left-sided paralysis, (3) a persistent chink across the entire length of the glottis during the closed phases of vibration, (4) mild recruitment of the ventricular folds during phonation efforts, and (5) lack of aerodynamic fluttering on the involved side.

CT scans of the head, neck, and chest were unremarkable, as was the rest of the clinical examination battery.

The diagnosis: unilateral left vocal fold paralysis. The etiology was unknown. A viral origin was considered, in view of all laboratory and clinical findings and the patient's history of the flu immediately preceding the onset of voice difficulty. A voice therapy program was prescribed at the outset instead of phonosurgery, for the following reasons: the patient was not suffering from signs of aspiration; the paralyzed vocal fold rested in the median position, which usually bodes well for compensatory voice exercises; and conservative treatment is usually best with patients who do not aspirate and who have a good chance of complete recovery of function because of the nature of the underlying (suspected) etiology.

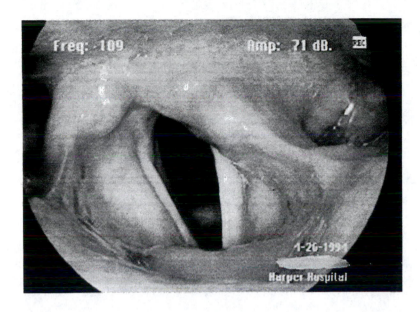

**FIGURE 6–6A.** This laryngeal photograph illustrates paramedian paralysis of the left true vocal fold in a 58-year-old male. Note the mild flaccidity of the overhanging arytenoid cartilage, which obscures view of the posterior one-third of the ipsilateral vocal fold.

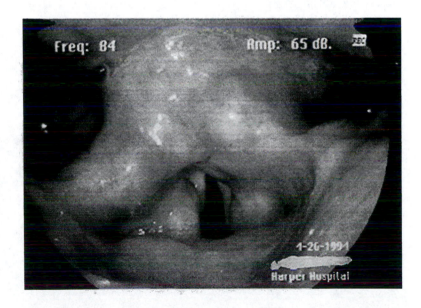

**FIGURE 6–6B.** This photograph illustrates the patient's attempts at phonation. Note the large glottal chink across the entire length of this mechanism. This accounts for the breathy-hoarse dysphonia and abnormal airflow dynamics.

## TREATMENT RESULTS

The next **voice sample** highlights the patient's voice after four 50-minute therapy sessions, one per week. Note the moderate improvement in overall voice ability, and that maximum phonation time has more than doubled. Acoustic analysis revealed (1) a gain in fundamental frequency of phonation to 125 Hz, (2) a near normal jitter level @ 0.66%, (3) a near normal shimmer level @ 0.50 dB, and (4) a gain in the H/N ratio @ 8.4 dB. These results indicate clinically significant improvements across the board.

Speech aerodynamic testing demonstrated dramatic improvements, but continued evidence of glottal incompetency and hypofunctioning. Mean airflow rate dropped from 2,694 to 365 cc/sec. Subglottal pressures remained unchanged, at normal levels. Glottal resistance improved moderately from 4 to 13 cmH$_2$O/lps.

Videostroboscopy also illustrated improvements over the pretherapeutic examinaton results, as shown in Figure 6–6C. Whereas the midline paralysis of the left vocal fold had not changed, flutter activity was now evident during phonation. The contralateral vocal fold establishes compensatory contact with the affected fold, across the midline of the glottis. Remaining, however, are intermittent periods of glottal incompetency during continuous phonation and running speech. Recruitment of the ventricular folds has subsided to a large extent. Additional therapy was prescribed, with hopes of making further gains. The patient was disinterested, and he was lost to follow-up.

## DISCUSSION

This patient presented with unilateral paralysis of the left vocal fold, probably of viral origin. In cases like this one, conservative approaches to management are usually most

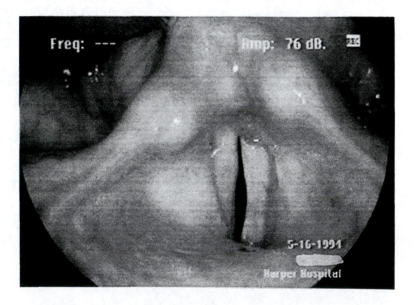

**FIGURE 6–6C.** This photograph demonstrates the patient's phonation efforts following a brief stint of voice therapy. Note the improved glottal competency, athough a persistent chink still exists in the midline of the glottis. The patient's voice is significantly improved as a result of therapy. Also note the improvement in the appearance of the overlying arytenoid cartilage on the left side.

efficacious. As long as the patient is not significantly dyspneic, and the airway is protected during swallowing, there is little justification to proceed with phonosurgery as the primary treatment modality. Instead, vocal fold valving exercises, including pushing, pulling, hard glottal attack phonation, and manual compression of the larynx on the paralyzed side, may be effectively employed. This type of exercise program was used with the current patient either to facilitate compensatory action of the uninvolved vocal fold, to stimulate functioning of the affected one, or both. The results obtained demonstrated that these exercises were responsible for the patient's voice improvements. The patient attended four sessions of biofeedback therapy, during which stimulated voice patterns were viewed on the Visi-Pitch® apparatus. This regimen was coupled to a home therapy maintenance program, which was designed by the voice therapist. The patient was instructed to practice various isolated vowels, vowel combinations, individual words, short phrases, sentences, and oral reading while simultaneously incorporating any one of the artificial vocal fold valving maneuvers. Whereas the paralyzed vocal fold did not show significant signs of physiologic recovery, the contralateral fold was trained to compensate as much as possible for this persistent deficit.

Whether or not the paralyzed fold would have eventually recovered in this case is impossible to predict with certainty. In many other cases of (probable) reversible vocal fold paralysis, full recovery is usually realized within 1 year. We believe that stimulative voice exercises, like those employed with the current patient, often speed this rehabilitation process. Phonosurgery options can always be explored at a later date if neither therapy nor time result in significant voice improvements.

When a patient presents with idiopathic vocal fold paralysis, diagnostic thoughts should turn to the possibility of a virus as the cause. Inquiries into the patient's recent medical history may shed light on this assumption.

# CASE 7
## *Laryngeal Leukoplakia*

## HISTORY

The patient is a 39-year-old female who presented with a 2-month history of persistent dysphonia. She had had no prior voice difficulties. She sang in a gospel choir and complained of chronic throat clearing and coughing activities. Although she did not use acid blocker medication, she struggled with severe signs and symptoms of gastric reflux. She reported a long-standing problem with asthma and associated shortness of breath and occasional chest pains; inhalant and steroid drug treatments provided moderate relief. She admitted to a long history of cigarette and alcohol product abuses, which persist to date. She sought help for her voice problem because it was interfering with her singing activities.

## EXAMINATION FINDINGS

Perceptually, the patient's voice was severely breathy-hoarse in quality, with a strained-harsh overlay. Pitch was mildly lower than normal, and she spoke with abnormally soft volume. Maximum phonation time was roughly 4 seconds, which is markedly reduced.

**CD1
Track 7**

The next **voice sample** highlights these dysphonia features.

Acoustic analysis revealed the followng: (1) fundamental frequency @ 211 Hz, (2) jitter @ 7.9%, (3) shimmer @ 1.8 dB, and (4) harmonic to noise ratio @ 1.2 dB. With the exception of the habitual pitch level, which is within normal limits, these data are all profoundly abnormal. There is a marked degree of instability and irregularity in the cycle-to-cycle vibratory characteristics of the vocal folds during voice production. The harmonics results suggest the presence of a substantial amount of noise in the voice signal.

Speech aerodynamic testing yielded the following: (1) mean airflow rate @ 470 cc/sec, (2) subglottal pressure @ 14 cm $H_2O$, and (3) glottal resistance @ 93 cm$H_2O$/lps. All of these data are moderately abnormal. Transglottal egress was roughly four times normal, suggestive of hypofunctional vocal fold valving and glottal incompetency. Tracheal pressure was moderately higher than normal, indicative of excess respiratory effort to generate voice. Laryngeal resistance was twice normal levels, which is in contradistinction to the hypothesis of a hypofunctional glottal valve.

Videostroboscopy was conducted next. Figures 6–7A and 6–7B illustrate the appearance of the laryngeal inlet during phonation and at rest. Note the presence of bilateral, diffuse swelling of the vocal folds. There is a white, leukoplakic patch on the middle third of the left true vocal fold. Granulation changes are also evident in the interarytenoid region, with bulbous extension into the glottis. At no time during phonation was complete glottal closure achieved. The ventricular folds are heavily recruited during most voice efforts, which periodically obstructs examination of true cord activity. Experimentation with clinical techniques to stifle these abnormal supraglottal behaviors was unsuccessful.

The diagnosis: laryngeal leukoplakia, with co-occuring pachydermia laryngis, and Reinke's edema.

## TREATMENT RESULTS

CT scans of the head, neck, and chest were ordered to rule out malignant disease. A pinch biopsy was scheduled to evaluate the histoloic status of the leukoplakic tissue.

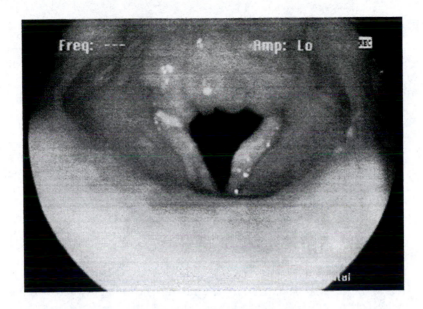

**FIGURE 6–7A.** This laryngeal photograph was obtained from a 39-year-old female with chronic leukoplakic changes throughout the laryngeal inlet. Note the significant amount of pachydermia laryngis in the interarytenoid region and the leukoplakic patches along the covers of the vocal folds.

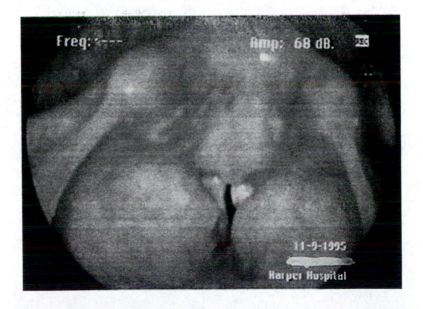

**FIGURE 6–7B.** Note on this photograph that the patient heavily recruits the ventricular folds to compensate for glottal incompetency. This perverse behavior exacerbates the dysphonia.

The patient was placed on a 6-week regimen of Zantac (150 mg b.i.d.) to combat the acid reflux symptoms. An intensive voice therapy program was prescribed to begin as soon as possible following the results of the CT studies and biopsy. The patient was urged to stop smoking and drinking and to begin taking the antacid medication. To date, she has failed to submit to these procedures and treatments.

## DISCUSSION

This patient presents with an interesting complex of laryngeal abnormalities. She misuses and abuses her vocal folds as a consequence of many different abnormal behaviors and conditions that have operated collectively. These include gospel singing, chronic throat clearing and coughing, untreated, persistent acid reflux, cigarette smoking, and excessive alcohol consumption. Singers and those who struggle with chronic throat clearing and coughing often present with diffuse edema of the vocal folds. It is well known that these types of activities have a traumatizing effect on this mechanism, especially when they occur in combination with one another. As in this case, the voice is usually hoarse in quality. In severe instances, breathiness may eventually contaminate the voice signal as glottal incompetency worsens with increased swelling of the vocal folds. Some patients begin to strain at phonation to overcome the problem, which often exacerbates the dysphonia. This scenario effectively characterizes our patient's voice disorder history. In fact, the higher than normal glottal resistance findings are likely secondary to her tendency to squeeze voice out in a strained-harsh manner.

The throat clearing and coughing difficulties exhibited by the current patient may have been secondary to the long-standing history of smoking, as well as the irritating effects of reflux material spilling over into the laryngeal inlet. Additionally, there is very high correlation between chronic gastro-esophageal reflux difficulties and the development of pachydermal (granulation) tissue in the interarytenoid region, and posterior vocal fold erythema and edema. Customary acid-blocker medication was prescribed for this patient to try to combat these symptoms and resolve the laryngeal side effects.

The suspected leukoplakia was of greatest concern, because these types of lesions can evolve into malignant neoplasms. They are observed in many patients who either smoke, abuse alcohol, or both. Moreover, a growing body of literature has emerged to demonstrate a high correlation between chronic gastro-espohageal-reflux disease and the formation of hyperkeratotic laryngeal growths. In the current patient, all of these potential causative agents may have operated collectively. Routine follow-up evaluations are essential to ensure early detection of any pathologic changes that may occur. Unfortunately, some patients are noncompliant and cavalier, despite these warning signs.

# CASE 8
## *T2N2c Glottic Carcinoma*

## HISTORY

The patient is a 72-year-old male who presented with a 6-month history of progressively deteriorating voice and a moderate degree of chronic obstructing pulmonary disease. Prior to these difficulties, he had been in excellent health, with no prior history of dysphonia. He was an avid bicyclist, having logged more than 10 miles per day for the past 10 years. He denied use of alcoholic products, and he quit smoking about 10 years ago.

## EXAMINATION FINDINGS

Perceptually, the patient's voice was severely breathy-hoarse in quality, with occasional pitch breaks and a shrill overlay. Maximum phonation time was 5 seconds, which is markedly low.

The next **voice sample** highlights these dysphonic features.

**CD1**
**Track 8**

Acoustic analysis revealed the following: (1) fundamental frequency @ 147 Hz, (2) jitter @ 5.3%, (3) shimmer @ 2.2 dB, and (4) harmonic to noise ratio @ 0.45 dB. With the exception of the habitual pitch level, which was within normal limits, these findings are significantly abnormal. The jitter and shimmer results point to substantial vibratory instability and variability from cycle to cycle. The harmonics data suggest the presence of a profound amount of noise in the voice signal.

Speech aerodynamic testing yielded the following: (1) mean airflow rate @ 1,374 cc/sec, (2) subglottal pressure @ 18 cm $H_2O$, and (3) glottal resistance @ 20 cm $H_2O$/lps. These data are also significantly abnormal. Transglottal egress was roughly 13 times the normal degree, which is indicative of a markedly hypofunctional laryngeal valve. The patient was utilizing excessive respiratory force to vocalize, as evidenced by the moderately higher than normal tracheal pressure level. The resistance results substantiate the hypothesis of glottal incompetency, as the patient generated approximately one half the normal degree of vocal fold compression force during phonation.

Videostroboscopy was performed next. Figure 6–8A illustrates the results, which included the following salient features: (1) ulcerative appearing lesions that extend bilaterally from the anterior commissure to the vocal processes of the arytenoids, (2) extension of these growths into the glottis off of the free edges of the vocal folds, more pronounced on the right side, (3) persistent glottal incompetency, (4) dysphasic vibratory patterns, (5) reduced amplitudes of excursion of the vocal folds, (6) overall hypomobility of the folds, (7) lack of mucosal waves bilaterally, and (8) intermittent hyperventricular vocal fold activity.

Clinical examination revealed bilateral, mobile neck nodes in levels II and III. CT scans of the head, neck, and chest were ordered, and a triple endoscopy was performed with laryngeal biopsy. Results revealed that the dimensions of the neck nodes were less than 6 cm each, and there was no evidence of cartilaginous invasion or disease spread outside of the larynx.

The diagnosis: T2N2cM0 well differentiated, invasive squamous cell carcinoma of the glottis. An organ preservation strategy was employed, wherein the patient was scheduled for full course radiation therapy (RT) @ 6000 cGy (30 fractions × 200/6 weeks). Voice laboratory analyses were conducted halfway through, at the completion of, and 4 months following this treatment protocol.

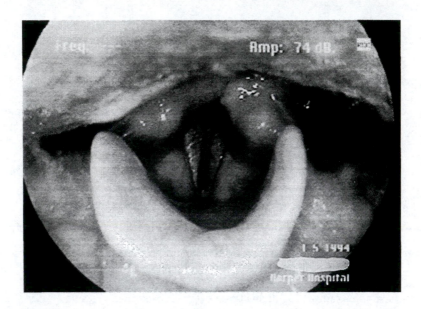

**FIGURE 6–8A.** This photograph represents the appearance of the laryngeal inlet of a 72-year-old male diagnosed with T2 squamous cell glottic carcinoma. Note the involvement of both vocal folds, more pronounced on the left side.

## TREATMENT RESULTS

### Halfway Through RT

Perceptually, the patient continued to exhibit a very high-pitched, shrill, breathy-hoarse voice, with periodic straining features. He complained of being unable to project his voice with sufficient loudness control. Maximum phonation time had significantly improved to within normal limits. Acoustic analysis revealed (1) Fo @ 432 Hz, (2) jitter @ 2.7%, (3) shimmer @ 0.77 dB., and (4) H/N ratio @ 0.70 dB. Whereas the jitter and shimmer findings were still abnormal, both measures showed moderate signs of improvement over the initial examination results. The habitual pitch level, however, had risen dramatically within the past few weeks.

Speech aerodynamic testing demonstrated (1) transglottal flow rate @ 1,027 cc/sec, which was a mild improvement over the original findings, (2) tracheal pressure @ 14 cm $H_2O$, which had also mildly improved, and (3) laryngeal resistance @ 30 cm $H_2O$/lps., which further illustrated the patient's mild voice and speech physiologic gains.

The next **voice ssmple** highlights his voice at this point in the treatment regimen.

**CD1
Track 8**

Figure 6–8B depicts the results of videostroboscopy. Note that the overall appearance of the vocal folds has greatly improved from that shown in the previous figure. The lesions have shrunk considerably, but the anatomy of the free margins of the vocal folds remains grossly irregular. Vibratory activities of the cords are still hypomobile and dysphasic; mucosal wave features are absent, and the ventricular folds are recruited during most phonation efforts.

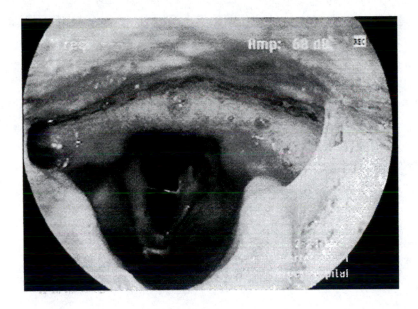

**FIGURE 6–8B.** This photograph was obtained from the same patient roughly halfway through the radiation therapy program. Note the persistent degree of erythema throughout the laryngeal inlet and the accumulation of saliva in the piriform sinuses. There is no discernable improvement in the appearance of the vocal folds themselves at this point in therapy.

## At completion of RT

Perceptually, the patient continued to exhibit high-pitched, breathy-hoarse dysphonia, with low volume output. These features represent no significant improvements since the initial evaluation 2 months earlier. The next **voice sample** highlights the patient's voice characteristics.

Maximum phonation time was within normal limits. Acoustic analysis revealed (1) $F_0$ @ 320 Hz, (2) jitter @ 1.1%, (3) shimmer @ 0.90 dB, and (4) H/N ratio @ 4.0 dB. Whereas these data are moderately abnormal, they nonetheless represent significant improvements over the preirradiation evaluation results, and moderate gains over the data obtained halfway through RT.

**CD 1**
**Track 8**

Speech aerodynamic studies revealed (1) mean airflow rate @ 273 cc/sec, (2) subglottal pressure @ 5 cm $H_2O$, and (3) glottal resistance @ 24 cm $H_2O$/lps. These findings also represent significant improvements over all previous examination results. Whereas transglottal airlfow is mildly excessive, tracheal pressure and laryngeal resistance have fallen to near normal levels.

Figure 6–8C illustrates the results of videostroboscopy. Note the anatomic irregularity of the free marginal surfaces of the true vocal folds, more pronounced on the left side. Also observe the widespread erythema of the laryngeal inlet, including the vocal folds. Mucositis changes are evident in the form of scattered white patches involving the ventricular and true vocal folds. During phonation, vibrations of the cords are moderately dysphasic. There is a persistent chink across the entire length of the glottis during voice output. Most striking is the conspicuous stiffness of the vocal folds, and the lack of mucosal wave dynamics bilaterally.

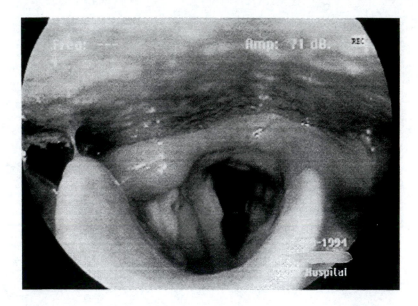

**FIGURE 6–8C.** This photograph was obtained from the patient at the completion of the radiation therapy program. Note that there is still a persistent degree of erythema throughout the laryngeal inlet. Also observe the irregular anatomy of the covers and free edges of the vocal folds.

## At 4 Months Post-RT

**CD1
Track 8**

These data were collected roughly 6 months after the initial, pretreatment evaluation. Perceptually, the patient continued to exhibit moderately hoarse-breathy quality, with intermittent periods of high-pitched, shrill features. The next **voice sample** highlights his voice at this point in time. Maximum phonation time remains within normal limits. Acoustic and speech aerodynamic testing revealed the following: (1) $F_0$ @ 194 Hz (2) jitter @ 1.3%, (3) shimmer @ 0.58 dB, (4) H/N ratio @ 12.3 dB, (5) mean airflow rate @ 600 cc/sec, (6) subglottal pressure @ 10 cm $H_2O$, and (7) glottal resistance @ 86 cm $H_2O$/lps. The harmonics and fundamental frequency data show mild improvements over the previous evaluation results. However, jitter, airflow rate, and laryngeal resistance are all moderately abnormal and excessive.

Figure 6–8D illustrates the videostroboscopy results. Overall, the laryngal inlet appears less erythematous and edematous than in all prior analyses. Mild mucositis is still evident, characterized by unpatterned white patchy lesions. Vibrations of the vocal folds remain stiff, without signs of mucosal waves. A small but persistent chink is observed across the midline of the glottis. The patient has a tendency to recruit the ventricular folds during most phonation efforts, perhaps accounting for the squeal-like vocal quality and increased jitter and laryngeal resistance findings. At this point in time, he was placed on a 6-month follow-up evaluation schedule. There was no gross evidence of disease in the larynx. Furthermore, clinical examination of the neck reflected no discernable nodal disease.

## DISCUSSION

Radiation therapy for T2 glottic cancer is curative in approximately 75% of individuals treated. With co-occuring nodal disease this rate is reduced by 10 or 15%. Throughout the world laryngologists and radiation oncologists generally agree that

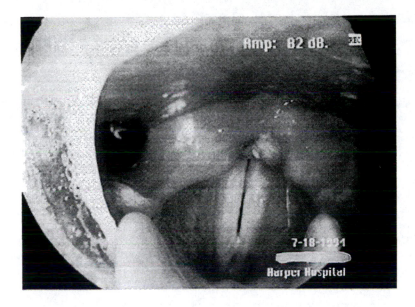

**FIGURE 6–8D.** This laryngeal photograph was obtained from the patient 4 months following the completion of radiation therapy. Note the marked improvement in the appearance of the laryngeal inlet. The covers and free edges of the cords are smooth and free of lesions. The substantial degree of erythema noted on the previous photographs has resolved. The patient was considered to be disease free at this examination.

the most efficacious treatment method for most glottic carcinomas, with the exception of those classified as T4, is full course RT. In most medical facilities within the United States, the standard radiation dose to the larynx ranges from 6000 to 7000 cGy, fractionated daily over the course of 5 to 6 weeks.

The literature is replete with qualitative reports on the treatment outcomes of RT for T1 and T2 glottic cancer. Most of the data regarding the effects of irradiation on the anatomy and physiology of the larynx are based on subjective opinions rendered by the investigators. These types of data argue strongly that RT not only provides a cure in the large majority of cases, but it ultimately improves voice to normal or near normal levels. Unfortunately, few voice laboratory studies have been published to substantiate these outcome conclusions with objective data. In fact, within this limited objective data base various researchers have shown that RT may cure the disease, but it often results in long-lasting, abnormal laryngeal tissue changes and lingering voice difficulties. These types of studies suggest that RT indeed may improve the patient's voice over pretreatment levels, but a normal or even near normal voice outcome should not be promised to the patient nor expected by team members.

For the current patient, we were very pleased with his responses to RT. At the time of this report, he exhibited no evidence of disease. His voice was better than it was prior to therapy, but nowhere near normal. Obviously, laryngeal preservation was the best choice for him, as it usually is for others with similar disease histories. In the low percentage of patients who may fail such treatment, surgery for salvage can be performed, but not without potential complications. Operating in a radiated bed of tissue often presents more difficulty for both the patient and surgeon, because of increased risks for wound healing problems and the formation of fistulas.

# CASE 9
## Parkinson's Disease (Vocal Fold Hypomobility)

### HISTORY

The patient is a 72-year-old male who presented with a 12-month history of progressively worsening dysphonia. Eighteen months ago he was diagnosed as having Parkinson's disease, with the usual assortment of physical signs and symptoms. Most notably, he exhibited strong pill-rolling tremors of the left hand, which were exacerbated by various bodily motor behaviors, including speech activities. He had a stooped posture, shuffling gait, and masklike facies. Speech articulation was only mildly imprecise, despite moderate degrees of lip, tongue, and jaw rigidity. Most pronounced, however, was prosodic insufficiency, as the patient spoke at a very slow rate, with excess and equal stress and monopitched features. He was referred by neurology service for chief complaints of voice difficulties, and occasional aspiration on thin liquids. A drug therapy regimen of trihexyphenidyl (Artane) and carbidopa-levodopa (Sinemet) was prescribed q.i.d.

### EXAMINATION FINDINGS

Perceptually, the patient's voice was moderately hoarse-breathy in quality and his volume was markedly reduced, almost to a whisper. Pitch variations were virtually impossible to detect, giving running speech a severely flat, monotone affect. Maximum phonation time was within normal limits.

**CDI**
**Track 9**

The next **voice sample** highlights the patient's speech and voice disorder.

Acoustic analysis revealed the following: (1) fundamental frequency @ 224 Hz, (2) jitter @ 0.87 %, (3) shimmer @ 0.65 dB, and (4) harmonic to noise ratio @ 6.9 dB. The jitter findings are mildly abnormal, suggestive of instability in the cycle-to-cycle vibratory characteristics of the vocal folds; likewise, the shimmer results point to irregular midline excursions during phonation efforts. The harmonics data show a moderate amount of excess noise in the voice signal.

Speech aerodynamic testing yielded the following salient findings: (1) mean airflow rate @ 336 cc/sec, (2) subglottal pressure @ 9 cm $H_2O$, and (3) glottal resistance @ 7.6 cm $H_2O$/lps. The transglottal egress findings are roughly three times the normal degree during phonation, suggestive of glottal incompetency and air wastage. The laryngeal resistance results are approximately one fifth the normal degree of compression force between the vocal folds during the closed phases of vibration. These data substantiate the hypothesis of a hypofunctional laryngeal valve.

Figure 6–9 illustrates the appearance of the laryngeal inlet, obtained during videostroboscopy examination. Note that the following abnormal anatomical and pathophysiological features were observed: (1) a relatively pronounced petiole of the epiglottis, which obscures visualization of the anterior commissure, (2) mild atrophic changes of the left true vocal fold, (3) persistent glottal incompetency, with an elliptically shaped chink in the middle third of this mechanism, (4) moderate to severe degree of stiffness in the pre-, post-, and para-phonatory activities of the vocal folds, and (5) severely rigid anteroposterior vocal fold stretching during efforts to alter pitch.

The diagnosis: hypokinetic dysarthria, secondary to Parkinson's disease, with involvement of the phonatory, articulatory, and prosody subsystems. Because the patient's chief complaints were focused on the dysphonic symptoms, he was enrolled in a twice per week voice therapy program for 2 months.

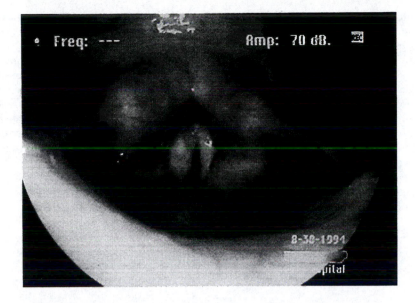

**FIGURE 6–9.** This laryngeal photograph was obtained from a 72-year-old male diagnosed with Parkinson's disease. Note the glottal incompetency caused by mild bowing of the left true vocal fold. The patient's voice was breathy-hoarse as a consequence, with reduced volume and pitch controls.

## TREATMENT RESULTS

The patient completed 15 sessions of therapy, which concentrated largely on increasing laryngeal resistance and loudness control utilizing various vocal fold medialization, clinical valving maneuvers. Techniques such as pushing on the arms of his chair, pulling up on the seat bottom, and squeezing the palms together while simultaneously generating voice were all quite helpful. The Visi-Pitch apparatus was also used for vocal loudness biofeedback. Treatment began with isolated vowel efforts and progressed, over the course of the program, to include simple words, phrases, sentences, and conversational speech activities. After 10 sessions, therapy focused on trying to teach the patient to fade the valving maneuvers and at the same time maintain the minimal improvements in voice output induced by these techniques. He was unable to do so with consistency, as his carryover from session to session was very poor. At the time of discharge he had made only marginal gains.

## DISCUSSION

In 1817 James Parkinson first described the clinical syndrome that now bears his name. This chronic, slowly progressive disease is caused by degeneration of the dopamine-rich cells and tracts of the basal ganglia and, in particular, the substantia nigra complex in the upper brainstem. Patients are afflicted with widespread muscle hypertonicity and rigidity, as well as unremitting rest tremors of the head and upper limbs. The cause remains unknown.

The speech disturbances in patients with Parkinson's disease are generically classified as hypokinetic dysarthria because of the underlying rigidity and reduced (hypo) mobility of involved speech musculature. The most prominent dysarthric features include short rushes of speech, hoarse-harsh vocal quality, monopitch, monoloudness, and imprecise articulation. These predictable patterns were indeed exhibited by the current patient. Clinical research has shown that many patients benefit from the aforementioned types of voice exercises, especially in the early stages of this disease. In fact, when the phonation subsystem responds favorably to these stimulative techniques, the other speech subsystems may automatically function at improved levels as well. This observed clinical result highlights the important contributions that the larynx may make to overall vocal tract output and integrity. Unfortunately, our patient did not do well in voice therapy, and he was disinterested in refocusing the program on the articulation mechanism.

Dopamine replacement therapy is the usual pharmaceutical treatment of choice. Currently, neurosurgical procedures to reduce profound tremors and associated motor disabilities have been reported to provide relief for some, but not, all patients.

# CASE 10
## Supraglottic Non-Hodgkin's Lymphoma

## HISTORY

The patient is a 73-year-old female who presented with a 2-month history of progressively deteriorating voice quality. With the exception of mild hypertension, which was well managed with medication, she did not report any significant medical background information. She admitted to having smoked cigarettes for more than 40 years at two packs per day, but maintained that she had quit within the last year. She complained of moderate-to-severe pain in her left neck in the region of levels III and VI. There was no associated dysphagia.

## EXAMINATION FINDINGS

Perceptually, the patient's voice was moderately breathy-hoarse, with lower than normal pitch characteristics. Most striking were her aggressive, forceful vocalizations, which resulted in a harsh vocal quality overlay. Maximum phonation time was within normal limits.

The next **voice sample** illustrates this patient's overall voice features.

**CD1
Track 10**

Acoustic analysis revealed the following: (1) fundamental frequency @ 208 Hz, (2) jitter @ 0.77%, (3) shimmer @ 0.35 dB, and (4) harmonic to noise ratio @ 12.5 dB. These data are all at the low end of normal with the exception of the jitter findings, which suggest a mild degree of cycle-to-cycle vocal fold vibratory instability.

Speech aerodynamic testing yielded the following: (1) mean airflow rate @ 159 cc/sec, (2) subglottal pressure @ 9 cm $H_2O$, and (3) glottal resistance @ 6.7 cm $H_2O$/lps. The flow data are roughly two times the normal amount of transglottal egress during phonation, suggestive of mild glottal incompetency. Although tracheal pressure was within normal limits, laryngeal resistance was approximately one-sixth the normal degree. This finding substantiates the hypothesis of a weak glottal valve.

Videostroboscopy results are illustrated in Figure 6–10A. Note the pronounced inflammation of the right ventricular fold. This area of swelling has a smooth, nonulcerative, erythematous appearance. It virtually obliterates views of the underlying true vocal fold. During phonation, the left vocal fold vibrated against this opposing mass; there was a small chink in the posterior third of the glottis during this activity. Whereas movements of only the left vocal fold were observable, normal rocking and tilting of both artyenoid cartilages were evident during voice efforts. This finding suggested that both true vocal folds were adequately mobile, even though actions of the right one were unobservable. Because of these viewing limitations, the overall vibratory characteristics and mucosal wave phenomena could not be assessed with confidence.

Triple endoscopy with biopsy, and CT studies of the head, neck, and chest were performed. Results of the latter measurements revealed isolated fullness of the right supraglottic, intraluminal region with mild encroachment of the airway. The neck and chest were clear, and no cartilaginous or bone invasion was evident. Endoscopy results corroborated the CT findings of a mass confined to the right ventricular fold. The histologic diagnosis was low grade, non-Hodgkin's lymphoma.

## TREATMENT RESULTS

The patient underwent six courses of chemotherapy as the definitive treatment method. She returned to the voice laboratory thereafter for reevaluation. Perceptually,

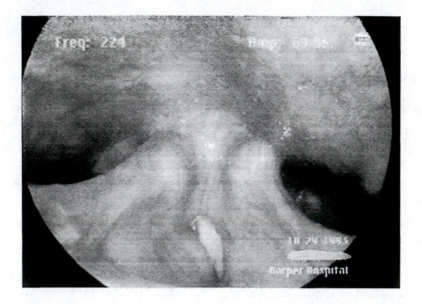

**FIGURE 6–10A.** This laryngeal photograph was obtained from a 73-year-old female diagnosed with non-Hodgkin's supraglottal lymphoma. Note the bulge across the midline of the glottis due to a lymphoma mass involving the right ventricular fold.

**CD1
Track 10**

her voice was within normal limits, which was a significant improvement over the pretreatment level. The next **voice sample** highlights this outcome. Acoustic analysis revealed completely normal findings on all parameters previously measured. Speech aerodynamic testing also revealed improvements to normal levels on all measures. Videostroboscopy results, illustrated in Figure 6–10B, included the following: (1) slight fullness of the right ventricular fold, which suggests at least a partial response to CT, (2) full and complete vibratory excursions of the vocal folds during phonation, (3) adequate mucosal wave dynamics, and (4) vascular changes in the piriform sinuses, more pronounced on the left side. Adjuvant radiation therapy was recommended to combat the small but persistent ventricular mass. The patient declined this option, and no additional treatment was rendered. Two months later she presented with recurrence of the lesion, as shown in Figure 6–10C.

## DISCUSSION

Isolated non-Hodgkin's lymphoma of the supraglottis is a very rare condition. Usually, patients present with similar tumors in other areas of the body as well. For the current patient, chemotherapy was chosen as the treatment modality. This is a common management approach for lymphomas in general. Success has also been reported in the literature with concurrent chemo- and radiation therapy, and with chemotherapy followed by irradiation in patients who are only partial responders.

Supraglottal and subglottal lesions do not always disturb phonation activities of the vocal folds. Such growths must either interfere with glottal closure, tether vocal mold mobility, or both for clinically significant dysphonia to result. It is not uncommon to discover large growths within the larynx in patients with normal or near normal voices. The current patient exhibited moderate dysphonic features. We believe that the

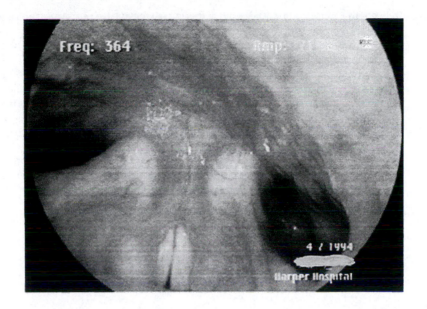

**FIGURE 6–10B.** This photograph was obtained from the patient following six courses of chemotherapy. Note the improvement in the size of the lymphoma mass. There is still a residual amount of fullness of the right ventricular fold.

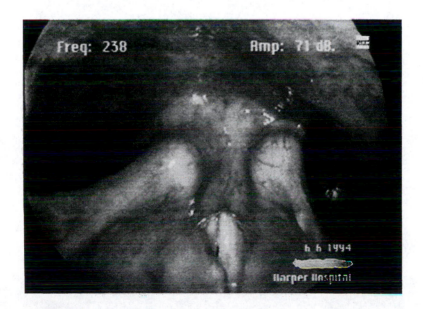

**FIGURE 6–10C.** Note that 2 months later the patient re-presented with recurrence of the lymphoma involving the right ventricular fold.

lymphoma caused a load-bearing, tethering effect on the right vocal fold, which reduced its mobility and fluidity of vibration. As a consequence, voice was adversely affected. Shrinkage of the mass released the underlying vocal fold to function more naturally. The patient's voice, in turn, was restored to within normal limits.

We remain concerned about this patient because of the aforementioned residual laryngeal mass following chemotherapy, and her refusal to undergo radiation therapy. Signs of disease persistence and locoregional metastases are commonly observed in patients with lymphoma histories, regardless of the initial treatment outcomes. She is being followed every 6 weeks. At the time of this report, 6 months postchemotherapy, the lesion site has not changed and there is no evidence of disease elsewhere in the body.

# CASE 11
## *Adductor Spasmodic Dysphonia*

## HISTORY

The patient is a 38-year-old female who presented with a 6-month history of strained-strangled voice quality. She suggested that this problem had worsened over the past 2 months. She was not a voice abuser, but reported that she smoked a pack of cigarettes per day for 20 years. Up until 3 years ago, she was addicted to heroin, which she injected in the neck, and crack cocaine. Otherwise, her medical background was clinically insignificant.

## EXAMINATION FINDINGS

Perceptually, the patient's voice was severely strained-strangled in quality. Running speech was plagued by intermittent arrests of phonation, and characteristics of adductor spasms of the vocal folds. As a consequence, and perhaps for compensatory purposes, she frequently lapsed into whispered speech patterns. Although these behaviors are abnormal, they produce fluent, more intelligible speech. Interestingly, vowel prolongations are less adversely affected than connected discourse. Maximum phonation time was 7 seconds, which is roughly one-third the normal length.

The next **voice sample** highlights the patient's voice profile.

Acoustic analysis revealed the following: (1) fundamental frequency @ 153 Hz, (2) jitter @ 0.74%, (3) shimmer @ 0.62 dB, and (4) harmonic to noise ratio @ 9 dB. These data quantify that the patient used a moderately low habitual pitch, and she suffered from abnormally increased cycle-to-cycle vocal fold vibratory variability and instability. The harmonics findings point to a mild amount of excess noise in the voice signal.

**CD1**
**Track 11**

Speech aerodynamic testing yielded the following: (1) mean airflow rate @ 584 cc/sec, (2) subglottal pressure @ 7 cm $H_2O$, and (3) glottal resistance @ 60 cm $H_2O$/lps. Transglottal flow was roughly 6 times normal, which is usually indicative of glottal incompetency or weak vocal fold valving. Laryngeal resistance was mildly elevated, and the tracheal pressure finding was within normal limits.

Videostroboscopy illustrated the following: (1) normal appearance of the vocal folds at rest, (2) mild incompetency at the midline of the glottis, resulting in a small chink anteriorly and posteriorly, (3) mildly prolonged vocal fold contact time during contextual phonation tasks, (4) adequate mucosal wave dynamics during vowel prolongation, and (5) unimpaired laryngeal-respiratory biomechanics. Figure 6–11 demonstrates some of these findings.

The clinical diagnosis: adductor spasmodic dysphonia. Neurology was consulted and the diagnosis was corroborated. All cranial nerves were intact. There were no signs of long tract disturbances, and all sensory and reflex testing yielded normal findings. With the exception of the focal laryngeal dystonic features, no other evidence of neurologic abnormality was identified.

The patient was enrolled in a voice therapy program at the outset. Discussions were held about the possibility of Botox injections into the vocal folds if behavioral exercises failed to induce significant improvements.

## TREATMENT RESULTS

The patient attended a total of eight 50-minute sessions of therapy. These included: (1) easy onset voice activities, (2) yawn-sigh phonation techniques, (3) humming, (4) ex-

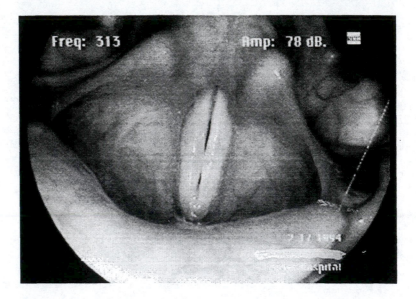

Freq: 313                    Amp: 78 dB.

**FIGURE 6–11.** This figure illustrates the appearance of the laryngeal inlet in a female patient with adductor spasmodic dysphonia. No gross lesions are evident across the length of the vocal cords and the surrounding soft tissue. There is a suggestion of a mildly edematous nodule on the middle one-third of the free edge of the right true vocal fold. This may be a sequela to the squeezing, adductory friction forces characteristic of the patient's spasmodic dysphonia.

perimentation with pitch and loudness variations, (5) laryngeal massage, and (6) an assortment of vowel prolongation, isolated word, phrase, sentence, and conversational speech productions. At the conclusion, no discernable voice improvements were obtained. Botox was recommended and described in detail. The patient was introduced to others who had experienced good to excellent results with similar treatment. Unfortunately, she was leery of this drug and the procedure itself, and refused to submit to the injections.

## DISCUSSION

This patient exhibited adductor laryngeal spasms, which resulted in severely strained-strangled voice quality. She did not display co-occurring bodily tremors, often observed in other patients with spasmodic dysphonia, nor did she suffer from spasms of other musculature. No signs of abductor laryngeal spasms were evident either. The diagnosis of isolated laryngeal involvement was relatively straightforward. The clinical neurologist confirmed this conclusion by classifying the problem as a form of focal laryngeal dystonia. This hyperkinetic movement disorder is thought to be attributable to disturbances within the extrapyramidal (nervous) system. At times, patients present with mixed signs and symptoms of adductor and abductor laryngeal spasms. When this occurs, voice may be mostly strained or breathy, depending on which pathophysiologic component is predominant.

In most instances, the diagnosis is reached through clinical examinations like those employed with the current patient. In her case, the perceptual impressions were striking. As we listened to the patient's voice samples there was little doubt that she suffered from adductor vocal fold spasms, which caused phonatory arrests and speech dysfluency. The acoustic and aerodynamic data collected did not shed great light on these impressions, as they rarely do in patients with spasmodic dysphonia. In fact, on the surface the transglottal airflow and laryngeal resistance findings were mildly contradictory. Whereas the former results suggested glottal hypofunctioning and a leaky valve, the latter results were consistent with vocal fold hyperfunctioning. This paradox may be, at least partially, explained by the intermittent nature of the laryngeal spasms in patients with this disorder. Vocal fold compression forces are abnormally increased during intermittent spasmodic episodes. When the spasms subside, bursts of transglottal airflow may be uncontrollably released into the vocal tract. Thus, mean airflow rate may be abnormally high, although measures of laryngeal resistance point to a tight glottal valve.

Adductor spasmodic dysphonia is caused by hyperexcitability of the intrinsic muscles of the larynx that regulate vocal fold closure. Voice therapy is rarely effective, perhaps with the exception of those cases considered to have a very strong psychogenic underpinning. Because it is impossible to know in advance whether or not such exercises would be beneficial, a trial therapeutic run should be permitted as the first treatment approach. If and when this behavioral program fails, our next treatment of choice is bilateral Botox injection into the vocal fold bodies that are formed by the vocalis muscles. This drug will weaken the adductory muscle forces by paralyzing the motor units, which in turn reduce the spasmodic behaviors of the vocal folds and the strained voice quality. Ultimate sprouting of the terminal nerve endings usually occurs within 3 to 6 months, resulting in gradual regression of the gains made. Reinjection is required to recycle the therapeutic effect. Because a very limited amount of the drug is used to achieve the desired result, and there have been no reports of systemic absorption, there is little concern that repeated injections places the patient at risk. Following the Botox procedure, patients may experience mild to moderate breathiness for a few days. Within a week or so voice output strengthens, without the prominent spasmodic overlay. In many cases, subtle or residual spasms are evident in contextual speech, but they are usually much less disruptive than they were prior to the injections. On occasion, a repeat injection is needed within a week or two after the inital injection if the voice result is less than acceptable. Some laryngologists inject only one vocal fold, whereas others always inject both. We routinely subscribe to the latter approach. Most recently, the research literature on this subject suggests that Botox injections that encompass both the vocalis and lateral cricoarytenoid muscles simultaneously produce the best voice results and the longest interval between injections. More research is needed to determine whether one method is better than the other. Unlike the current patient, most individuals do not object to the Botox treatment recommendation.

# CASE 12
## *Psychogenic Aphonia*

## HISTORY

The patient is a 48-year-old female who presented with a 1-month history of whispering. She had been unable to phonate at all within this period of time, necessitating an extended leave of absence from her employment as a secretary. When questioned about her voice prior to this breakdown she suggested that it was perfectly normal. However, she admitted to episodic voice difficulties over the past several years, but on each occasion the aphonia never lasted more than a few days. She denied significant emotional, professional, or financial stress. With the exception of chronic heartburn symptoms for many years, for which she took over-the-counter antacid medication, her overall medical background was unremarkable. She did not smoke, use alcoholic beverages, or abuse her voice.

## EXAMINATION FINDINGS

Perceptually, the patient whispered throughout the evaluation period. She was oriented to time and place, and possessed normal language and prosody skills. Despite the voiceless utterances, speech was 100% intelligible. Maximum (whispered) phonation time was 8 seconds.

The next **voice sample** highlights this behavior.

Neither acoustic nor speech aerodynamic testing was indicated in view of the presenting problem. When instructed to clear her throat and deliberately cough, the patient generated appropriate vocalizations. A brief session of experimental voice therapy ensued.

**CD1
Track 12**

## TREATMENT RESULTS

The patient was taught to mold the coughing and throat clearing sounds into prolonged vowels. This took about 10 minutes to master. Humming activities were introduced next, wherein the patient was requested to hum up and down the scale, and to hum the "Happy Birthday" tune. Next, she practiced simple words in isolation, and progressed to simple phrases, such as "One Monday morning." Longer sentences were then rehearsed, followed by conversational speech interaction. For the first 20 minutes of this stimulation period the patient was requested to sit with her eyes closed. The therapist sat behind her with both hands gently on her shoulders as instructions and voice demonstrations were given. Within approximately 30 minutes from the start of this exercise regimen the patient had regained her ability to phonate normally.

The next **voice sample** illustrates this improvement.

Videostroboscopy was conducted next, the results of which are shown in Figure 6–12. Note that during phonation there is a persistent small chink in the posterior third of the glottis. The interarytenoid region is edematous, with pachydermal granulation changes, perhaps as sequelae to the aforementioned chronic history of gastroesophageal reflux symptoms (heartburn). Vibrations of the cords are within normal limits with respect to phase symmetry, amplitude of movement, pre- and postphonatory adjustments, and mucosal wave dynamics.

**CD1
Track 12**

The diagnosis: psychogenic aphonia and reflux laryngitis.

The patient was urged to enroll in a comprehensive voice therapy program, and to seek psychologic counseling to discuss the factors that may be contributing to the

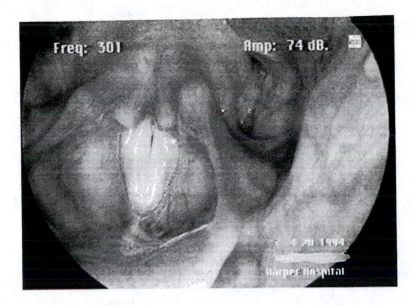

Freq: 301    Amp: 74 dB.

Harper Hospital

**FIGURE 6–12.** This photograph illustrates the laryngeal appearance of a patient diagnosed with psychogenic dysphonia. Note that the cords are within normal limits relative to their anatomy. There are no gross lesions within the laryngeal inlet. There is a small chink in the posterior glottis during the closed phases of vibration associated with voice.

episodic loss of voice. She concurred that these recommendations were appropriate, but to our knowledge never sought either form of intervention. She was lost to follow-up.

## DISCUSSION

Aphonia occurs when the vocal folds fail to make contact with one another during speech efforts. The persistent glottal incompetency not only causes whisper-like verbal communication patterns, but vocal fatigue and limited syllables per breath as well.

The patient with psychogenic aphonia, sometimes referred to as a hysterical or conversion disorder, often presents with aphonia. The inability to phonate is usually consistent during speech efforts, but adequate vocalizations may occur involuntarily when the patient coughs, clears the throat, or laughs. This paradox should signal the examiner that the aphonia is not likely to be caused by laryngeal pathology, such as bilateral adductor paralysis of the vocal folds.

Therapy is usually helpful in restoring voice to within normal limits. This improvement is often dramatic and immediate, despite the length of time that the patient may have been struggling with dysphonia/aphonia. In many cases, consultation with a clinical psychologist or psychiatrist is indicated to explore personal factors that are often causally related to this unusual voice disorder.

# CASE 13
## *Chronic Reflux Laryngitis and*
## *Recurrent Vocal Fold Granulomas*

## HISTORY

The patient is a 62-year-old female whose voice difficulties began 4 years ago. She did not seek medical advice until last year, when she was rushed to a local emergency room (ER) because of profound dyspnea. At that time, an emergency tracheotomy was performed, and a #4 Shiley, (cuffless) tracheotomy tube was placed. She was transferred to another hospital and otolaryngology was consulted for detailed appraisal of large, obstructive laryngeal growths that were identified by the ER attending physician. Prior to their removal, biopsies revealed that they were granulomatous lesions. Although she did not follow through with recommended postoperative voice therapy, lifestyle modifications, or antireflux medications, she reported that both her preoperative dyspnea and hoarse vocal quality had improved significantly.

Because of progressive recurrence of these difficulties over the past 2 months, she presented for examination. Historically, she has struggled with symptoms of gastroesophageal reflux disease for more than 30 years, but has never used prescription drugs for this condition. She admitted to chronic throat clearing and coughing behaviors, which she ascribed to daily sinus drainage problems and her long-standing history of cigarette smoking at more than a pack per day. She denied any form of voice abuse patterns. With the exception of a tonsillectomy as a child, the patient had never been hospitalized until the aforementioned tracheotomy. She had mild hypertension and diabetes, both of which were treated successfully with oral medications.

## EXAMINATION FINDINGS

Perceptually, the patient's voice was severely breathy-hoarse, with limited pitch and loudness control. Maximum phonation time was 13 seconds, which is moderately low.

The next **voice sample** highlights the patient's voice features.

**CD1**
**Track 13**

Acoustic analysis revealed the following: (1) fundamental frequency @ 183 Hz, (2) jitter @ 3.6%, (3) shimmer @ 3.25 dB, and harmonic to noise ratio @ 0.17 dB. These data are markedly abnormal. In particular, the jitter and shimmer findings suggest profound degrees of asynchrony, instability, and variability in the cycle-to-cycle vibratory characteristics of the vocal folds. The harmonics data point to a substantial amount of noise in the voice signal.

Speech aerodynamic testing yielded the following: (1) mean airflow rate @ 176 cc/sec, (2) subglottal pressure @ 13 cm $H_2O$, and (3) glottal resistance @ 55 cm $H_2O$/lps. The transglottal flow and subglottal pressure findings were only mildly higher than normal. Laryngeal resistance was within normal limits.

Videostroboscopy results are illustrated in Figure 6–13A. Note the presence of a large granulated lesion on the posterior third of the right true vocal fold, which protrudes across the midline of the glottis. Also note the irregular medial and longitudinal surfaces of the left vocal fold, perhaps sequelae to the biopsy and phonosurgery a year earlier. Pachydermia laryngis and mild erythema are evident in the interarytenoid region. Throughout all voice efforts profound hyperactivity of the ventricular vocal folds was observed (Figure 6–13B), which obscured views of the vibratory characteristics of the underlying true cords.

The diagnosis: hyperplastic laryngeal abnormalities, likely secondary to gastroesophageal reflux disease and chronic vocal fold abuse and misuse. A confirmatory

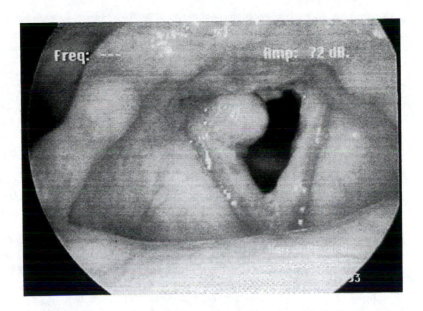

**FIGURE 6–13A.** This laryngeal photograph was obtained from a 62-year-old female with the diagnosis of laryngeal granuloma and gastro-esophageal-reflux disease. Note the large granulation mass in the posterior glottal region. Also note the irregularity of the free edges of the true vocal folds, more pronounced on the left side.

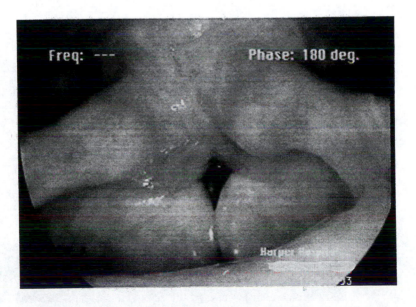

**FIGURE 6–13B.** This illustration demonstrates the profound hyperactivity of the false vocal folds during all phonation efforts.

biopsy was prescribed with surgical excision of the residual lesion. The patient was placed on a 3-month course of H2 blocker medication (Zantac, 150 mg/b.i.d.), and voice therapy was scheduled to begin 10 days postoperatively.

## TREATMENT RESULTS

The biopsy revealed nonspecific hyperplastic histopathology, consistent with granulo-matous disease. Laser excision of the lesion was performed without complication. Voice laboratory reevaluation of the patient was conducted roughly 6 weeks postoperatively and prior to the initiation of voice therapy. The patient requested the delay because of important family matters.

Perceptually, her voice was mildly hoarse-breathy in quality, with lower than average pitch features. Maximum phonation time was within normal limits. These were moderate improvements over the preoperative condition. The next **voice sample** demonstrates these gains.

**CD1
Track 13**

Acoustic and speech aerodynamic testing revealed the following: (1) Fo @ 176 Hz, (2) jitter @ 1.0%, (3) shimmer @ 0.22 dB, (4) H/N ratio @ 9.3 dB, (5) mean airflow rate @ 180 cc/sec, (6) subglottal pressure @ 9 cm $H_2O$, and (7) glottal resistance @ 59 cm $H_2O$/lps. The Fo finding corroborated perceptual impressions of a persistently low pitched voice. Although the jitter data illustrate significant improvements over the preoperative level, a mild to moderate disturbance remains. Both the shimmer and harmonics features had almost fully recovered to within normal limits. The aerodynamics findings showed an improvement in tracheal pressure associated with phonation, to within normal limits. However, a mild degree of increased transglottal airflow during phonation was still evident, which correlates with the hoarse-breathy quality of the patient's voice.

Figures 6–13C and 6–13D illustrate the anatomic status of the larynx observed during videostroboscopy. Note the fullness of the right true vocal fold, which may be sec-

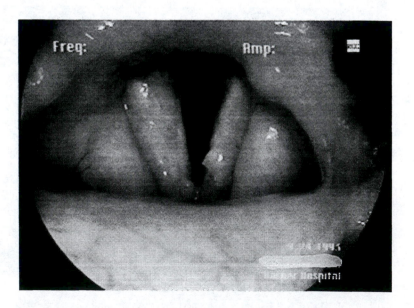

**FIGURE 6–13C.** This figure was obtained following laser excision of the granuloma in the posterior glottis. Note the widespread erythema of the laryngeal inlet and the mild irregularity of the free edges of the vocal folds.

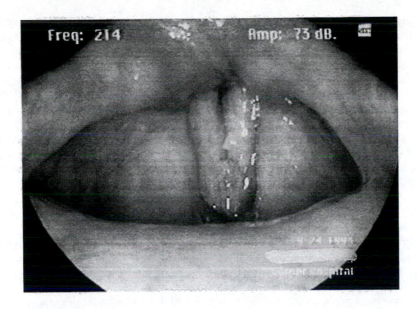

**FIGURE 6–13D.** This figure demonstrates the full glottal competency that the patient achieves during phonation postsurgically. Note that there is still a mild degree of irregularity along the free edges of the cords. Also note that the hyperactivity of the false vocal cords has substantially subsided.

ondary to the recent surgical procedures. Also note the mild irregularity in the free margin anatomy of the left true vocal fold. The ventricular folds were significantly less hyperactive during phonation efforts, which enabled study of the movement dynamics of the underlying true cords. The mucosal wave on the right was stiff. Vibration of the left fold was within normal limits with respect to mucosal wave features and pre- and postphonatory adjustments. However, there was a mild degree of asynchrony in the overall cycle-to-cycle vibratory patterns of both vocal folds. Notwithstanding this abnormality, relatively consistent midline glottal closure was evident throughout most of the examination.

The patient thereafter attended twice weekly voice therapy sessions for a total of 3 months. Focus was placed on increasing her Fo to 225 Hz and improving the range of pitch and loudness control. The Visi-Pitch® apparatus was instrumental in providing biofeedback of the patient's voice signals during most treatment sessions. Only minimal phonation gains were realized at the conclusion of this therapy program. The patient continued to smoke on a daily basis, despite warnings to the contrary, and she struggled with intermittent throat clearing behaviors. However, her reflux symptoms had improved dramatically as a consequence of the daily use of Zantac and moderate diet alterations. Overall, she was pleased with the treatment outcomes.

## DISCUSSION

This patient presented with severe signs and symptoms of progressive gastro-esophageal reflux disease. She had neglected this condition until granulomatous vocal fold lesions had formed and obstructed her airway. She was ultimately rushed to the ER, unable to breathe. She admitted that she had been dyspneic for several months prior to this event. The stridorous behaviors that she exhibited were interpreted by her family physician as signs and symptoms of a persistent upper respiratory infection. She was then placed on an antibiotic therapy program over the course of 6 weeks, without success. In the interim, the patient continued to smoke, cough, clear her throat, and struggle with breathing.

This scenario is not uncommon. Obstructive laryngeal lesions cause dyspnea and stridor. Stethoscopic examination of the patient with such signs and symptoms must include placement of the instrument on the larynx and trachea. As the patient is instructed to alternate normal and deep breaths, restricted airflow dynamics will be easily detected at this level of auscultation. This salient diagnostic finding should lead to, at least, mirror examination of the laryngeal inlet. Unfortunately, many general medical practitioners and internists do not perform laryngoscopic procedures as part of their routine evaluation. Had the current patient undergone such testing at the outset of her chief complaints, perhaps early signs of granulation changes would have been identified. This finding would have triggered follow-up referral to an otolaryngologist for definitive diagnosis and management. The institution of H2 blocker medication early on in the course of this disease process may have been especially facilitative as a first-line treatment approach. It is likely that the ER experience and tracheotomy would have been entirely avoided. Perhaps only a single biopsy and phonosurgical procedure would have been necessary in the final analysis.

Postoperative voice therapy may have resulted in greater gains; perhaps less vocal fold scarring and fibrosis would have resulted, enabling the patient to respond even more favorably to the voice exercises employed. In most cases of chronic reflux laryngitis and associated vocal fold hyperplasia, a combination of pharmacologic management, lifestyle changes, and voice therapy works well to combat this common disease entity. Phonosurgical alternatives should be delayed until and unless this conservative initial treatment approach fails to induce functional voice improvements and resolution of the abnormal tissue growth.

The current patient achieved a reasonably good management outcome, as evidenced by the pre- and posttreatment laboratory findings. We believe that her gains would have been much more impressive if she had been treated sooner and able to stop smoking.

# CASE 14
## *Systemic Lupus Erythematosis, Multiple Sclerosis, and Gross Histopathologic Vocal Fold Changes*

## HISTORY

The patient is a 45-year-old female who presented with a 10-year history of systemic lupus and a 12-year struggle with multiple sclerosis (MS). She received intermittent Prednisone therapy (20 mg qd) for the lupus condition, and Tylenol #4 and Librium had been effectively used to quell the symptoms of MS and depression. The patient suggested that at the time of this evaluation the MS symptoms had been in remission for approximately 1 year. She was hospitalized 2 weeks prior for persistent sleep apnea over a 2-month period, characterized by chronic dyspnea, choking, vomiting, and coughing spells that aroused her frequently in the middle of the night. She admitted to a three-pack per day smoking habit for 30 years, as well as occasional snorting of cocaine. She denied voice abuse, allergies, gastric reflux, or any other significant past medical background.

## EXAMINATION FINDINGS

Perceptually, the patient's voice was moderately to severely aphonic, with intermittent periods of whispered/hoarse vocal quality. The next **voice sample** highlights this difficulty. Note that the other speech subsystems are not impaired in their functioning, as the patient is 100% intelligible despite severe phonatory involvement. Because of the paucity of phonation, the initial voice laboratory examination was confined to videostroboscopy of the larynx.

**CD1
Track 14**

Figures 6–14A and 6–14B illustrate the results of this procedure. Note the leukoplakic appearing lesions on the surfaces of both vocal folds. The interarytenoid zone is grossly irregular in its appearance. There is mild atrophy of the posterior third of the vocal folds, which causes an associated chink in the glottis during all voice attempts. The true folds have a pearly gray, translucent appearance, characteristic of submucosal fluid retention; there is a subtle erythematous overlay. Vibratory patterns of the vocal folds were asymmetrical and asynchronous. Movements to the midline of the glottis were incomplete, owing largely to slow action of the vocal fold. Mucosal waves were absent bilaterally. Intermittent but strong actions of the ventricular vocal folds were observed throughout the examination.

The diagnosis: laryngeal lupus, compounded by multiple sclerosis and vocal fold leukoplakic lesions. Recommended treatment included increasing the patient's daily Prednisone level to 40 mg qd, instituting a voice therapy program at once, and consulting with a psychiatrist relative to the history of illegal drug use, profound sleep apnea, and continuous cigarette smoking.

## TREATMENT RESULTS

The patient readily complied with the pharmacologic adjustment. However, she was unwilling to schedule appointments with the psychology and voice clinics. She was subsequently lost to follow-up.

## DISCUSSION

Lupus is a generic term that is used diagnostically for many different diseases characterized mostly by skin lesions. Systemic lupus erythematosus (SLE) is a chronic,

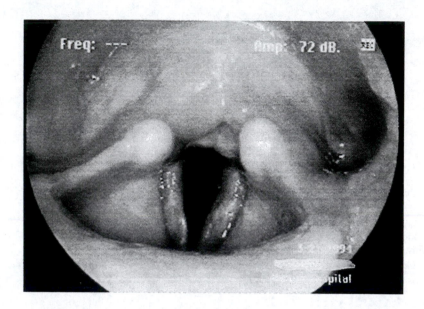

**FIGURE 6–14A.** View of the laryngeal inlet of a patient with systemic lupus erythematosus. Note the widespread erythema and edema of the true vocal folds bilaterally. Also observe the irregularity in the free edge anatomy of both vocal folds.

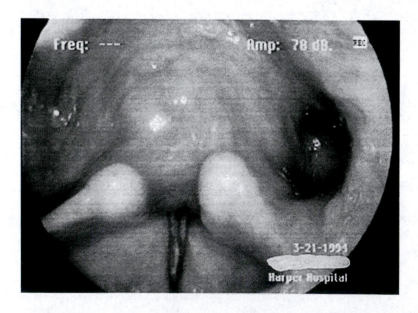

**FIGURE 6–14B.** This illustration demonstrates the hyperventricular activity during phonation efforts.

autoimmune condition with diffuse involvement of vascular and connective tissue. Approximately 25% of patients with SLE exhibit laryngeal abnormalities as part of the symptom complex. Virtually all of these individuals are complete responders to corticosteroid therapy (i.e., methylprednisolone [Prednisone] 50–200 mg/d). Degenerative reactions may occur at different levels of the larynx: mucosal, submucosal, synovial, vasculitic, and neuromuscular. Submucosal nodules, diffuse thickening, atrophy, ulcerations, hyperemia, and necrotic changes may occur either singly or in various combinations. Voice therapy is necessary only if the patient's response to the drug regimen is less than satisfactory.

Multiple sclerosis is a demyelinating neurologic disease. It unpredictably and episodically attacks the long tracts of the central nervous system as well as specific cerebellar pathways. The etiology is unknown, and close to 10,000 new cases are reported in the United States each year. The pathophysiology in most patients includes both spastic and ataxic movement disturbances, which may afflict virtually all body parts. The severity level may range from subtle to profound across different individuals with MS. Many patients experience prolonged periods of remission, during which they may realize significant improvements of their overall symptoms. When the phonation subsystem is involved the dysarthria that results may be characterized by a mixture of strained-harsh-tremorous vocal quality, due to spastic-ataxic disturbances of the vocal fold musculature. These features are often compounded by co-occurring articulation, resonation, and prosodic abnormalities. Both corticosteroids and corticotropin (ACTH) pharmacologic agents have been used for short-term relief of these symptoms, with mixed results.

The current patient suffered from a combination of problems, each of which alone would have been sufficient to affect adversely functioning of the vocal folds. The SLE probably accounted for most of the anatomical abnormalities observed during videostroboscopy of the larynx. The leukoplakic patches on the vocal fold covers were interpreted as premalignant lesions, secondary to the long and profound smoking habit. The pathologic vibratory patterns were likely manifestations of MS as well as these degenerative anatomical changes.

Voice therapy would have focused on vocal fold valving exercises to reduce the breathy vocal quality component. This clinical technique would have to be balanced against the patient's tendency to recruit the ventricular folds to compensate for underlying glottal incompetency. Whereas coupling vigorous pushing and pulling maneuvers with vocal efforts invariably induces a tight glottal seal, these activities may also exacerbate preexisting hyperactivity of the false vocal folds. Visual biofeedback of the laryngeal inlet during these exercises often helps the patient to relax this interruptive, supraglottal activity. However, the prognosis is usually guarded for the patient whose dysphonia is complicate by an underlying neuromuscular disorder.

# CASE 15
## *Vertical Hemilaryngectomy*

## HISTORY

The patient is a 41-year-old male who underwent a left vertical hemilaryngectomy, left modified neck dissection, and adjuvant radiation therapy at another institution 10 years prior to the present examination. At that time, the diagnosis of moderately differentiated squamous cell carcinoma of the larynx was rendered, and staged as a T3N1 condition. At the level of the glottis, the lesion was confined to and fixed the left vocal fold. Both clinical appraisal and CT scans revealed a 2 cm positive node in level III of the ipsilateral neck. Because of intermittent dysphagia, characterized by variable aspiration symptoms since these surgical procedures, the patient had been wearing a #6 Shiley (cuffless) tracheotomy tube. Until recently, he had tolerated full-time plugging of the tube for speaking purposes. Within the prior 3 months, he had experienced progressive breathing difficulty, particularly when he exerted himself or engaged in physical activities. This necessitated frequent removal of the plug to ease respiration. He presented for examination of these symptoms.

## EXAMINATION FINDINGS

Perceptually, the patient's voice was moderately hoarse-harsh in quality with reduced volume dimensions. Maximum phonation time was within normal limits.

**CD1
Track 15**

The next **voice sample** highlights these voice characteristics.

Acoustic analysis revealed the following: (1) fundamental frequency @ 127 Hz, (2) jitter @ 7.8%, (3) shimmer @ 2.9 dB, and (4) harmonic to noise ratio @ 0.5 dB. These data are moderately to severely abnormal. The jitter and shimmer results suggest a significant degree of instabiity and variability in both the frequency and amplitude of cycle-to-cycle vocal fold vibratory activity. The harmonics data point to a pronounced amount of noise in the voice signal.

Speech aerodynamic testing yielded the following: (1) mean airflow rate @ 1,570 cc/sec, (2) subglottal pressure @ 16.2 cm $H_2O$, and (3) glottal resistance @ 13.7 cm $H_2O$/lps. These data represent significant abnormalities across the board. Transglottal flow was roughly 15 times the normal degree, suggestive of glottal incompetency. Subglottal pressure was twice normal levels, indicative of increased respiratory effort to initiate and sustain phonation. Laryngeal resistance was one third the amount normally observed, which is consistent with the hypothesis of weak glottal valving forces.

Videostroboscopy results are illustrated in Figures 6–15A and 6–15B. Note the anatomical abnormality caused by the left hemilaryngectomy. There is a decided 120 degree tilt to the glottal configuration. Observed on the left side was a small lip of reconstructed soft tissue, which fluttered during phonation efforts. A small but persistent chink existed along the length of the glottis throughout the evaluation. Patency of the airway was compromised by a bulbous mass that had the appearance of scar tissue. This growth occupied the area immediately inferior to the glottis. Respiratory biomechanics of the right true vocal fold were within normal limits.

Fiberoptic endoscopic evaluation of swallowing ability revealed intermittent, trace degrees of aspiration on both liquid and pureed food substances. This disturbance was considered the result of the aforementioned glottal incompetency. When these items were thickened no signs of aspiration were evident. Semisolid and solid foods were swallowed without significant difficulty.

Recommendations: (1) Surgical excision of the subglottal scar band to facilitate breathing with the tracheotomy tube plugged, (2) behavioral therapy to improve

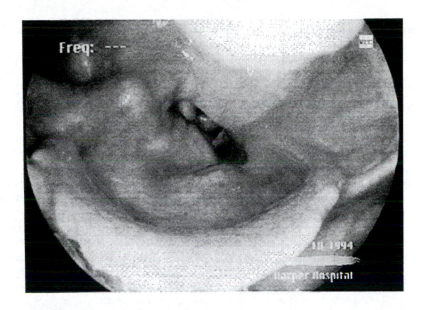

**FIGURE 6–15A.** View of the laryngeal inlet of a 41-year-old male who underwent a vertical hemilaryngectomy. Note the marked anatomical abnormality and 120 degree tilt to the glottal configuration.

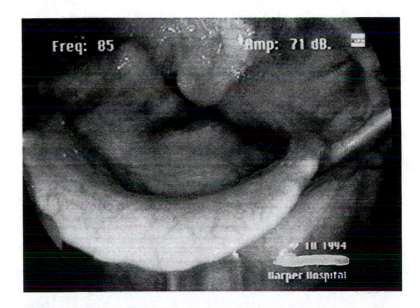

**FIGURE 6–15B.** This photograph illustrates the patient's attempts at phonation. Note the abnormal anatomy of this mechanism and the difficulty defining the anatomical boundaries of its components.

glottal valving during voice and swallowing activities. To date, the patient has not complied with either of these treatment recommendations.

## DISCUSSION

Laryngologists and radiation oncologists disagree considerably with respect to the best method of managing T3 glottic carcinoma with palpable lymph nodes in the neck. In general, there are three primary treatment approaches that might be employed: (1) total or near total laryngectomy, with neck dissection, if the tumor involves both vocal folds; (2) partial or hemilaryngectomy, with neck dissection, if the tumor is confined to one vocal fold; or (3) full course radiation therapy, with planned neck dissection if necessary. Most laryngologists prescribe adjuvant radiation therapy postoperatively. The cure rates for all of these treatment options are roughly equivalent: a 5-year disease-free survival of approximately 60%. For those who elect radical radiation therapy as the primary method of management, approximately 50% retain an intact larynx without the need for salvage surgery for persistent or recurrent disease. Posttreatment voice is usually mildly to moderately hoarse-harsh. Swallowing is rarely adversely affected, and unless salvage surgery is required, the need for a tracheotomy is remote.

The current patient elected to undergo a vertical hemilaryngectomy and neck dissection followed by adjuvant radiation therapy. He has been disease-free for 10 years. However, he has struggled with several persistent functional difficulties throughout this period of time. He remains dependent on a tracheotomy because of dyspnea, due to the formation of a postsurgical subglottal scar band. He experiences episodic aspiration on thin liquids and pureed food as a consequence of reconstructed glottal incompetency. His voice is moderately hoarse-harsh in quality, and he exhibits several anatomical and physiological laryngeal abnormalities that disturb the aerodynamics of speech production. It is impossible to predict with certainty if the patient would have realized greater benefits had radiation therapy been employed as the initial method of treatment. However, we have speculated that he would probably be (1) less hoarse, (2) able to swallow without aspirating, and (3) able to breathe comfortably without a tracheotomy. Had he presented more recently with the same T3 glottic lesion, he might have been dissuaded from laryngeal surgery in favor of such an organ preservation strategy. Unfortunately, he has not agreed to the recommended secondary surgical procedure to remove the subglottal scar band, nor has he submitted to voice and swallowing therapy. Without these treatments, it is unlikely that he will ever be decannulated.

# CASE 16
## *Essential Tremor Syndrome*

## HISTORY

The patient is a 69-year-old female who presented with a 10-year history of head, upper limb, and voice tremors. She suggested that these symptoms had progressively worsened in degree over the past 3 years. She reported that her father suffered from similar difficulties, but neither her brother nor her sister exhibited signs of tremor. With the exception of infrequent aspiration of thin liquids, she had no other medical concerns. Recent evaluation by a neurologist yielded the diagnosis of heredofamilial essential tremor syndrome, with predominant laryngeal involvement. She was referred by that practitioner for voice evaluation and treatment. She had been using antihypertensive medication for 5 years, and nasal steroids for seasonal allergic rhinitis. The neurologist did not prescribe any beta-blocking agents for tremor relief.

## EXAMINATION FINDINGS

With the exception of confirming the aforementioned tremor syndrome, the physical examination of the head and neck proved unremarkable.

Perceptually, the patient's voice quality was severely tremorous. During connected discourse there was evidence of a mild adductor spasmodic overlay. Pitch was lower than normal for the patient's sex and age. During prolongation of a vowel for maximum phonation time assessment, which amounted to 13 seconds, the tremor feature was most pronounced. She was noted to exhibit mild rest tremors of the head and upper right limb.

The next **voice sample** clearly demonstrates these voice abnormalities.

Acoustic analysis revealed the following: (1) fundamental frequency @ 125 Hz, (2) jitter @ 1.7%, (3) shimmer @ 0.76 dB, and (4) harmonic/noise ratio @ 1.6 dB. The fundamental frequency finding correlates positively with perceptions of a low pitched voice. The abnormal jitter and shimmer results are consistent with the pronounced degree of vocal tremor. The harmonics data point to a severe amount of noise in the voice signal.

**CD1**
**Track 16**

Speech aerodynamic testing yielded the following: (1) mean airflow rate @ 75 cc/sec, (2) subglottal pressure @ 13.5 cm $H_2O$, and (3) glottal resistance @ 162 cm $H_2O$/lps. Whereas transglottal flow was within normal limits, the tracheal pressure finding was mildly elevated, suggestive of increased respiratory effort to vocalize. Laryngeal resistance was roughly three times normal, indicating tight glottal compression forces during phonation. These results were consistent with our perceptual impressions of intermittent adductor spasmodic dysphonia features.

Videostroboscopy illustrated unremarkable laryngeal anatomy, as shown in Figure 6–16. However, profound and persistent tremors and clonic contractions of the true vocal folds and supraglottic mechanism were observed both at rest and during phonation activities. Involvement of the ventricular folds intermittently obstructed views of the underlying true vocal folds during this examination. Vibratory abnormalities included the following: (1) variably prolonged closure times, (2) absence of mucosal waves bilaterally, (3) markedly limited lateral excursions, and (4) episodic glottal incompetency. The diagnosis: hyperkinetic dysarthria: essential tremor syndrome.

Recommendations: Bilateral Botox injections into the true vocal folds, followed by a stint of voice therapy.

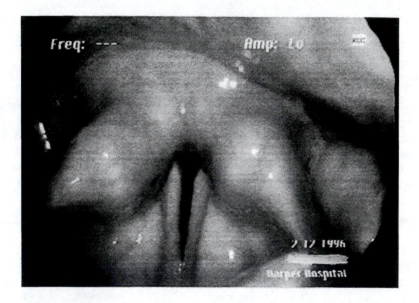

**FIGURE 6–16.** This photograph was obtained from a 69- year- old with the diagnosis of essential tremor syndrome, with a strong voice component. There are no gross lesions in the laryngeal inlet nor on the vocal folds themselves. However, the patient exhibited intermittent glottal incompetency like that shown in the illustration during most phonatory efforts.

## TREATMENT RESULTS

**CDI**
**Track 16**

The patient received four units of Botox, two in each vocal fold. She returned 3 days later for reevaluation. Perceptually, she exhibited signs of moderate voice improvement. The degree of vocal tremor had been reduced, and the spasmodic features were significantly less perceptible. However, the patient complained of mild hoarseness. The next **voice sample** highlights these posttreatment changes. Maximum phonation time was 14 seconds, which did not differ significantly from the initial evaluation score. Acoustically, her Fo increased to 171 Hz, and jitter, shimmer, and H/N ratio levels had improved minimally. No significant differences were obtained during reassessment of her speech aerodynamic characteristics. Videostroboscopy illustrated mild improvements of the true vocal fold tremors and clonic contractions, both at rest and during phonation efforts. Although the vibratory patterns remained moderately impaired, they were more fluid, symmetrical, and complete at the midline than had been originally observed.

The patient was immediately enrolled in voice therapy for five 50-minute sessions. Upon discharge she had not made any additional gains.

## DISCUSSION

Essential tremor is a slowly progressive, nonfatal, neurologic disease of unknown origin. The dentato-rubro-olivary tract of the extrapyramidal system has been implicated as the primary lesion site. There is a hereditary predisposition for contraction of this disease; hence, the diagnostic term "heredofamilial" tremor. Although some patients experience simultaneous tremors of the limbs, head, and larynx, others may suffer from isolated involvement of one of these bodily regions. This is especially true in the early stages of the disease. In moderate to severe forms of essential voice tremor, adductor spasms of the vocal folds may co-occur. This pathophysiologic overlay gives the voice a choking, strained-strangled quality that exacerbates the effects of the underlying tremor disorder. The current patient exhibited this dysphonic combination with perceptually predominant tremor features. However, the voice laboratory measurements helped to quantify both components of this disorder. Beta-blocking pharmacologic agents such as propranolol (Inderal) or ethanol have been used with some success to relieve limb tremors. The phonation subsystem is considerably less responsive to such treatment.

The spastic dysphonia of essential voice tremor can be treated with periodic intramuscular botulinum toxin (Botox) injections to lessen the severity of the phonatory arrests during running speech. Although this treatment technique generally does not impact the underlying voice tremor, reducing the spasmodic overlay often improves speech fluency and facilitiates overall communication effectiveness.

This treatment method was employed for the current patient. Botox injections were administered using a transthyroid cartilage approach, in which the hypodermic needle pierces the thyroid cartilage at the level of the vocal fold for drug delivery. The entire procedure takes less than 10 minutes, including time spent outlining the injection locations on each side of the larynx. Whereas in the past electromyographic feedback was used to guide needle placement, we agree with other clinicians that this ancillary technique is unneccesary. The patient responded as anticipated. Because the spasmodic characteristics of her voice were largely suppressed, the fluidity of running speech was considerably improved. Adjuvant voice therapy did not augment the Botox effects. Although she continued to struggle with a pronounced degree of voice tremor, she was very pleased with the overall treatment outcome.

# CASE 17
## *Bilateral Hemorrhagic Vocal Fold Polyps*

### HISTORY

The patient is a 46-year-old female who presented with a 1-year history of episodic shortness of breath and persistent hoarseness, which had progressively worsened during the prior 6 months. She had smoked a pack of cigarettes per day for 30 years, and she admitted to chronic voice abuse in the home environment. She was a single parent, rearing 10-year-old twin boys. There were no apparent hearing or speech-language difficulties. Her internist had requested a comprehensive voce evaluation and recommendations for treatment.

### EXAMINATION FINDINGS

Results of the head and neck physical examination were unremarkable. Perceptually, the patient's voice was moderately to severely hoarse in quality, with significantly lower than normal pitch and reduced loudness dimensions. Maximum phonation time was 15 seconds.

**CD1**
**Track 17**

The next **voice sample** illustrates these dysphonic features.

Acoustic analysis revealed the following: (1) fundamental frequency @ 136 Hz, (2) jitter @ 2.95%, (3) shimmer @ 0.68 dB, and (4) harmonic/noise ratio @ 1.8 dB. These data are markedly abnormal. The Fo finding correlates highly with the perceptual impression of a low pitched voice. The jitter and shimmer results point to a profound degree of cycle-to-cycle vocal fold vibratory instability and variability. The H/N ratio substantiates the perception of excess noise in the voice signal, as evidenced by the level of hoarse vocal quality exhibited by the patient.

Speech aerodynamic testing yielded the following: (1) Mean airflow rate @ 1,085 cc/sec, (2) subglottal pressure @ 11 cm $H_2O$, and (3) glottal resistance @ 48 cm $H_2O$/lps. Although the latter two measures fell within normal limits, transglottal airflow was roughly nine times the normal amount, suggestive of substantial glottal leakage during phonation.

Videostroboscopy results are illustrated in Figures 6–17A and 6–17B. Note the presence of large hemorrhagic polyps on both vocal folds, more pronounced on the right side. These masses partially obstruct the airway at rest and during deep inhalatory maneuvers, which likely accounts for the aforementioned symptoms of dyspnea. Also observe the diffuse erythema of the vocal folds, most notably in the anterior commissure region, which extends supraglottally onto the ventricular folds. During phonation efforts, there is persistent glottal incompetency across the length of the mechanism. The associated escape of unphonated air through this glottal leak helps explain the hoarse vocal quality and excessive transglottal airflow results. Vocal fold vibrations are limited with respect to phasic symmetry and amplitudes of excursion, which underscores the patient's difficulty with loudness control. Mucosal waves are virtually absent bilaterally due to the load effects of these growths.

The diagnosis: bilateral vocal fold polyps, probably due to chronic abuse and misuse of the vocal folds.

Recommendation: surgical removal of the growths, followed by voice therapy.

### TREATMENT RESULTS

The patient underwent a bilateral polypoidectomy procedure, using the minimicroflap phonosurgical technique described in Chapter 4. She was restricted from cigarette

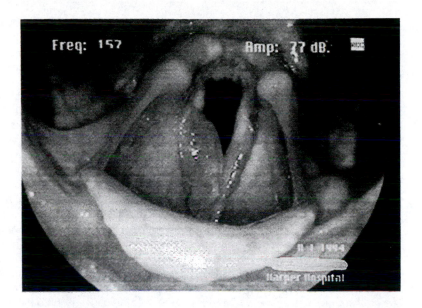

**FIGURE 6–17A.** View of the laryngeal inlet of a 46-year-old female with a history of chronic voice abuse. Note the large hemorrhagic polyp emanating off of the right true vocal fold and ventricle region. Mild polypoid changes are also seen on the left vocal fold.

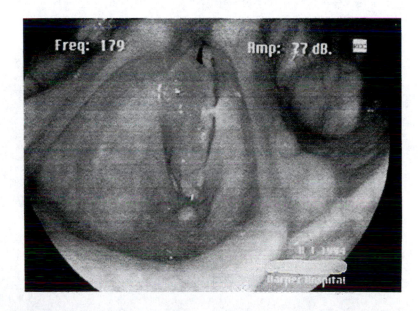

**FIGURE 6–17B.** This photograph illustrates the patient's efforts at phonation. Note how the bulbous polyp obscures views of the underlying true vocal fold.

smoking, placed on a 2-week period of total voice rest and scheduled for voice laboratory reevaluation on the 14th day postoperatively.

On reexamination the patient admitted that she could neither adhere to the total voice rest requirement nor discontinue smoking. She engaged in occasional yelling episodes and experienced frequent coughing and throat clearing spells. Perceptually, her voice was moderately to severely hoarse-harsh in quality, with low pitch features. She complained of inability to generate sufficient loudness control. Maximum phonation time was 14 seconds. These abnormalities were not significantly different from the preoperative voice characteristics. The next **voice sample** highlights the patient's voice 14 days after surgery. Both the acoustic and speech aerodynamic test results were remarkably similar in severity to the levels obtained during the preoperative evaluation. Figure 6–17C illustrates the appearance of the larynx following this surgical procedure. Videostroboscopy revealed marked anatomic irregularity of the marginal free edges of both true vocal folds. Whereas there was no evidence of gross lesions within the laryngeal inlet, mild erythema and edema were observed, especially in the anterior commissure region. The patient no longer struggled with a compromised airway, as removal of the polyps afforded easy air exchange through the patent glottis. During the closed phases of vibration associated with voice, there was a persistent chink along the entire length of the glottis. At no time during this examination was full and complete glottal competency evident. Vibrations of the vocal folds were stiff, relative to mucosal wave dynamics, and the amplitudes of excursion and phase symmetry were moderately abnormal. These disturbances were judged to be sequelae to vocal fold edema, caused by the surgery as well as unrelenting voice abuse and misuse behaviors.

The patient was enrolled in a once per week voice therapy program, which focused on eliminating these behaviors and specific vocal exercises. We targeted a higher habitual pitch of 175 Hz, and easy onset voice activities were incorporated to reduce strained-harsh phonatory features. Although the patient's gains in therapy were in-

**CD1
Track 17**

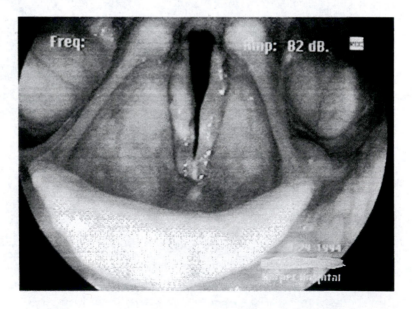

**FIGURE 6–17C.** This view of the larynx was obtained postsurgically. Note that the free edges of the cords are mildly irregular, but that the massive polyp abnormalities have largely improved.

significant, as she continued to exhibit moderate dysphonia after five treatment sessions, the anatomical status of her larynx did improve. Figure 6–17D was obtained at this point in time. Note that the free edges and covers of the cords are much less irregular in appearance than was observed in the previous evaluation. When the patient generated higher pitched voice, glottal competency was consistently complete; lower pitched habitual speech patterns induced variable glottal incompetency. Because the patient was unable to master additional gains with therapy, she was discharged. At that time, she continued to abuse her voice regularly, and she refused to quit smoking.

## DISCUSSION

This patient was a chronic voice abuser. Additionally, she had smoked for more than 30 years, and she struggled with habitual coughing and throat clearing difficulties. It is likely that the roots of her dysphonia dated back more than 1 year, although she did not agree with this hypothesis. The size of her hemorrhagic polyps would support a lengthy period of chronic voice abuse and dysphonia. She neglected the symptoms of dysphonia for quite some time prior to our initial evaluation. Had it not been for the co-occurring dyspnea, which was caused by the airway-obstructing effects of these growths, the patient might have adapted to her hoarse vocal quality without concern.

Hemorrhagic vocal fold polyps usually occur as a result of a violent vocal incident or they form and enlarge in response to aggressive and persistent voice abuse. When these types of lesions involve both vocal folds, they may cause significant stridor and dyspnea. The purplish appearance highlights the extreme level of submucosal vascularity. When patients present with advanced stages of this condition, as in the current case, surgical intervention is almost always required followed by therapy. A microflap or mini-microflap surgical approach is indicated to limit the degree of vocal fold inva-

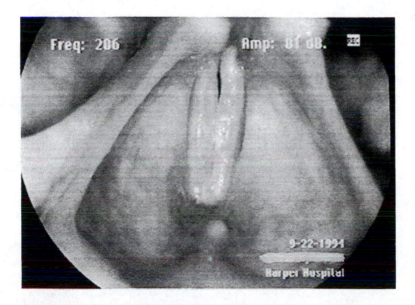

**FIGURE 6–17D.** In this illustration the patient is phonating. Note that she achieves nearly complete glottal competency across the length of this mechanism. There is still a mild degree of swelling of both true vocal folds.

sion and secondary scarring. This method was employed for our patient. Some laryngologists would not have operated on both vocal folds at the same time, for fear of anterior commissure web formation. Because of this patient's level of anxiety, and her personal lifestyle, she would not have submitted to a staged surgical approach. In the final analysis, she did not develop a web, and she realized an improved airway. Her vocal folds healed reasonably well over the course of 2 months postoperatively, but she continued to struggle with moderate to severe dysphonia.

This is a classic example of the extent to which habitually abusive vocal fold behaviors may threaten the prognosis for voice improvement, regardless of the technical success of phonosurgery. For patients like this one, both voice therapy and psychological counseling may be necessary to maximize the effects of surgery. Unfortunately, our patient rejected the latter treatment suggestion.

Patients who present with large vocal fold lesions may never develop normal voice production, even if they learn to abandon all abusive speaking habits. Surgery rarely results in a perfectly normal vocal fold mechanism. Postoperative scarring and surgically induced tissue asymmetry are potential side effects, which may linger forever, disrupt vibratory dynamics, and cause persistent dysphonia. Adjuvant voice therapy is designed to reduce these residual difficulties. Patients who are compliant often make further improvements. Those who are not generally end up with disappointing surgical and therapeutic results.

# CASE 18
## *Abductor Spasmodic Dysphonia*

## HISTORY

The patient is a 45-year-old female who presented with a 1-year history of progressively worsening voice difficulties. She complained that, without forewarning, her voice would become breathy in the middle of words and sentences. During the prior 3 months this problem had become noticeable to her professional associates, which prompted questions about her health status. She reported that ordinarily she was required to communicate verbally with many different individuals in her daily work. She was unable to carry out these responsibilities for fear that her voice would fade during these conversations. Her past medical history was relatively unremarkable, though she admitted to occasional migraine headaches, difficulty with vocal fatigue, and shortness of breath. Over the prior 6 months she had been under a considerable amount of emotional stress related to a recent divorce. She had been consulting with a psychiatrist for the past 12 months. This medical practitioner referred the patient to neurology and our service for a comprehensive evaluation. Results of the clinical neurologic examination were within normal limits.

## EXAMINATION FINDINGS

Results of the physical examination of the head and neck region were unremarkable. Perceptually, the patient exhibited intermittent but moderately to severely breathy-hoarse dysphonia. There were periods of normal phonation embedded within this overall abnormal voice profile. Maximum phonation time was 5 seconds. However, the patient was able to prolong nonvocalized exhalation for 13 seconds, which is within normal limits. This performance suggests that the substantially low maximum phonation time is probably attributable to disturbances at the level of the glottis, and not the respiratory subsystem.

The next **voice sample** highlights this unusual voice pattern.

Acoustic analysis revealed the following: (1) fundamental frequency @ 186 Hz, (2) jitter @ 4.9%, (3) shimmer @ 1.3 dB, and (4) harmonic to noise ratio @ 1.8 dB. The jitter and shimmer results are severely abnormal. They suggest the presence of significant instability and abnormal degrees of variability in the cycle-to-cycle vibratory characteristics of the vocal folds. The harmonics data point to a profound amount of noise in the voice signal, in concert with the aforementioned perceptual characteristic of extreme breathiness.

**CD1**
**Track 18**

Speech aerodynamic testing yielded the following: (1) mean airflow rate @ 145 cc/sec, (2) subglotal pressure @ 8 cm $H_2O$, and (3) glottal resistance @ 24 cm $H_2O$/lps. Transglottal flow was mildly high, and laryngeal resistance was mildly reduced, suggestive of a weak and incompetent glottal valve.

Figure 6–18 illustrates the relatively normal anatomical appearance of the laryngeal inlet, obtained during videostroboscopy. During connected discourse episodic abductor spasms of the true vocal folds were evident, which resulted in abnormal breathy voice interludes.

The diagnosis: Abductor spasmodic dysphonia. Botox injections into the posterior cricoarytenoid and cricothyroid muscles were recommended, followed by a stint of voice therapy.

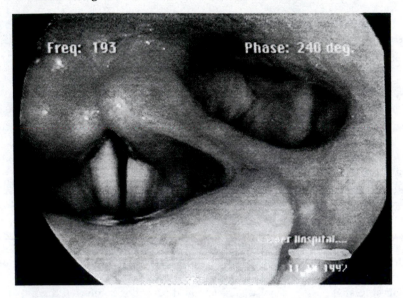

**FIGURE 6–18.** This photograph was obtained from a 45-year-old female with the diagnosis of abductor spasmodic dysphonia. Note that there are no gross lesions involving the laryngeal inlet or the vocal folds themselves. The patient does exhibit intermittent spasmodic action of the abductory musculature, which causes momentary chinks in the glottis during phonation. This causes the breathy interludes in voice quality.

## TREATMENT RESULTS

The patient submitted to this treatment paradigm. However, she did not experience any clinically significant improvements in voice. Therapy was discontinued after five 1-hour sessions.

## DISCUSSION

Abductor spasmodic dysphonia is characterized by intermittent breathiness and arrests of phonation. The breathy interludes usually occur more frequently on words produced in succession, and voiceless consonants are most susceptible to these abnormal events. Recent research has shown that patients with abductor spasmodic dysphonia also exhibit increased sentence articulation and prolonged voice onset times. These hyperkinetic phonatory breakdowns are considered the result of episodic spasms of the posterior cricoarytenoid musculature, which normally regulates abduction of the vocal folds. Clinical researchers presently view this condition as a neurologic disorder; a sequela of focal laryngeal dystonia or essential tremor. Psychogenic or idiopathic factors have also been implicated as possible causes.

Botulinum toxin (Botox) injections are currently the standard treatment for spasmodic dysphonia secondary to laryngeal dystonia. This drug inhibits release of acetylcholine at the level of the neuromuscular junction, causing weakness and paresis of the recipient musculature. However, within approximately 3 months nerve sprouting occurs, which reinnervates the muscle. At that point, Botox reinjection is usually indicated to combat recurring muscle spasms. Generally, patients with abductor spasmodic dysphonia are more resistant to such treatment than their counterparts with the adductor form of this disorder. Explanations for this discrepancy in treatment efficacy and outcomes are unclear.

The current patient did not respond to the Botox injections. We used EMG biofeedback to ensure needle positioning within the target muscles, and to counter potential arguments that the drug was not delivered effectively. Voice therapy served only to educate the patient about this complex disorder, which was an important objective of the program. However, no discernible improvements in voice were obtained.

# CASE 19
## *Systematic Lupus Erythematosus*

### HISTORY

The patient is a 24-year-old female who presented with complaints of pharyngitis, laryngitis, odynophagia (painful swallows), morning stiffness, and intermittent arthralgias of the hands, feet, and large joints. These symptoms had persisted for approximately 6 weeks. She revealed a recent history of cutaneous vasculitis of the chest and malar regions and bouts of intraoral ulcers.

Rheumatology service rendered an empiric diagnosis of systemic lupus erythematosus (SLE). Salient examination findings included the following: (1) restricted range of movement of both shoulders, knees, and left elbow; (2) pain, warmth, and swelling of virtually all extremity joints; (3) papular rashes on the forehead and malar areas; and (4) erythema multiforme of the right breast. The patient was started on Prednisone drug therapy @ 40 mg qd, nabumetone 1 g b.i.d., and hydroxychloroquine 200 mg b.i.d. Insulin was prescribed 5 weeks later because of steroid-induced diabetes mellitus. The daily prednisone dosage was gradually decreased to 25 mg qd and supplemented with titrated doses of Immuran (50–150 mg qd) over the course of 3 months. Because of persistent hoarse-breathy dysphonia, episodic aspiration of all food types, nonproductive coughing spells, and wheezing on deep inhalation, the patient was referred to otolaryngology service for comprehensive examination and treatment recommendations.

### EXAMINATION FINDINGS

The head and neck physical examination revealed localized, nontender cervical adenopathy along the upper and middle jugular nodal chains.

Perceptually, the patient's voice was profoundly breathy-aphonic, with intermittent shrill-like vocal outbursts. Maximum phonation time was 3 seconds, which was markedly reduced.

The next **voice sample** highlights these abnormal features.

**CD1**
**Track 19**

Most acoustic and speech aerodynamic testing could not be performed with confidence because of the profoundly aperiodic voice signal. However, mean airflow rate was assessed @ 2,138 cc/sec, roughly 20 times normal. This finding is compatible with a hypothesis of glottal incompetency, and it is consistent with the breathy voice quality exhibited by the patient.

Figure 6–19A illustrates the results of videostroboscopy. Note the severe irregularity in the surface and free margin appearances of the true vocal folds. Submucosal nodules appear evident in the middle third region of both vocal folds. Observe the hemorrhagic, inflammatory, and ulcerative changes in the area of the anterior commissure. Also note the dense vascularity of the ventricles. During phonatory efforts severe incompetency was consistent along the entire length of the glottis, as vocal fold vibrations were hampered by inelastic, stiff, and slow movement variations. The mucosal wave feature was absent bilaterally.

The diagnosis: SLE with phonation subsystem disturbances.

Voice therapy was initiated on a twice per week basis for 1 month. Direct vocal exercises were employed, utilizing biofeedback of voice signals on the Visi-Pitch to stimulate voice improvements. Various pushing, pulling, and laryngeal compression techniques to increase glottal valving efficiency were unsuccessful. The next **voice sample** highlights the patient's persistent dysphonia at the completion of eight therapy sessions.

**CD1**
**Track 19**

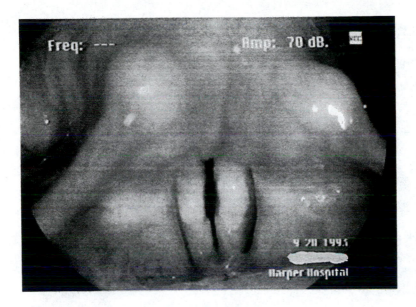

**FIGURE 6–19A.** This is a view of the larynx obtained from a 24-year-old female with the diagnosis of systemic lupus erythematosus with widespread bilateral vocal fold abnormality. Of greatest significance are the submucosal nodules on the covers of both cords as well as the free edge irregularities. Note the substantial chink in the glottis during phonation effort.

Recommendations: Phonosurgical management: An Isshiki type I thyroplasty on the right side of the larynx.

## TREATMENT RESULTS

Figure 6–19B illustrates the anatomical results, obtained during videostroboscopy on the 38th postoperative day. When compared to the preoperative figure, note the following beneficial surgical effects: (1) the submucosal nodules have markedly diminished, (2) the free margins and covers appear more symmetrical and smooth, and (3) the vasculitic changes in the ventricles and anterior commissure regions have significantly resolved. However, phonatory efforts continued to be plagued by residual glottal incompetency, although to a lesser degree. There was a persistent glottal chink and only a hint of mucosal wave activity. Vibrations of the vocal folds were seemingly stiff with limited amplitudes of excursion. Perceptually, the patient continued to exhibit breathy-hoarse dysphonia, but the severity level had improved from profound to moderate. She struggled with intermittent pitch breaks and reduced volume control. Maximum phonation time was 10 seconds, which represented a threefold increase over the preoperative level.

Mean airflow rate reassessment yielded 676 cc/sec during vowel prolongation. This compared to the 2,138 cc/sec result obtained prior to surgery. Whereas this most recent finding represented a significant improvement, transglottal flow was still moderately excessive. The previously mentioned voice therapy program was reinitiated for 10 sessions to increase glottal valving efficiency and improve voice quality and control.

Results of therapy were impressive. Figure 6–19C illustrates the progressive improvement in the appearance and functional status of the vocal folds, obtained with

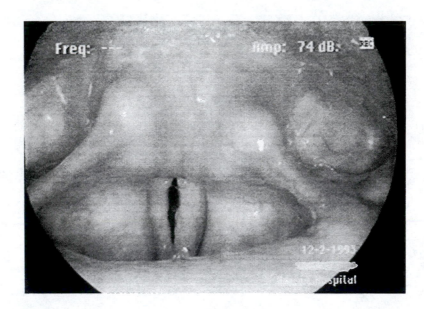

**FIGURE 6–19B.** This photograph was obtained following the Isshiki medialization thyroplasty on the right side. Note the mild improvement in the appearance of the vocal cords as well as the glottal chink.

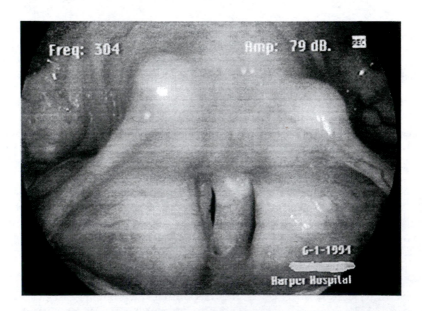

**FIGURE 6–19C.** This illustration was obtained following voice therapy after the aforementioned thyroplasty. Note the substantial improvement in the appearance of the vocal folds. The submucosal nodules have significantly resolved and glottal competency has improved.

stroboscopy at the completion of this second round of voice therapy. Note that only a narrow chink in the midline of the glottis occurs during the closed phases of vibration. Bilateral mucosal waves were evident and phase symmetry was near normal. Perceptually, the patient exhibited mild dysphonia, characterized mostly by hoarse-breathy vocal quality. The next **voice sample** highlights these gains.

Acoustic analysis revealed the following: (1) fundamental frequency @ 240 Hz, (2) jitter @ 2.0%, (3) shimmer @ 0.33 dB, and (4) harmonic to noise ratio @ 12 dB. Maximum phonation time was 15 seconds. With the exception of the jitter data, which reflect a moderate degree of instability in the cycle-to-cycle vibratory activities of the vocal folds, these findings were within normal limits. Speech aerodynamic measures yielded the following: (1) mean airflow rate @ 375 cc/sec, (2) subglottal pressure @ 9.8 cm $H_2O$, and (3) glottal resistance @ 20 cm $H_2O$/lps. The transglottal airflow result reveals moderate improvement over the prevoice therapy level, indicative of less waste of air through the glottis during phonation. Laryngeal resistance was roughly one-half the normal amount, also suggestive of mildly persistent glottal incompetency. The tracheal pressure result was near normal. Upon discharge the patient had made substantial gains.

**CD1
Track 19**

## DISCUSSION

In some ways the laryngeal abnormalities exhibited by this patient resemble those detected in Case 14. Both of these individuals suffered from SLE. Patients with dysphonia secondary to this autoimmune condition usually improve when corticosteroid medications are administered. However, the present patient did not benefit from this standard treatment approach. In fact, her voice deteriorated despite use of these drugs. Voice therapy as a first-line defense strategy was ineffective. The literature on SLE provided no alternative voice rehabilitation suggestions. Phonosurgical options were considered, and the medialization thyroplasty technique was judged to be potentially advantageous in view of the patient's profound glottal incompetency. This approach had in its favor reversibility if poor or counterproductive results were obtained. Precedence had already been established in the laryngology literature for use of this procedure with nonparalyzed, incompetent vocal folds. For example, many patients with pronounced degrees of bowing secondary to presbylaryngis benefit from the Isshiki type I thyroplasty.

The current patient initially presented with complex collagenous abnormalities in the deep layers of both vocal folds. Significant improvements in laryngeal tissue appearance and functioning occurred following phonosurgery and adjunctive voice therapy. This treatment combination positively influenced the vibratory efficiency, compliance, phasic symmetry, and glottal competency of the vocal folds. Not only did the patient demonstrate dramatically improved phonation skills, she suggested that it was much easier to vocalize. She no longer suffered from extraordinary laryngeal muscle tension and respiratory fatigue during conversational speech.

It is reasonable to speculate that the anatomical and physiological gains experienced by the patient were directly attributable to the treatments rendered. Once the midline compression forces were improved through phonosurgery, the intrinsic mucosal, elastic, collagenous, and muscle fibers, which run parallel to the edges of the vocal folds, were stimulated to facilitate vibratory movements. Blood vessels that lace through the mucosa of the free margins and covers of the vocal folds also received compression stimulation, which in turn may have contributed to the improved vibration patterns, voice output, and overall healing process observed. At the time of this report, approximately 2 years following surgery, the patient continued to struggle with mild dysphonia. Although additional phonatory gains are not likely, she was very pleased with her "functionally useful" voice.

# CASE 20
## *Bilateral Abductor Vocal Fold Paralysis*

## HISTORY

The patient is a 22-year-old male. Twelve months ago he was involved in an automobile accident that resulted in a closed head injury. At the scene of the accident he was in a comatose state, vital signs were moderately depressed, but stable, and no penetrating wounds or broken bones were detected by the paramedics. After arriving at the ER he remained comatose and nonresponsive. He exhibited conjugate, random eye movements without signs of papilledema. All superficial facial wounds were cleaned and full scale neurologic testing was ordered. The patient was admitted to the hospital.

Computerized tomography revealed moderate-to-severe right intracerebral frontal and parietal lobe edema, without signs of hemorrhaging. The patient was placed on a ventilator, and transferred to the head trauma unit. He remained comatose for 7 days, and gradually became arousable shortly thereafter. EEG analysis illustrated right frontal and parietal lobe dysrhythmia grade II. Repeat CT studies showed a decreased degree of cerebral edema. Low grade pneumonia developed ith spiking fevers. Ten days later he was taken off of the respirator, and he was decannulated. With the exception of mild language confusion, short-term memory disturbances, and articulatory imprecision, the patient exhibited no other discernable neurologic deficits. He was discharged from the hospital and scheduled for outpatient speech and language therapy. He attended eight sessions and was discharged with no residual communication difficulties.

Six months ago he developed an upper respiratory infection, which caused severe dyspnea and stridor. He was treated with antibiotics and cough suppressant medication. Two days later, he was rushed to the ER because he was struggling for breath. Bilateral abductor vocal fold paralysis and edema were identified. An emergency tracheotomy was performed, and a #6 cuffless Shiley tracheotomy tube was placed. The patient was admitted to the hospital for observation and otolaryngology consultation.

## EXAMINATION FINDINGS

Results of the physical examination of the head and neck were unremarkable, except that a mild degree of rhinorrhea was observed. To speak, the patient used his finger to occlude the tracheotomy tube opening. Placing a cap on the tube caused significant respiratory distress and stridor, especially during deep-breathing tasks.

Perceptually, the patient's voice and speech proficiency were within normal limits. Maximum phonation time was also unimpaired.

**CD I**
**Track 20**

The next **voice sample** highlights these normal features.

Acoustic analysis revealed the following: (1) fundamental frequency @ 100 Hz, (2) jitter @ 0.40%, (3) shimmer @ 0.20 dB, and (4) harmonic to noise ratio @ 13.6 dB. These data are all within normal limits.

Speech aerodynamic testing yielded the following: (1) mean airflow rate @ 274 cc/sec, (2) subglottal pressure @ 9 cm $H_2O$, and (3) glottal resistance @ 47 cm $H_2O$/lps. The transglottal airflow result was mildly higher than normal, suggestive of underlying glottal incompetency. The remaining data were within normal imits.

Figure 6–20 illustrates the status of the laryngeal inlet, as observed during videostroboscopy. Note the mild irregularity in the anatomy of the free margins of the vocal folds. There is suggestion of a small nodule on the anterior third of the left fold. Of greatest significance were the characteristics of bilateral abductor vocal fold paralysis. At no time during the examination were the folds seen to abduct. The laryngeal

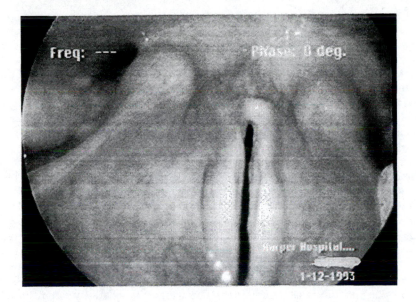

**FIGURE 6–20.** This laryngeal photograph was obtained from a 22-year-old male diagnosed with bilateral vocal fold paralysis. In this view the patient is attempting deep inhalation. Note the severely restricted airway. Also note the mild erythema of the true vocal fold free edges.

photograph represents the full extent of glottal opening as the patient attempts deep inhalation with the tracheotomy tube plugged. The airway is severely compromised. During phonation, complete adduction at the midline of the glottis is evident.

The diagnosis: bilateral abductor vocal fold paralysis.

Treatment recommendation: laser cordotomy to increase the glottal opening and enable decannulation. The patient did not agree to this treatment, due to his fear of the possible adverse effects on swallowing and voice functioning.

## DISCUSSION

The patient with bilateral abductor vocal fold paralysis usually presents with near normal phonation and uncompromised swallowing skills because the folds typically rest very close to the midline of the glottis. However, this abnormally constricted airway often causes dyspnea and stridor, the extent of which varies from patient to patient. In patients whose symptoms are mild, medical help may not be sought and the condition may go undetected because the voice is virtually normal and breathing is only minimally impaired. Those whose dyspnea and stridor symptoms are moderately disabling may be erroneously treated by their family physicians for asthma, bronchitis, or a common cold. We occasionally see patients who have been struggling on antibiotic, antihistamine, and inhalant medications for months without relief as a consequence of such misdiagnoses. Sometimes it is not until the patient actually experiences an upper respiratory infection that differential diagnosis of bilateral abductor vocal fold paralysis is reached As associated coughing and vocal fold edema cause a narrowing of the compromised airway, the patient suffers from progressively worsening respiratory distress. The current patient was rushed to the ER for this reason, and an emergency tracheotomy was necessary.

When patients present with dyspnea and stridor, routine placement of a stethoscope on the larynx is a simple but valuable examination technique. The results obtained may provide important information relative to the potential source of these signs and symptoms. Pulmonary auscultation results generally are within normal limits, and laryngoscopy substantiates the diagnosis. Bilateral abductor vocal fold paralysis is most often caused by either damage to the recurrent laryngeal nerves or profound trauma of the vocal folds. In the latter case, the disturbance is often temporary (neurapraxia). Less common etiologies include severe cricoarytenoid jointitis, mechanical fixation of the vocal folds secondary to an interarytenoid scar band, and invasive (T3) glottic carcinoma.

In the current patient, vocal fold paralysis was probably induced when the first tracheotomy was performed and a ventilator was placed immediately following his car accident. The diagnosis was not reached until several months later, for the previously mentioned reason. Until that time, he thought that his (mild) breathing difficulty was due to the closed head injury and its adverse effects on his overall energy level. Every year in the United States, more than 7 million individuals sustain head injuries. Of these, approximately two thirds are admitted to the hospital for treatment. Most of these injuries are mild to moderate in degree, necessitating brief hospitalizations. The remainder, however, are severe, with potentially long-lasting mental, physical, emotional, social, and financial complications. Our patient was relatively fortunate, in that he did not experience severe brain damage despite having lapsed into a coma for more than a week following his head injury.

Treatment for bilateral abductor vocal fold paralysis is not straightforward. Surgical intervention, to create a wider glottal aperture for more comfortable respiratory exchange, may induce counterproductive swallowing and voice abnormalities.

# CASE 21
## *Apraxia of Phonation*

## HISTORY

The patient is a 66-year-old female who presented with a long standing history of dysphonia. She reported that 27 years ago she experienced a left CVA with resulting right hemiplegia, and recurrent seizures to date. Since the stroke she had struggled with mild aphasia, apraxia of speech, agraphia, and dyslexia. Of greatest concern to the patient was her predominant voice difficulty, which had become progressively more disabling over the previous 12 months. She was referred by her neurologist for laryngeal examination and treatment recommendations. The patient was otherwise in very good health.

## EXAMINATION FINDINGS

The head and neck physical exam was within normal limits, except that the patient was edentulous.

Perceptually, running speech was characterized by mild articulatory groping and sound transposition errors, especially on multisyllable words. The patient was alert and oriented to the conversation, and she used appropriate language in response to the interview questions and examination tasks. Phonation was moderately to severely abnormal. Throughout testing she exhibited frequent pitch and loudness breaks, with tendencies toward squeal-like outbursts. Pitch fluctuated from high to low levels throughout contextual speech efforts. The patient was able to phonate a prolonged vowel without significant difficulty. Strings of contiguous vowels and conversational voice patterns, however, were plagued by these abnormal phonation phenomena. There was a mild to moderate hoarse vocal quality overlay. She denied voice abuse or misuse, gastric reflux disturbances, or use of tobacco or alcohol products.

The next **voice sample** highlights tshe patient's significant voice motor control disorder.

**CD1**
**Track 21**

We confined the remainder of our initial examination to videostroboscopy of the larynx. Figure 6–21 illustrates the appearance of the laryngeal inlet, which was within normal limits. Simple vowel prolongation was unremarkable relative to vibratory activity of the vocal folds. Running speech induced groping actions of the vocal folds, which resulted in intermittent glottal incompetency, abnormally prolonged closed and open phases of vibration, and numerous voiced/voiceless production errors.

The diagnosis: the patient exhibited fluctuating voice and speech articulation abnormalities, which were characteristic of apraxia of speech and phonation. The phonatory difficulties were most pronounced, as they were judged to interfere with speech intelligibility and overall communication effectiveness more than the coexisting articulatory error patterns. These disturbances were likely sequelae to the aforementioned left CVA, which the patient suffered many years ago.

Treatment recommendations: she was enrolled in a voice therapy program at the outset to improve voice motor control and programming skills.

## TREATMENT RESULTS

The patient attended ten 45-minute therapy sessions over the course of 2 months. Focus was placed on voice motor timing, coordination, and initiation exercises. A metronome was used throughout the program to regulate and pace all voice activities.

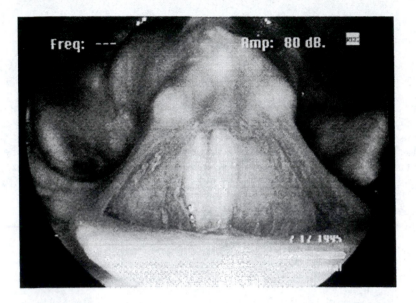

**FIGURE 6–21.** View of the laryngeal inlet of a 66-year-old female with the diagnosis of apraxia of phonation. Note the overall normal appearance of the vocal folds and surrounding soft tissue.

The pendulum was set to swing at 30 beats per minute at the outset, and it was progressively increased to 60, 90, and 120 beats per minute as the patient demonstrated improved performances at the slower speeds. Exercises began with isolated vowels, and became more complex as the patient showed the ability to generate normal voice characteristics (100% correct) or near normal voice output (acceptable production on 90% or more of the trial utterances) at the fastest speed (120 bpm) on the simpler stimuli. Additional practice material included: (1) 2, 3, and 4 vowel combinations; (2) monosyllable, bisyllable, trisyllable, and multisyllable words; (3) brief phrases; and (4) contextual speech. All of these were practiced sequentially to the target beats of the metronome.

By the fourth treatment session, the patient had progressed beyond the vowel stimuli. By the conclusion of the sixth session, she had mastered productions of the individual word hierarchy. The tenth session marked the conclusion of the program, as the patient demonstrated appropriate voice motor control behaviors in virtually all speaking situations. She continued, however, to exhibit mild articulatory errors, most predominantly on individual words with complex sound combinations, such as "catastrophe." Error patterns were not symptomatic of faulty control of the phonation subsystem. Rather, they were characteristic of disturbed articulator posturing and sequential movement control. The next **voice sample** highlights the gains made by the patient following the therapy program.

**CD1**
**Track 21**

## DISCUSSION

Apraxia of speech is caused by damage to Broca's area in the left frontal lobe of the brain. This motor speech disorder is observed in many patients who have had a stroke, and it often coexists with other sequelae such as aphasia and hemiplegia. Apraxia is characterized largely by disturbances of articulation and prosody, which result from faulty programming of speech musculature positioning and sequential movement patterns. Perhaps the most commonly occurring apraxic features include the following: (1) slow rate of speech; (2) greater number of phonetic errors as syllable complexity increases; (3) abnormal phoneme prolongations and intersyllabic pausing; (4) groping behaviors to posture speech musculature accurately, which cause false starts, restarts, and part and whole word repetitions; (5) transpositions of sounds within words and words within sentences; and (6) variability of performances with repeated attempts of same stimuli. These error patterns occur without evidence of associated speech musculatre weakness, paresis, or tonal alterations.

Laboratory studies of the acoustic parameters of apraxia have demonstrated significant levels of mis-timing and temporal dyscoordination of the phonation and articulation subsystems. In this vein, many apraxic speakers struggle to initiate and sustain phonation, exhibit more difficulty producing voiced stops and fricatives, use more voiceless than voiced sounds in connected discourse, and experience uncontrollable pitch and loudness outbursts. The current patient certainly suffered from many of these articulatory and phonatory disturbances, and she presented with milder signs of aphasia and right hemiplegia.

Clinical studies have shown that rhythmic stimulation exercises, which impose a form of rate control, may facilitate both articulation and phonation activities in apractic patients. Some clinical researchers have suggested that rhythm is a predominant element in the foundation of all motor behaviors; that the spatiotemporal events underlying motor speech activities may be regulated by central timing mechanisms at several different neurologic levels. It may be that pairing of speech activities with repetitive beats of the metronome therapeutically stimulates this overlying central rhythm generator or oscillatory mechanism. The positive responses of the current patient to this exercise paradigm are supportive of the metronome as a tool in the treatment of voice motor programming difficulties. Additionally, the metronome probably served several other clinical functions: (1) it prompted the patient to attend to, focus, and concentrate on the therapeutic targets; (2) it induced a slow, deliberate speaking rate, which appeared to facilitate control, regulation, timing, and temporal sequencing of volitional voice efforts; and (3) the beating pendulum provided visual and auditory cues that likely helped to "jump-start" voice initiation disturbances.

Our patient achieved significant improvements in voice motor control. She quickly responded to the exercise pogram, and she reported that carryover to her home environment was excellent. No further treatment was administered. On follow-up examination, 6 months after discharge from therapy, the patient demonstrated maintenance of all gains obtained.

# CASE 22
## *Adductor Spasmodic Dysphonia*

## HISTORY

The patient is a 24-year-old female who presented with a 4-month history of dysphonia characterized by complaints of arrests of phonation, vocal tremors, and strained-strangled vocal quality. She suggested that these difficulties had progressively worsened over the previous 2 months. She also complained that when she engaged in conversation she experienced profound headaches and vocal fatigue. She denied experiencing symptoms of blepharoclonus, blepharospasm, oromandibular dystonia, jaw pain, bruxism, tongue biting, or writer's cramp. Further, she did not report a past history of neuroleptic drug exposure, hospitalization, surgery, or chronic medical illness.

Neurologic examination revealed the following: (1) the patient was alert and oriented to person, place, and time, (2) judgment and reasoning skills were within normal limits, (3) there was no evidence of language disturbances, (4) recent and remote memory were intact, (5) all cranial and spinal nerve sensory and motor functions were within normal limits, (6) there was no evidence of pyramidal system or cerebellar impairment, (7) there was an absence of orofacial dystonia, and (8) bodily reflexes were normal.

Magnetic resonance imaging (MRI) of the brain demonstrated no evidence of a space-occupying mass lesion either above or below the tentorium. The gray/white matter differentiation and periventricular white matter were within normal limits. The ventricles were normal in size and in the midline position. Neither the basal cisterns, brainstem, nor corpus callosum were compromised. MRI examination of the Circle of Willis revealed satisfactory patency of all major vessels.

The neurologist concluded that the patient's spasmodic voice difficulty was due to focal laryngeal dystonia.

## VOICE LABORATORY EXAMINATION FINDINGS

Perceptually, the patient's voice was moderately to severely strained-strangled in quality, with intermittent arrests of phonation. There was a subtle tremor quality to the voice as well. Because of the severe aperiodicity of the acoustic signal, neither acoustic nor speech aerodynamic measurements were conducted during the initial evaluation session. Maximum phonation time was 8 seconds, which is moderately reduced.

The next **voice sample** highlights these abnormal voice features.

**CD I**
**Track 22**

Figure 6–22 illustrates the appearance of the laryngeal inlet, obtained during videostroboscopy. Note the normal anatomy of the vocal fold mechanism. No gross lesions were observable, and the tissue coloration and surface textures were within normal limits. During phonation efforts, a small chink in the posterior glottis was evident. Signs of periodic, abnormal prolongations of the closed phases of vibration occurred throughout the examination. Characteristics of intermittent but tight adductory forces of both the true and false vocal folds were observed, especially during running speech production. These abnormal activities correlated significantly with the underlying strained-strangled voice quality. Mild tremors of the soft tissue structures that compose the laryngeal inlet were also appreciable, both at rest and occasionally during phonation. Mucosal waves of both vocal folds were mildly stiff and restricted with respect to the amplitudes of excursion.

**Clinical Diagnosis:** Adductor spasmodic dysphonia, with a mild organic voice tremor overlay.

**Treatment Recommendation:** Because the patient was not interested in Botox injections into the vocal folds, we enrolled her in a voice therapy program.

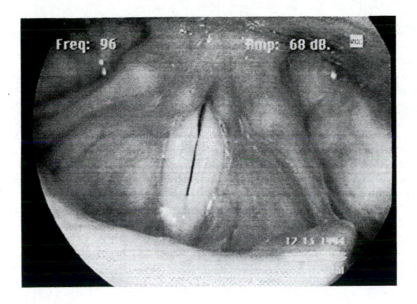

**FIGURE 6–22.** This laryngeal photograph was obtained from a 24-year-old female with the diagnosis of adductor spasmodic dysphonia. Note the overall normal anatomical appearance of the mechanism.

## TREATMENT RESULTS

Therapy focused on raising the patient's fundamental (habitual pitch) level from 170 to 220 Hz. The Visi-Pitch apparatus provided biofeedback of all voice signals relative to pitch, loudness, and inflection patterns. A melodious stimulation paradigm was employed, wherein the patient was required to generate short phrases, sentences, and contextual speech using a sing-song manner of voice production. She was also encouraged to hum familiar tunes, but to remain within the targeted pitch range of 200 to 260 Hz throughout all efforts. After five treatment sessions, each lasting approximately 1 hour, the patient demonstrated notable voice improvement. The next **voice sample** highlights these gains. The patient was discharged from the program two sessions later, and she was lost to follow-up.

**CD1**
**Track 22**

## DISCUSSION

Most clinical researchers, voice scientists, and otolaryngologists consider spasmodic dysphonia to be a manifestation of laryngeal dystonia. Many patients with this disorder exhibit coexisting tremors of the voice, limbs and/or head. Co-occurring oromandibular or generalized dystonias are much less common. From a generic point of view, dystonia is a (slow) hyperkinetic movement disorder. When speech musculature is adversely affected, the resulting articulatory, phonatory, and prosodic disturbances are diagnostically classified as "hyperkinetic" dysarthria. Although dystonias have been associated with lesions of the basal ganglia (extrapyramidal system), there is little quantitative evidence to support this hypothesis. Biochemical studies have suggested that the bizarre features of dystonia may be caused by a dopaminergic-cholinergic imbalance. Focal dystonias, including spasmodic dysphonia, spasmodic torticolis, Meige's syndrome, and writer's cramp, are often construed as early isolated signs of a more widespread movement disorder.

The current patient exhibited focal laryngeal abnormalities. Because of the severity of the condition we recommended Botox injections into both vocal folds as the primary method of treatment. We were convinced from the outset that voice therapy alone would not yield clinically significant results. The patient surprised us with her indisputable voice improvements, which were attributable to the behavioral exercises that we employed. Some clinical researchers have commented that, for those patients who respond to voice therapy in lieu of Botox, there may be a strong psychogenic component to the disorder. The fact that our *young* patient suffered from severe frontal headaches and emotional despair may lend support to this hypothesis. The MRI studies were conducted to rule out specific neurologic abnormalities to which these disabling symptoms may have been attributed.

We have discovered that elevating the patient's pitch and practicing voice and speech with a deliberate melodious, sing-song pattern of production induces fluidity of vocal fold vibration in many patients with adductor spasmodic dysphonia. This result often improves the quality of the voice and reduces the frequency and degree of phonatory arrests. For those patients disinterested in Botox injections, or for patients with very mild symptoms, this treatment approach may be worth considering as a first-line defense against this disorder.

# CASE 23
## *Essential Tremor Syndrome*

## HISTORY

The patient is a 69-year-old male who presented with a 10-year history of progressive difficulty with voice, head, and limb tremors. He also suffered from intermittent choking sensations and aspiration symptoms on various food items. He had recently noticed mild tongue, lip, and jaw muscular incoordination and weakness, which caused occasional articulatory imprecision. For at least 2 years he had been taking, with moderate success, both Inderal and Mysoline to alleviate the tremors. He was referred for voice management suggestions by his neurologist, who diagnosed the condition as heredofamilial-essential tremor syndrome.

## EXAMINATION FINDINGS

Perceptually, the patient's voice quality was moderately to severely tremorous with a pronounced spasmodic overlay. Speech intelligibility was 100%. Maximum phonation time was 12 seconds.

The next **voice sample** highlights the patient's voice profile.

Acoustic analysis revealed the following: (1) fundamental frequency @ 147 Hz, (2) jitter @ 0.50%, (3) shimmer @ 0.29 dB, and (4) harmonic to noise ratio @ 1.7%. Of these data, only the harmonics findings were abnormal, suggestive of a severe amount of noise in the voice signal.

**CD1**
**Track 23**

Speech aerodynamic testing yielded the following: (1) mean airflow rate @ 374 cc/sec, (2) subglottal pressure @ 7.5 cm/$H_2O$, and (3) glottal resistance @ 241 cm $H_2O$/lps. The transglottal flow result was roughly twice the normal degree, indicative of glottal incompetency. Laryngeal resistance was six times normal, which points to excessive adductory forces of the true vocal folds during ongoing phonation. These results are consistent with the perceptual impressions of voice tremor and intermittent adductor spasmodic dysphonia.

Figure 6–23 illustrates the appearance of the laryngeal inlet, as obtained with videostroboscopy. Anatomically, the vocal folds and surrounding structures were within normal limits; no gross abnormalities were detected. At rest, a profound degree of continuous tremors and gross shaking activities of the entire larynx, pharynx, and base of tongue were observed. During voice efforts, similar degrees and types of uncontrollable vocal fold movement abnormalities were evident. Only the anterior two-thirds of the folds were seen to vibrate, whereas the posterior third was held in an adducted position throughout phonation.

**Clinical Diagnosis:** Predominantly an organic voice tremor, with a less severe adductor spasmodic component.

**Treatment Recommendation:** Voice therapy was recommended as the first line of treatment, followed by planned Botox injections, if indicated. Because of the guarded prognosis with either one or both of these treatment options for this type and severity of dysphonia, the patient decided to think about the recommendations. He has since been lost to follow-up.

## DISCUSSION

This patient exhibited the classic voice features of essential tremor syndrome, a hyperkinetic movement disorder. The pronounced tremorous vocal quality is due to involvement of the phonation subsystem. It is not uncommon for patients with this con-

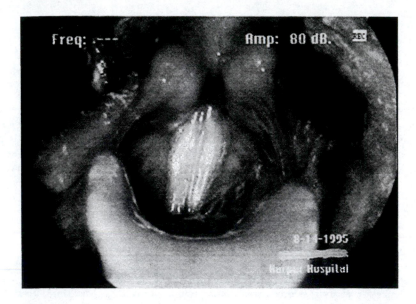

**FIGURE 6–23.** This photograph was obtained from a 69-year-old male with essential tremor syndrome. Note the normal anatomy of the laryngeal inlet.

dition to present with orofacial, head, arm, and hand tremors as well. The motor speech diagnosis is hyperkinetic dysarthria. If lip, tongue, and jaw tremors coexist, articulation and prosodic difficulties may compound the effects of the dysphonia.

Essential tremor syndrome is a neurologic disorder, thought to be due to degenerative changes within the extrapyramidal system. The pathogenesis is variable, and the movement disturbances progressively worsen. There may be a familial predisposition to development of the disease. The dentato-rubro-olivary tract network has been implicated as the possible site of lesion responsible for the signs and symptoms of this condition. On occasion, essential tremor is misdiagnosed as Parkinson's disease or parkinsonism because of associated limb, orofacial, and neck musculature rigidity. Unfortunately, unlike these other disorders, essential tremor does not respond to dopaminergic drug agents such as Sinemet. However, the beta blocker Inderal has been shown to provide some degree of limb and head tremor relief for many patients; no drug has been used with confidence to ameliorate the pronounced voice tremor problem.

As with the current patient, when predominant laryngeal tremors are discovered they average a rate of 4 to 6 Hz. This abnormal voice feature is obvious during running speech, but most evident when the patient is requested to prolong a vowel. The tremors usually occur in synchrony with the disturbed movements of other body parts. These correlated hyperkinetic events are considered pathognomonic of essential voice tremor; they are indispensable differential diagnostic indicators. Voice arrests may or may not co-occur.

Methods of treatment for this voice disorder are not clear-cut. Botox injections may reduce any coexisting spasmodic component, which may in turn amplify the tremor effects. Voice therapy, including laryngeal stabilization techniques and melodic intonation exercises, may be attempted experimentally to determine their potential value. In most cases, the prognosis is very poor for clinically significant voice improvements regardless of the types of medico-surgical and/or behavioral treatments that may be rendered.

# CASE 24
## *Spastic Dysarthria*

## HISTORY

The patient is a 55-year-old female who suffered a cerebral vascular accident (CVA) 18 months prior to this evaluation, which resulted in profound dysarthria without apraxia or aphasia. She did not exhibit sensory or motor disturbances of the limb or trunk musculature. At the time of the stroke, CT scan results revealed two hypodense lesions involving the internal capsule, bilaterally. Three months following the stroke the patient underwent an MRI of the brain. A single punctate area of increased density was discovered in the area of the white matter of the anterior corona radiatum on the right side. This abnormality was consistent with a hemorrhagic infarct. A bilateral duplex cerebrovascular doppler scan was also conducted, which proved to be within normal limits. Metabolic spect technetium-99 ceretec scan studies showed hemispheric defects in the right frontal, right temporal, and right parietal lobe regions. All other laboratory measures, including blood tests, liver and kidney function analyses, and electrocardiography yielded normal findings. The patient was considered neurologically and medically stable, and she was placed on daily vitamin, calcium, hormonal, cholesterol, and analgesic medications: Zestoretic, Calan, Premarin, Mevacor, and Ascriptin. Because of her persistent inability to communicate verbally, she was referred by her neurologist for speech and voice evaluations and treatment recommendations.

## EXAMINATION FINDINGS

The patient was virtually unintelligible. Informal nonverbal measures of language and cognitive functioning demonstrated near-normal abilities; the patient resorted to writing all of her thoughts. Perceptually, all volitional speech efforts were plagued by profound articulatory imprecision, strained-strangled voice quality, hypernasal resonance, and prosodic insufficiency. On numerous occasions, she exhibited uncontrollable and unprovoked emotional outbursts of both laughter and crying. The next **voice sample** highlights this motor speech disorder.

**CD1**
**Track 24**

Clinical examination of the oral mechanism revealed the following: (1) bilateral severe weakness, paresis, and hypertonicity of the lips, tongue, velopharyngeal and jaw musculature, (2) moderately to severely hyperactive gag reflex, and (3) intractable drooling out of both corners of the mouth. The severity of these pathophysiologic and perceptual findings prohibited meaningful acoustic and speech aerodynamic analyses. Figure 6–24 illustrates the appearance of the laryngeal inlet, obtained with videolaryngoscopy. Phonation efforts were characterized by tight, adductory forces of the vocal folds, bilaterally. The patient intermittently recruited the ventricular folds during vocal efforts. Voice output was marred by marked degrees of vocal fold stiffness and limited amplitudes of excursion. Mild erythema was evident on the covers of both vocal fold covers, likely as a consequence of the strained-strangled phonatory activity. Respiratory biomechanics of the vocal folds, however, appeared unimpaired.

**Clinical Diagnosis:** Profound spastic dysarthria, with involvement of all speech subsystems, secondary to CVA.

**Treatment Recommendation:** Intensive speech therapy was prescribed, and consultation with a prosthodontist for fitting of a palatal lift appliance was arranged. The prognosis was very poor.

## TREATMENT RESULTS

The patient was fitted with a palatal lift device prior to the institution of the speech

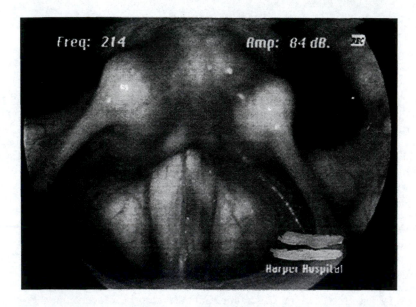

**FIGURE 6–24.** This laryngeal photograph was obtained from a 55-year-old female who was diagnosed with spastic dysarthria following a cerebral vascular accident. Note that there are no gross lesions in the laryngeal inlet or on the vocal cords themselves. There is a mild degree of hyperemia on both covers of the cords. The patient achieves tight adductory forces during the closed phases of vibration associated with voice effort.

therapy program. Several adjustments were made to the lift to establish the best fit possible. Throughout these modifications, the speech pathologist employed a desensitization program to reduced the gag response so that the patient could tolerate wearing the lift appliance. This involved finger pressure and massage stimulation of the soft palate musculature. The patient was given homework assignments for self-stimulation and massage of the palate. Within three treatment sessions the patient was able to insert the palatal lift without interruptive gagging activity. At the completion of the final lift adjustment, roughly 2 weeks after the initial fitting, the patient could wear the appliance throughout the day without discomfort. With the appliance in position, primitive vowel utterances were less hypernasal, and abnormal nasal air emission was less pronounced than without the prosthesis.

Speech therapy began at this point in time, with initial focus on facilitating functioning of the resonation subsystem, followed in order by exercises designed to improve phonation, articulation, and prosody skills. These included: (1) nasal airflow and nasal resonance biofeedback activities using speech and nonspeech stimuli; (2) various phonation and artificial larynx exercises to stimulate verbal speech output; and (3) tongue, lip, and jaw strengthening, tone reduction, and force physiology exercises to improve overall motor control, coordination, and speech production capabilities of these important articulatory structures. Tight evaluation and discontinuation criteria were adopted at the outset of this treatment regimen to avoid prolonging therapy for any subsystem without evidence of treatment efficacy. After 3 months of twice weekly 1-hour therapy sessions, the patient demonstrated no discernable motor speech gains. A hand-held typewriting device was introduced at this point in time to facilitate nonverbal communication. The patient appreciated this tool in place of the pencil and paper technique that she had been using since the stroke, almost 2 years prior. She was discharged from therapy one session later.

## DISCUSSION

The patient exhibited classic signs and symptoms of pseudobulbar palsy and associated severe spastic dysarthria, most likely sequelae to infarcts at the level of the internal capsule. The higher cortical (right hemisphere) lesions, discovered with MRI of the brain, may have exacerbated the motor speech difficulties, but they did not result in clinically significant language, cognitive, perceptual, or appendicular sensorimotor disabilities. Pseudobulbar palsy is a medical diagnostic term used to classify the widespread neuromusclar abnormalities (spastic paresis, weakness, hypertonicity, and hyperreflexia) of the speech mechanism caused by bilateral upper motor neuron (corticobulbar tract) damage. The resultant pathophysiology falsely resembles some of the abnormal signs of bulbar palsy, due to lower motor neuron (cranial and spinal nerves) damage; hence the prefix "pseudo." If parallel corticospinal tracts are unimpaired, the patient will not struggle with co-occurring limb or trunk musculature disturbances. The patient with pseudobulbar palsy usually presents with a complex motor speech disorder, which is generically classified as spastic dysarthria. Although the severity of involvement will vary from patient to patient, most if not all of the following abnormal verbal communication features will likely be detected during the differential diagnosis: (1) hypernasality, (2) strained-strangled phonation, (3) articulatory imprecision, and (4) slow-labored rate of speech. As with the current patient, many others with pseudobulbar palsy are prone to episodes of emotional lability, wherein they may inappropriately laugh or cry. These behaviors are normally governed, inhibited, and modulated by various subcortical and cortical nuclei. Signs of their abnormal release or disinhibition provide additional important diagnostic clues.

Muscles that are profoundly weak, paretic, and hypertonic do not usually respond dramatically to neurorehabilitation exercises. Our patient was virtually anarthric because of widespread speech musculature pathophysiology. Involvement of the resonation subsystem was addressed initially by fitting the patient with a palatal lift prosthesis to reduce hypernasality and excess nasal air emission. Without such improvements, there would be little chance of facilitating speech intelligibility through subsequent phonation, articulation, and prosody exercises. We achieved reasonably good results with this appliance, which justified proceeding with stimulation of these other speech subsystems. In the final analysis, the patient did not make clinically significant gains in verbal speech ability, despite her diligence to succeed. These poor therapeutic results are not uncommon when working with severely disabled spastic dysarthric patients. It continues to be our experience with this population that the phonation subsystem tends to be the most difficult one of all speech mechanism components to rehabilitate.

Recently, we have injected Botox into the vocal folds of other less severely involved spastic dysarthric patients with hopes of reducing glottal resistance and improving supralaryngeal airflow dynamics for speech purposes. In patients with at least fair prospects for obtaining compensatory articulation skills, we have had good success with this phonation subsystem treatment approach.

# CASE 25
## *Hyperkinetic Dysarthria-Huntington's Disease*

### HISTORY

The patient is a 48-year-old male who resided in a local nursing home. He presented with a profound hyperkinetic movement disorder, characterized by quick, jerky, uncontrollable activities of the head, orofacial, trunk, and limb musculature. He used a walker to ambulate. Because of progressively deteriorating speech, voice, language, and swallowing functions, he was referred to us by his attending physician at the nursing home for comprehensive evaluations and treatment recommendations. The medical diagnosis was late stage Huntington's disease. Daily medications included Haldol and Prolixin for palliative relief of the choreiformic movements and signs of dementia.

### EXAMINATION FINDINGS

Perceptually, the patient was moderately to severely unintelligible. Throughout testing he demonstrated pronounced irritability and intermittent periods of noncompliance with certain examination procedures. Connected discourse was characterized by a mixture of the following abnormal speech subsystem features: (1) moderate articulatory imprecision, (2) intermittent hypernasality, (3) moderately harsh-strained vocal quality, and (4) prosodic insufficiency marked by excess and equal stress within and between words. These disturbances were compounded by profound speech breathing difficulties; maximum phonation time was 2 seconds, and the patient was unable to generate more than two syllables per breath during running speech.

Tests of language formulation, vocabulary, syntax, short- and long-term memory, commission and omission, and reading and auditory comprehension revealed severe, generalized deficits. The oral mechanism examination yielded the following results: (1) contortions, tics, and choreiformic movements of the lips, jaw, and tongue musculature, both at rest and during volitional speech and nonspeech activities, and (2) articulator weakness, paresis, and slow-labored diadochokinetic rates.

The next **voice sample** highlights the patient's speech characteristics.

**CD I**
**Track 25**

Acoustic analysis revealed the following: (1) fundamental frequency @ 170 Hz, (2) jitter @ 0.75%, (3) shimmer @ 0.42 dB, and (4) harmonic to noise ratio @ 2.4 dB. The Fo finding is moderately elevated, and there is a profound degree of noise in the voice signal.

Speech aerodynamic testing showed the following: (1) mean airflow rate @ 850 cc/sec, (2) subglottal pressure @ 10 cmH$_2$O, and (3) glottal resistance @ 11 cmH$_2$O/lps. Transglottal flow was roughly eight times normal, suggestive of glottal incompetency. The laryngeal resistance result also suggests a hypofunctional laryngeal valve, with approximately one-third the normal degree of vocal fold compression forces.

The patient was on a pureed food diet because he could not masticate solid foods. He required assistance during feeding as a consequence of poor fine and gross motor control of the upper limbs. Multiple swallows were usually necessary to process each spoonful of food.

Videostroboscopy illustrated bilateral recruitment of the ventricular folds during most phonation efforts, as shown in Figure 6–25. A persistent chink existed throughout the length of the glottis during all voice tasks. The free edge of the left vocal fold was irregularly shaped, contributing to glottal incompetency. Bilateral vocal fold vibratory activity was hampered by intermittently stiff mucosal waves and reduced amplitudes of excursions.

**Clinical diagnosis**: Severe quick hyperkinetic dysarthria, involving all speech subsystems. The etiology: Late stage Huntington's disease.

**Treatment Recommendation:** Cognitive, memory, and language stimulation exercises.

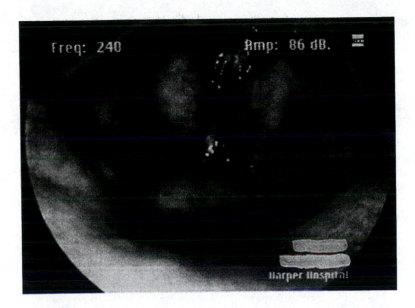

Freq: 240      Amp: 86 dB.

Harper Hospital

**FIGURE 6–25.** This laryngeal photograph was obtained from a 48-year-old male with the diagnosis of Huntington's disease. Note the recruitment of the left false vocal fold during phonation. Also note the irregular anatomical appearance of the free edge of the right true vocal fold. There is a persistent chink in the glottis during phonation.

## DISCUSSION

Huntington's disease is an autosomal dominant progressive neurologic disorder that usually appears in the fourth decade of life. The average course of the illnesss is 15 to 20 years. Early signs of basal ganglia degeneration include choreiform movements, characterized by quick, involuntary, random, and jerky activities of the head, orofacial, limb, and trunk musculature. In the middle to late stage of the disease process, cortical degeneration occurs. This eventually results in psychosis and dementia. At this advanced stage, patients are most often placed in nursing homes or chronic care hospital facilities. They are usually prescribed large doses of neuroleptic drugs to palliate the movement and mental disturbances. Unfortunately, many patients develop tolerances to such medication and need larger doses for symptomatic relief. This treatment approach may result in undesirable extrapyramidal side effects, including an exacerbation of dysphagic and dysarthric symptoms. This may result in the need for gastric feeding tubes and nonverbal, augmentative communication devices. Ultimately, patients are unable to recognize others.

The current patient exhibited the classic mixture of speech abnormalities observed in most individuals with the hyperkinetic dysarthria of Huntington's disease. He also suffered from higher cortical degenerative changes that caused numerous language, cognitive, and perceptual disturbances. This combination of moderate to severe signs and symptoms placed him at the beginning of the final phase of the disease process. We concluded that, at this stage, speech therapy would be most advantageous if focus was placed on facilitating language usage, memory, and cognition, so that he might interact more effectively with family members, friends, and staff. It was felt that in-depth motor speech exercises would prove physiologically taxing and counterproductive, in light of the severity of his movement disorder. No adjustments in the pureed diet were considered necessary at this time. Because the prognosis for clinically significant gains was very poor, the patient chose not to invest the time and energy required to engage in this treatment program.

# CASE 26
## *Bilateral Vocal Fold Nodules*

## HISTORY

The patient is a 45-year-old non-English-speaking female who presented with an 18-month history of persistent dysphonia. One year prior to this evaluation she underwent a vocal fold nodulectomy procedure at a foreign medical facility. She suggested (through an interpreter) that following surgery her voice had improved somewhat, but severe hoarseness recurred within 2 months postoperatively. Unfortunately, she never received voice therapy. She admitted to chronic voice abuse patterns, and she was an avid cigarette smoker for more than 20 years. She struggled daily with bouts of coughing, throat clearing, and gastric reflux symptoms. She was referred by an outside otolaryngolgist for a second opinion relative to the need for surgery and/or voice therapy. There was no other significant past medical history.

## EXAMINATION FINDINGS

The head and neck physical examination was unremarkable. Perceptually, the patient's voice was moderately hoarse-breathy in quality, with low pitch and volume dimensions.

The next **voice sample** highlights the dysphonia.

We confined the remainder of the evaluation to videostroboscopy of the larynx. Figure 6–26A illustrates the existence of a relatively large nodular-like mass lesion on the anterior third of the left true vocal fold. This growth causes deformation of the opposing fold and a substantial chink in the glottis during phonation efforts. The free margin appearance of this cord is irregular, which contributes to the glottal incompetency. Also note the presence of a (reaction) nodule on the anterior third of the right vocal fold free edge. The right ventricular fold compensates partially across the midline to make contact with the opposing (left) true vocal fold during phonation. This activity caused partial obstruction of the underlying right true vocal fold. The mucosal waves and diadochokinetic rates of the vocal folds were respectively stiffened and slow-labored as a consequence of the load effects of the nodules. The amplitudes of vibration, bilaterally, were similarly disturbed. Adequate biomechanical abductory respiratory movements were observed, however.

**CD1**
**Track 26**

**Clinical Diagnosis:** Bilateral vocal fold nodules.

**Treatment Recommendation:** Bilateral excision, using a microflap approach, followed by voice therapy. The severity of the pathology, its adverse effects on vocal fold vibratory activity, and the patient's non-English-speaking background collectively precluded voice therapy as the intial treatment of choice. It was also recommended that the patient undergo dietary lifestyle modification, and that antireflux medication be prescribed to limit the amount of gastro-esophageal reflux.

## TREATMENT RESULTS

The patient elected to have the surgery performed by her referring physician. Bilateral vocal fold strippings, instead of microflap excisions, were conducted without intraoperative complications. The patient was then placed on 10 days of total voice rest. She returned for reevaluation in the voice lab approximately 6 weeks postoperatively, despite a preoperative warning to schedule this exam 2 weeks after surgery. Unfortunately, no antireflux therapy was prescribed.

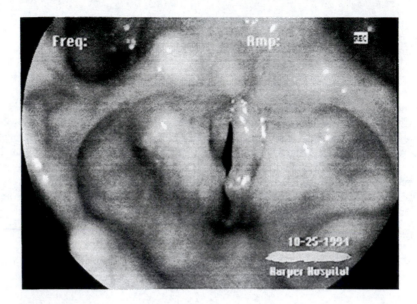

**FIGURE 6–26A.** This laryngeal photograph was obtained from a 45-year-old female with the diagnosis of bilateral vocal fold nodules. Note the hourglass-like chink in the glottis during the closed phases of vibration associated with voice. Note the nodular formation on the anterior one-third of the left true vocal fold. There is a mild reactive nodule on the opposing cord as well.

The patient admitted to complete voice rest for 10 days following surgery. She complained, however, that her coughing, throat clearing, and symptoms of indigestion and heartburn had not abated since surgery. Perceptually, her voice was severely hoarse-breathy in quality, which represented a decline in functioning over the preoperative voice status.

**CD1**
**Track 26**

The next **voice sample** highlights this disappointing surgical outcome. Jitter was 2.6%, shimmer was 0.92 dB, and mean airflow rate was 831 cc/sec. These data revealed severe instability and abnormal variability in the cycle-to-cycle vibratory characteristics of the vocal folds, as well as eight times the normal degree of transglottal egress during phonation. Maximum phonation time was less than 10 seconds. Videostroboscopy results are illustrated in Figures 6–26B and 6–26C. Note the persistence of a prominent chink throughout the length of the glottis during phonation, owing in part to a divot formation in the free margin of the right true vocal fold. Both cords appeared erythematous and edematous. At no time was complete glottal competency demonstrated, which accounts for the hoarse-breathy voice. The mucosal waves and amplitudes of vibration of both vocal folds were severely depressed, with features of profound stiffness. An intensive voice therapy program was prescribed, but the patient failed to follow through with the appointments.

## DISCUSSION

Vocal fold nodules usually result from persistent vocal fold abuse and misuse. If detected early, and the nodules are soft or immature, these benign, callous-like lesions usually respond completely to voice therapy as the primary treatment modality. In most cases, these types of nodules resolve with the adoption of appropriate voice hy-

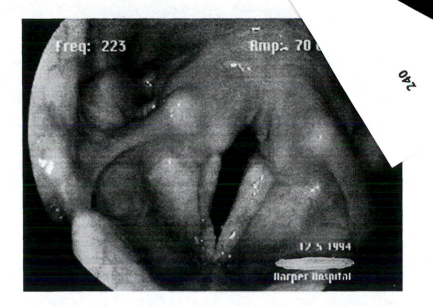

**FIGURE 6–26B.** This is the open phase view of the larynx postoperatively. Note that the nodule on the left has been successfully removed. Unfortunately, there is a divot in the right true vocal fold following the nodulectomy on that side.

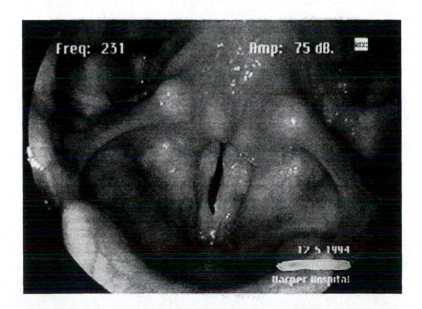

**FIGURE 6–26C.** This laryngeal photograph was also obtained postoperatively and illustrates the closed phases of vibration associated with voice effort. Note the persistent chink in the glottis as a consequence of the irregularity in the free marginal surfaces of the vocal folds. This anatomical disturbance accounts for the persistent voice difficulties exhibited by the patient.

giene and behavioral modification techniques. Cessation of chronic throat clearing activities and voice abuse patterns, coupled with specific vocal exercises, diet adjustments, and possible pharmacologic management of gastric reflux symptoms, are among the common objectives and methods of the nonsurgical treatment program. Fibrotic or hardened growths are usually more mature and resistant to therapy as the initial treatment approach. For these lesions, surgical excision is indicated first, followed by voice therapy.

The current patient suffered from recurring nodules, probably because her chronic voice abuse, throat clearing, coughing, and gastric reflux behaviors were never modified following the first phonosurgery procedure. It is impossible to know whether she actually required surgery as the initial treatment of choice. Certainly, she needed voice therapy after surgery to learn how to protect her larynx from the ill effects of these abuse and misuse factors. She suggested that her surgeon never recommended postoperative therapy. If this is true, it was a major clinical oversight or mistake. When she presented to our service for examination, the bilateral nodules detected were rather mature, and they caused significant vocal fold vibratory stiffness. Her voice was very poor. Therapy alone would not have helped her.

Unfortunately, her laryngologist stripped the vocal folds, notwithstanding our recommendation to use a mucosa sparing approach. The anatomical and physiological results were extremely disappointing. The patient's voice was actually worse following surgery. We cannot attribute this outcome entirely to her persistent voice abuse behaviors. Rather, the negative result was probably due to the type of surgery performed, and it was compounded by the patient's lifestyle, personality, and overall poor vocal hygiene. Today, stripping is considered counterproductive by most surgeons and voice therapists. This is an especially important caveat when operating on vocal folds that have been surgically treated before.

The patient did not keep her postoperative therapy appointments; however, we are not convinced that she would have made significant voice improvements had she been a conscientious patient. Perhaps at best she would have learned to avoid engaging in those vocal behaviors that got her in trouble in the first place and that could exacerbate her existing dysphonia.

# CASE 27
## *Bilateral Vocal Fold Bowing: Presbylaryngis*

## HISTORY

The patient is an 80-year-old female who presented with a 6-month history of progressively deteriorating voice quality. Sixteen months earlier she underwent a left thyroidectomy at another facility without complications. She suggested that her voice difficulty actually began more than 3 years prior, with chronic hoarseness as the chief symptom. At the time of this examination, she also complained of episodic aspiration on thin liquid material and pronounced degrees of vocal fatigue and shortness of breath. With the exception of 25 mg of Synthroid daily, the patient did not use any medication and her general health was excellent. She was referred by an outside laryngologist for a full scale voice evaluation and treatment recommendations. Left vocal fold paralysis was suspected.

## EXAMINATION FINDINGS

The head and neck physical examination was relatively unremarkable. No signs of lymphadenopathy were evident, and the extrinsic laryngeal region was within normal limits with the exception of the changes caused by the left thyroidectomy, and there were no edentulous spaces in either dental arch. Gross motor and sensory functions of the orofacial complex were also within normal limits.

Perceptually, the patient's voice was severely breathy-hoarse with a shrill quality overlay. Maximum phonation time was 7 seconds. The next **voice sample** highlights these disturbances.

Acoustic analysis revealed the following: (1) fundamental frequency @ 369 Hz, (2) jitter @ 1.2%, (3) shimmer @ 0.62 dB, and (4) harmonic to noise ratio @ 1.5 dB. These data are markedly abnormal. The shrill voice component likely contributes to the high-pitched fundamental finding. The jitter result points to a substantial amount of instability and variability in the cycle-to-cycle vibratory activities of the vocal folds. There is a significant amount of excess noise in the voice signal, as exemplified by the harmonics data.

**CD1**
**Track 27**

Speech aerodynamic testing yielded the following results: (1) mean airflow rate @ 496 cc/sec, (2) subglottal pressure @ 10.6 cm $H_2O$, and (3) glottal resistance @ 200 cm $H_2O$/lps. Transglottal flow was roughly five times the normal amount, suggestive of significant glottal incompetency. The laryngeal resistance finding highlights the presence of four times the normal degree of glottal (or supraglottal) compression forces during phonation efforts.

Figure 6–27A illustrates the appearance of the laryngeal inlet obtained with videostroboscopy. Note that both vocal folds are bowed, more pronounced on the left side. This causes a significant chink across the entire length of the glottis during phonation, and accounts for the voice quality disturbances exhibited by the patient. At no time during vigorous vocal and nonvocal laryngeal valving activities was complete glottal closure observed. Both vocal folds were symmetrically mobile in their biomechanical respiratory and pre- and postphonatory adjustments; no signs of adductory or abductory paresis or paralysis were evident.

**Clinical Diagnosis:** Bilateral presbylaryngis: bowed vocal folds.

**Treatment Recommendation:** Unilateral medialization of the left vocal fold, followed by voice therapy. Because of the size of the glottal chink, an Isshiki thyroplasty rather than vocal fold injection of autologous fat or collagen was considered the appropriate choice. A unilateral approach was viewed as a conservative but acceptable

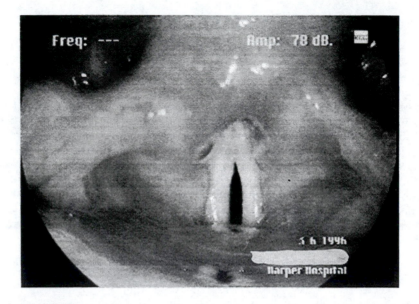

**FIGURE 6–27A.** This laryngeal photograph was obtained from an 80-year-old female with the diagnosis of presbylaryngis. Note the bilateral bowing of the true vocal folds and the persistent elliptical-shaped chink in the glottis during phonation.

initial method of treatment. Less than optimal results would permit a contralateral thyroplasty or intramuscular injection to facilitate phonation and swallowing skills.

## TREATMENT RESULTS

The patient underwent a left medialization thyroplasty. Figures 6–27B and 6–27C illustrate the results. Note the marked improvement in glottal competency across the midline of this mechanism. There is mild compromise of the airway secondary to this surgical procedure, and the left vocal fold is moderately erythematous. The right fold remains bowed, as can be seen. Perceptually, the patient's voice was significantly improved, and she no longer complained of severe vocal fatigue. The next **voice sample** highlights these gains, though the patient continued to struggle with a moderate degree of dysphonia. Plans were made to enroll her in a voice therapy program to facilitate further improvements in voice output.

**CD1**
**Track 27**

## DISCUSSION

Bowed vocal folds most often occur as a consequence of the normal aging process and progressive atrophy of the vocalis musculature. Bowing may also be exhibited by patients with longstanding weakness, paresis, and atrophy of the vocal folds, secondary to recurrent and/or superior laryngeal nerve injuries. Bilateral bowing, whether developmental or acquired, results in a spindle-shaped glottal chink. The size of the gap usually dictates the degree and nature of the associated dysphonia.

The treatment of choice will vary from patient to patient, depending upon the underlying etiology, involvement of one or both vocal folds, and degree of glottal incompetency. In most cases, surgery is indicated as the first-line method of intervention.

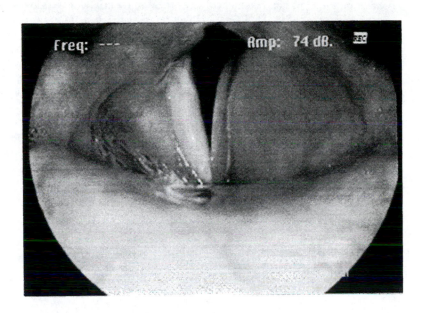

**FIGURE 6–27B.** This photograph was obtained from the same patient roughly one week following the medialization thyroplasty on the left side. Note the erythematous appearance of the ipsilateral vocal fold. Also note the mild compromise of the airway during inhalation.

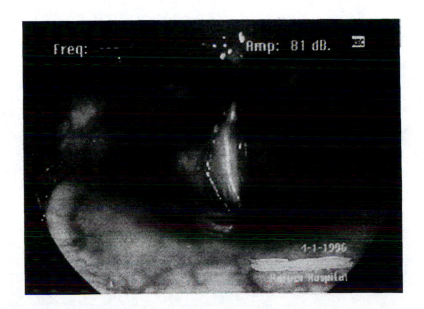

**FIGURE 6–27C.** This photograph was obtained from the same patient during the closed phases of vibration associated with voice effort. Note that she achieves full glottal competency across the entire length of this mechanism. There is some mild bowing of the contralateral cord as was observed in the preoperative examination.

Behavioral exercises alone are usually insufficient, especially if the glottal chink causes aspiration symptoms. Unilateral or bilateral medialization thyroplasty offers an advantage over intramuscular vocal fold injection in the patient with a large glottal chink. For small chinks, autologous fat or collagen may be used to plump and medialize the affected vocal fold. Following surgical treatment, vocal fold valving exercises may be indicated for any residual glottal incompetency. Pushing, pulling, head turning, and laryngeal compression techniques may help to strengthen the glottal seal, reduce excess transglottal airflow, increase maximum phonation time, and reduce vocal fatigue.

Because presbylaryngis is a degenerative disorder, the patient may experience a recurrence of symptoms at some point in time following successful phonosurgery and voice therapy. A revision thyroplasty is always possible to facilitate voice and swallowing potential. Repeat fat, collagen, or Teflon injections may pose vocal fold load effect difficulties and counterproductive phonation results.

# CASE 28
## *Mixed Hyperkinetic-Spastic Dysarthria*

## HISTORY

The patient is a 53-year-old female who presented with a 1-year history of breast cancer that required a left radical mastectomy. Three months prior she developed distant metastasis to the posterior brainstem and subcortex, which necessitated neurosurgery. Following this procedure she suffered from bilateral resting and intention tremors of the upper limb, orofacial, and laryngeal musculature. She struggled with articulatory and phonatory difficulties. With the exception of these medical problems, the patient was in good health, and clean margins were obtained during neurosurgery. She was referred by her neurologist largely for voice/speech evaluations and management recommendations.

## EXAMINATION FINDINGS

Physical examination of the head and neck yielded numerous neuromuscular abnormalities, including the following salient findings: (1) severe resting and intention tremors of the facial, labial, lingual, and mandibular musculature, bilaterally; (2) mild to moderate hypertonicity, weakness, and paresis of these muscle groups; and (3) moderate to severe labial and lingual dysdiadochokinesia. Perceptually, articulation was moderately imprecise and slow-labored, and phonation was severely tremorous in quality, with intermittent whispering and breathiness. Maximum phonation time was markedly reduced. The next **audiotape sample** highlights these grave communication difficulties.

**CD1**
**Track 28**

Figure 6–28 illustrates the results of videostroboscopy using a flexible fiberoptic endoscope because of pronounced gagging with the rigid instrument. There were no detectable anatomic anomalies of the laryngeal or supraglottal structures. However, profound tremors of the arytenoid cartilages, aryepiglottal folds, true vocal folds, and ventricular folds were observed, both at rest and during various phonatory efforts. Intermittent glottal incompetency occurred during vowel prolongation and running speech tasks, owing to the adverse vocal fold tremor effects. These abnormal behaviors correlated with and accounted for the aforementioned voice quality disturbances.

**Clinical Diagnosis:** Mixed hyperkinetic-spastic dysarthria, secondary to metastatic brain disease.

**Treatment Recommendation:** Speech and voice therapy. The prognosis was very poor, in light of the severity and etiology of the condition.

## TREATMENT RESULTS

The patient attended twice weekly 50-minute therapy sessions for a total of 10 weeks. Focus was placed on improving functions of the phonation, articulation, and prosody subsystems. Various clinical techniques were employed to reduce the profound voice tremor, including visual biofeedback of the voice signal during pitch, loudness, and vocal fold valving exercises. The most dramatic phonation gains were achieved by manual bracing of the larynx, humming of melodies, and breath support treatment methods. Articulation precision was facilitated by a variety of tongue, lip, and jaw force physiology exercises, which emphasized improving tone, strength, range, speed, and variable force control of these articulators. Prosody was stimulated through a modified melodic intonation therapy program, wherein voice inflection and melodi-

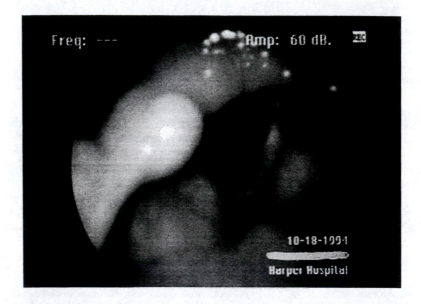

**FIGURE 6–28.** This laryngeal photograph was obtained from a 53-year-old female with mixed hyperkinetic-spastic dysarthria, secondary to neurosurgery for metastatic malignancy. Note the normal anatomy of the laryngeal inlet. No gross lesions are seen on the vocal folds or the surrounding soft tissue. Most impressive was the profound degree of tremors involving the entire mechanism during phonation.

ous speech patterns were utilized to decrease the interruptive speech subsystem tremors. At the conclusion of these treatments the patient demonstrated unexpected, excellent gains in voice and overall motor speech fluency and control.

The next **voice sample** illustrates these dramatic improvements.

**CD1
Track 28**

## DISCUSSION

This unfortunate young patient developed a severe motor speech disorder secondary to neurosurgery for metastatic brain carcinoma. The clinical examination findings suggested that the neuroanatomic sites of involvement included the extrapyramidal and pyramidal systems. Orofacial, laryngeal, and appendicular tremors have been ascribed to lesions of the dentato-rubro-olivary tract, a component of the extrapyramidal system located in the posterior brainstem from the level of the midbrain to the medulla. Hypertonic, slow-labored, weak, and paretic speech musculature may be caused by lesions of the corticobulbar tracts. These components of the pyramidal system originate in the primary motor strips of the frontal lobes and descend through the internal capsule enroute to cranial nerve motor nuclei along the brainstem. Our patient suffered damage to these extrapyramidal and pyramidal pathways at both the subcortical and brainstem levels, which resulted in the mixed hyperkinetic (tremors)-spastic speech musculature pathophysiology that she exhibited.

Voice tremor is not an easy disorder to treat. Neither pharmacologic agents nor phonosurgical alternatives have been shown to be consistently helpful for this disabling problem. Conversely, our past experiences with behavioral voice exercises, like those described here, have been occasionally successful. For the current patient, the manual bracing technique, wherein the larynx and surrounding strap muscles are firmly grasped with one or both hands, was very facilitative. She did not respond initially to vocal exercises alone. Once the bracing maneuver was employed, the tremors were subdued and she began to demonstrate better voice motor control. This response afforded her the opportunity to practice and benefit from these voice activities. The patient was delighted with her improvement. At the beginning of therapy we proceeded with great caution and little hope, therefore, we were somewhat surprised when she made such sharp gains. In the past we have been fortunate to realize moderate levels of success using these techniques with others, but none who presented initially with such a guarded prognosis.

We have speculated that the manual bracing method may serve to reduce the overall laryngeal shimmy caused by the tremors. If this stabilizing effect occurs, the patient may be taught to improve voice output with less uncontrollable acoustic and speech aerodynamic interruptions. We are especially enamored of *gentle* humming, using familiar tunes or songs as stimuli, as the initial exercise following successful bracing. We cannot overemphasize the importance of the term "gentle." Excessively loud, forceful vocalizations tend to exacerbate voice tremors, whether bracing is used or not. Unfortunately, we are unable to offer a scientifically sound explanation for the observed advantage of this gentle, rhythmic, and melodious treatment approach.

# CASE 29
## *Bilateral Vocal Fold Polyps*

## HISTORY

This patient is a 23-year-old male who presented with a chief complaint of acute onset of hoarseness which occurred while shouting at a music concert. His voice remained unchanged during the following 6 months before he sought the help of an otolaryngologist. His medical history was significant for allergy-induced rhinosinusitis, chronic cough, and continual throat clearing behaviors. He admitted to smoking one pack of cigarettes per day for the last 2 years and longstanding voice abuse patterns at work.

## EXAMINATION FINDINGS

**CDI
Track 29**

Perceptually, the patient's voice was moderately to severely hoarse-breathy in quality with reduced volume and pitch control. Maximum phonation time was only 10 seconds. The next **voice sample** highlights these dysphonic features.

Acoustic analysis revealed the following: (1) fundamental frequency @ 137 Hz, (2) jitter @ 0.81%, (3) shimmer @ 0.34 dB, and (4) harmonic to noise ratio @ 16 dB. These data are moderately abnormal, suggestive of instability in the cycle-to-cycle vibratory characteristics of the true vocal folds.

Figure 6–29A illustrates the appearance of the vocal folds using videostroboscopy. Note the appearance of a pronounced polyp on the middle third of the right true vocal fold, which compresses the opposite fold and reduces glottal competency across

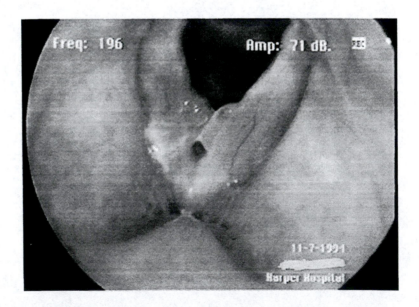

**FIGURE 6–29A.** Appearance of the laryngeal inlet in a 23-year-old male with a diagnosis of bilateral vocal fold polyps. In addition to the bulbous swellings on the anterior one-third of both true vocal folds, note the widespread erythema on the covers and surrounding ventricular regions.

the entire length of the glottic inlet. A reactive polyp has evolved over the left true vocal fold. Under stroboscopic visualization, the vibratory mucosal wave is restricted bilaterally owing to the load effect of these masses. Glottal incompetence at the midline is noted during all phases of vibration.

The clinical diagnosis: bilateral vocal fold polyps secondary to chronic voice abuse. Because of the size of these lesions and chronicity of symptoms, surgical removal was recommended followed by voice therapy.

## TREATMENT RESULTS

The patient underwent surgical excision of the bilateral vocal fold polyps. Postoperatively, the patient was placed on H2 blocker therapy and oral antibiotics. He was asked to maintain complete voice rest for 10 days. One month following surgery his voice was of good quality with normal volume and pitch control. Figure 6–29B shows the postoperative results. Note the mild persistent erythema and edema of the vocal folds. A chink in the posterior glottis during the closed phases of vibration is also observed. The patient was started on voice therapy to limit voice abuse behaviors.

## DISCUSSION

Acute onset of hoarseness associated with voice abuse may be the result of submucosal vocal fold hemorrhage caused by forceful and traumatic closure of the vocal folds during phonation. This hemorrhagic lesion may resolve completely with no resultant dysphonia. However, if voice abuse patterns and repeated vocal fold trauma persist, scar-

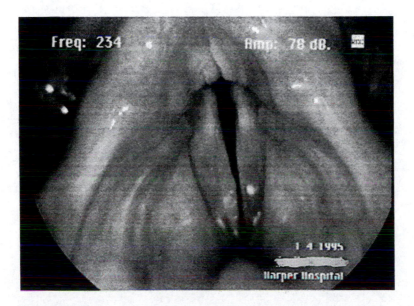

**FIGURE 6–29B.** This illustration was obtained following phonosurgery for removal of the polyps. Note the relatively smooth and clean appearances of the surgical site. There is some mild irregularity of the free edges of both true vocal folds. A persistent degree of hyperemia exists on the covers of both cords.

ring and polypoidal changes of the mucosal cover may occur. Reactive changes of the opposite fold may result from repeated contact trauma with this mass lesion during phonatory efforts. Such mucosal changes will usually result in a hoarse-breathy voice quality that may never revert to normal despite appropriate therapy.

Treatment for such disorders centers on correcting vocal abuse behaviors through speech therapy. This may be sufficient to reverse early and mild mucosal changes of the vocal folds. Surgery is indicated for those patients with larger, well organized, fibrotic, or chronic vocal fold polyps because the mucosal changes associated with these lesions are relatively irreversible, despite cessation of voice abuse behaviors. Often, removal of the original polyp will allow resolution of mucosal changes of the opposite fold without surgical intervention. Once the lesion is removed it is imperative to continue proper vocal behaviors or the disease process will usually reoccur. Postoperative voice therapy is of paramount importance for this reason. Occasionally, a clinical psychology consultation is indicated when a deep-seated emotional problem is evident and considered causally related to the voice abuse behavior.

# CASE 30
## *Overinjection of Teflon Left Vocal Fold*

## HISTORY

This patient is a 78-year-old female who presented with a chief complaint of persistent dysphonia following Teflon injection. Apparently, the patient suffered a left true vocal fold paralysis following a carotid endarterectomy procedure 2 years prior to this visit. A Teflon injection of the paralyzed fold was performed 6 months after the vascular procedure, without improvement in voice. The patient was intubated for an elective surgical procedure 6 months prior to this visit. She developed acute airway obstruction following extubation and a tracheotomy was placed. The patient's medical history was significant for emphysema and gastro-esophageal reflux disease.

## EXAMINATION FINDINGS

Perceptually, the patient's voice was moderately to severely hoarse-harsh in quality with low pitch and volume dimensions. Maximum phonation time was less than 5 seconds. The next **voice sample** highlights these disturbances.

**CDI**
**Track 30**

Acoustic analysis revealed the following: (1) fundamental frequency @ 329 Hz, (2) jitter @ 4.6%, (3) shimmer @ 0.36 dB, and (4) harmonic to noise ratio @ 2.4 dB. These data are significantly abnormal. Jitter findings suggest a marked degree of instability in the cycle-to-cycle vibratory characteristics of the true vocal folds associated with phonation. The noise data point to a marked amount of excessive noise in the voice signal. Maximum phonation time was less than one third the normal degree expected for the patient's age and sex.

Figure 6–30 illustrates the appearance of the vocal folds using videostroboscopy. Note the pronounced bulging of the left true vocal fold, which causes a bowing effect of the normal fold during the vibratory phases of phonation. Also note the prominence of the left false fold. During the closed phase of phonation a persistent chink exists over the entire glottal inlet region. During deep inhalation, only the posterior glottis opens; no anterior opening is evident during deep inhalatory maneuvers. During phonation the right true vocal fold adducts and abducts adequately, although restricted in part from achieving good compensatory action with the opposing paralyzed side by the bulging nature of the left Teflon injected fold. The left true vocal fold was immobile during phonation efforts.

The clinical diagnosis: left vocal fold paralysis with overinjection of Teflon into the vocal fold and improper placement of Teflon into the false fold. These abnormalities likely resulted in poor phonatory quality and obstructive airway symptoms. Suggested treatment included excision of Teflon from the true and false folds to provide a better glottic airway. Postoperative speech therapy was recommended. The patient elected not to proceed with either recommendation.

## DISCUSSION

Vocal fold paralysis is an unfortunate complication of a number of surgical procedures, especially thyroid operations. This disorder results from injury to the laryngeal nerve (superior and/or recurrent laryngeal branches of the Xth cranial nerve). Depending on the nature of the injury, vocal fold paralysis may be temporary or permanent. Patients will present with breathy dysphonia and possibly dysphagia, especially for liquids. However, compensatory action of the opposite vocal fold and/or sphincteric supraglottic adjustments may reduce the degree of dysphonia and dysphagia.

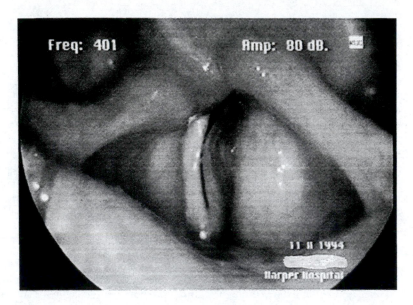

**FIGURE 6–30.** This laryngeal photograph was obtained from a 78-year-old female who underwent Teflon injection for left true vocal fold paralysis. Note the convexity of the injected cord, which causes distortion of the glottis and the opposing vocal fold during phonation.

When symptoms persist, phonosurgery may help provide adequate glottic closure. Teflon injection of a paralyzed vocal fold was once the most widely used augmentation procedure. Recently, other techniques have been described that may result in better voice with a lower incidence of postoperative complications. These techniques were described in Chapter 4.

The fundamental principle behind successful injection of Teflon is accurate placement of the material into the thyroarytenoid muscle complex, as far laterally as the inner thyroid perichondrium. Proper placement will allow for more normal mucosal wave characteristics, thus, better voice. When Teflon is injected improperly, or overinjected, it may result in abnormal stiffness of the vocal fold, granuloma formation, or airway compromise. Unfortunately, Teflon is not biodegradable and removal is extremely difficult.

# CASE 31
## *Bilateral Recurrent Laryngeal Nerve Paralysis*

## HISTORY

This is a 42-year-old female who presented to the emergency room with progressive hoarseness, stridor, and dyspnea for the past 2 days. Her symptoms were preceded by an upper respiratory tract infection. Past medical history was significant for a thyroidectomy at age 11 for an unknown etiology. She claimed to suffer from chronic, mild "wheezing" and shortness of breath, but had never suffered such severe symptoms. She denied tobacco, alcohol, or illicit drug abuse behaviors.

## EXAMINATION FINDINGS

Upon examination in the voice laboratory the patient exhibited pronounced inspiratory stridor and dyspnea. Perceptually, the patient's voice was mild to moderately hoarse in quality. Maximum phonation time was 11 seconds. The next **voice sample** highlights these dysphonic features.

**CD1**
**Track 31**

Acoustic analysis revealed the following: (1) fundamental frequency @ 195 Hz, (2) jitter @ 0.91%, (3) shimmer @ 0.33 dB, and (4) harmonic to noise ratio @ 1.6 dB. These findings are moderately abnormal, exemplified by instability in the cycle-to-cycle activity of the true vocal folds with a significant degree of excess noise in the voice signal.

Speech aerodynamic testing revealed the following results: (1) mean transglottal airflow rate during phonation @ 189 cc/sec, (2) subglottal pressure estimate @ 9.7 cm $H_2O$, and (3) glottal resistance @ 142 cm $H_2O$/lps. The latter findings suggest seven times the normal degree of compression forces between the vocal folds during phonation, indicating hyperadduction.

Figure 6–31A illustrates the appearance of the vocal folds using videostroboscopy. Note severe compromise of the airway due to bilateral abductor vocal fold paralysis. The true vocal folds are resting in a near midline position, thus allowing vibration for a relatively good quality voice. Mild edema and erythema of both folds is evident. The arytenoids are virtually motionless.

The clinical diagnosis: bilateral recurrent laryngeal nerve paralysis likely resulting from injury to the nerves at the time of her original thyroid procedure. The patient has suffered from chronic, mild upper airway symptoms since the procedure, but the recent upper respiratory infection caused enough glottic edema to transform a relatively stable airway into a severely compromised one. Recommended treatment included a tracheotomy, followed by a laryngeal procedure to provide a better airway at the level of the glottis.

## TREATMENT RESULTS

The patient underwent a tracheotomy to provide an immediate airway, thus bypassing the glottic obstruction. Subsequently, a left-sided laser cordotomy was performed to open the posterior glottis for better airflow.

The patient presented 2 months following the cordotomy procedure for reevaluation of her laryngeal status. She had a #4 uncuffed Shiley tracheotomy tube in place. During quiet breathing, with the tracheotomy tube plugged, she continued to struggle with airflow at the glottic level.

Perceptually, the patient's voice was significantly worse compared with her preoperative vocal quality. She demonstrated moderate to severe breathy-hoarse dysphonia with low-pitched features.

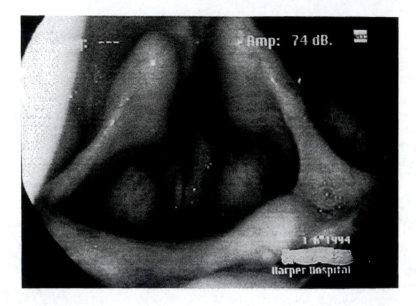

**FIGURE 6–31A.** View of the laryngeal inlet of a 42-year-old female with bilateral vocal fold paralysis. Note the markedly restricted airway during deep inhalation.

Acoustic analysis revealed the following: (1) fundamental frequency @ 235 Hz, (2) jitter @ 2.4%, (3) shimmer @ 0.55 dB, and (4) harmonic/noise ratio @ 12.0 dB. The jitter and shimmer findings suggest moderate instability in the vibratory cycles of the true vocal folds. These findings are mildly poorer than that which was observed before surgery.

The next **voice sample** demonstrates the patient's postoperative voice.

**CD1**
**Track 31**

Speech aerodynamic testing yielded the following: (1) mean airflow rate @ 433 cc/sec, (2) subglottal pressure estimate @ 8.0 cm $H_2O$, (3) glottal resistance @ 14.9 cm $H_2O$/lps. In comparison to the preoperative data, these results suggest that the airway is less compromised, as exemplified by the decrease in airflow resistance.

Videostroboscopic examination (Figure 6–31B) illustrates the following: (1) a markedly compromised airway during deep inspiratory efforts with a limited chink across the entire glottal length during quiet breathing, (2) mild inflammatory changes of the left true vocal fold area with some unusual subglottal bulking on that same side, and (3) irregular vibratory behaviors during phonation efforts, accounting for the aforementioned perceptual, acoustic, and aerodynamic disturbances.

Overall, the patient demonstrated persistent airway compromise and dysphonia, despite an initial surgical attempt at relieving this obstruction. The patient underwent a revision laser cordotomy with improved airflow dynamics. However, the voice remained poor. To date, she has not returned for follow-up evaluation.

## DISCUSSION

Bilateral vocal fold paralysis is an uncommon complication of thyroid surgery. The condition is caused by injury to the recurrent laryngeal nerves while dissecting the thyroid gland from the larynx. Usually, the patient will present immediately with airway compromise necessitating reintubation and eventual tracheotomy. Uncommonly,

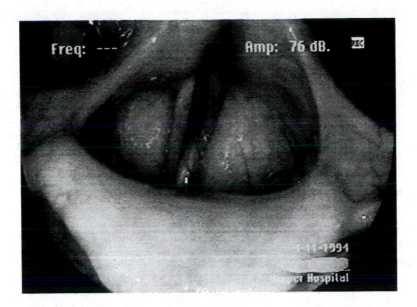

Freq: ---      Amp: 76 dB.

1-11-1994

Hospital

**FIGURE 6–31B.** This photograph was obtained postoperatively. Note that there is no discernable difference in the degree of glottal opening during deep inhalation from that seen in the previous photograph.

there are mild or no symptoms of airway compromise and voice is normal, due to the median position assumed by the paralyzed folds (unopposed action of the cricothyroid muscles, innervated by the superior laryngeal nerves, will result in a median or paramedian position of the folds). The current patient lived more than 30 years without severe respiratory symptoms and had a relatively normal voice. Her history of mild, chronic "wheezing" was likely not caused by a lower respiratory tract abnormality, but rather by bilateral vocal fold paralysis. Indeed, many patients suffering vocal fold paralysis are erroneously treated for "asthma" or "bronchitis." The recent upper respiratory tract infection caused enough glottic edema to cause this patient's severe upper airway symptoms.

Treatment for bilateral vocal fold paralysis with airway compromise includes performance of an emergency tracheotomy to establish an immediate airway. If the paralysis is thought to be irreversible, specialized laryngeal procedures may be performed to provide a better airway at the level of the glottic inlet. Such methods include arytenoidectomy or cordotomy. These techniques are designed to improve airflow and eventually allow removal of the tracheotomy tube, in exchange for poorer voice outcome and occasional dysphagic symptoms. The cordotomy procedure attempted on this patient was performed endoscopically using a $CO_2$ laser to release the vocal fold from its attachment to the vocal process of the arytenoid, thus establishing a larger diameter posterior airway. If the incision is not carried far enough laterally (i.e., to the inner thyroid cartilage perichondrium) an inadequate glottic opening will result once healing has occurred. This patient likely required a revision procedure because of this problem.

# CASE 32
## *Vocal Fold Nodules (Singer's Nodules)*

## HISTORY

This patient is a 60-year-old female who presented with a chief complaint of persistent hoarseness lasting for 6 weeks. She underwent excision of bilateral vocal fold nodules with postoperative voice therapy 15 years prior to this presentation. Voice results after surgery were excellent according to the patient. During the past few years she engaged in a number of choir activities and admitted to frequent voice abuse behaviors.

## EXAMINATION FINDINGS

**CDI
Track 32**

Perceptually, the patient's voice was moderately hoarse-breathy in quality with low pitch features. The next **voice sample** highlights this problem.

Videostroboscopic findings are shown in Figure 6–32. Note the presence of nodules on the middle third of both vocal folds. These tiny masses interfere mildly with closure of the vocal folds during phonatory efforts, resulting in a persistent chink in the glottis. This gap allows for escape of unphonated air and accounts for the hoarse-breathy quality exhibited by the patient. Some signs of posterior vocal fold and interarytenoid irritation are also evident, perhaps suggestive of mild gastro-esophageal-reflux disease. The clinical diagnosis: recurrent bilateral vocal fold nodules. The patient exhibited moderate dysphonia characterized by hoarse breathy voice quality. These symptoms were likely secondary to chronic vocal abuse. The recommended treatment for such lesions is voice therapy to eliminate these pathologic behaviors.

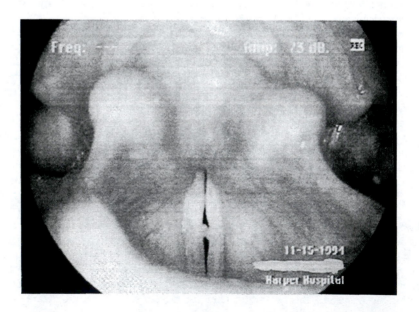

**FIGURE 6–32.** This photograph illustrates the presence of bilateral nodules on the middle one-third of the true vocal fold free edges. Note the hourglass-shaped chink caused by these compressing masses. Also note the mild degree of erythema in the anterior half of both true vocal folds.

## DISCUSSION

Vocal fold nodules develop as a result of chronic voice abuse. They a
ed at the medial free margin of the anteroposterior midpoint of the m
vocal fold. They are typically bilateral, white, small, sessile lesions tha
perficial layer of the lamina propria.

Because vocal fold nodules are behaviorally induced, they should
ed with voice therapy. The majority of patients will be cured with th
those lesions resistant to voice therapy, surgical excision is the treatment of choice.
However, it is imperative for the patient to undergo pre- and postoperative voice therapy to prevent recurrence. The patient presented in this case history developed recurrent vocal fold nodules after surgery because of failure to alter her vocal behaviors, despite postoperative voice therapy. She was relieved that the dysphonia was not due to
a more serious condition, such as glottic cancer. She elected to delay all forms of treatment at this time.

# CASE 33
## *Vocal Process Granulomas*

## HISTORY

This is a 65-year-old male with a significant smoking history who presented with 4 months of mild hoarseness, sore throat, and globus sensation. Upon more indepth questioning, he was noted to suffer from frequent heartburn symptoms, acid regurgitation, and chronic throat clearing behaviors. He enjoyed spicy foods, although they caused reflux symptoms, teas, colas, and late night snacks.

## EXAMINATION FINDINGS

**CD I**
**Track 33**

Perceptually, the patient's voice was mildly hoarse-harsh in quality, as can be heard in the next brief **voice sample,** which reveals trace degrees of hoarseness.

Figure 6–33A illustrates the appearance of the vocal folds using videostroboscopy. Noted are two large, smooth, rounded, pearl-colored masses which emanate from the vocal processes of the arytenoids. They interdigitate in a "key in lock" manner during phonatory efforts. These lesions inhibit complete posterior glottic closure during phonation, thus accounting for the aforementioned dysphonic features. The arytenoids are erythematous and the posterior commissure displays signs of pachydermia laryngis; the mucosa is hyperplastic and hyperkeratotic.

The clinical diagnosis: bilateral vocal process granulomas secondary to chronic reflux laryngitis. The patient was instructed on dietary and lifestyle changes to help decrease gastroesophageal reflux. He was also prescribed Prilosec (Omeprazole), 20 mg orally every 12 hours, to inhibit gastric acid secretion.

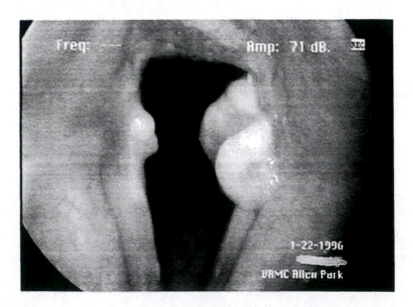

**FIGURE 6–33A.** This photograph illustrates the presence of bilateral contact granulomas in a 65-year-old male. Note the bulbous masses emanating off of the vocal process regions of both true vocal folds.

## TREATMENT RESULTS

The patient returned for a repeat videostroboscopy 4 weeks after instituting antireflux therapy. Subjectively, the voice was improved and reflux symptoms had nearly completely subsided.

Videostroboscopic examination (Figure 6–33B) illustrates near complete resolution of the right vocal process granuloma. The left sided mass has not changed in size, but appears less sessile and more rounded. The arytenoid erythema and posterior commissure mucosal changes have improved significantly.

## DISCUSSION

Chronic gastro-esophageal reflux can manifest as laryngeal disease. Most patients with laryngeal complaints will also describe heartburn symptoms. However, up to 34% will present with isolated laryngeal symptoms including morning dysphonia and sore throat, globus sensation, excess "phlegm," chronic throat clearing, acid regurgitation, dysphagia, and paroxysmal nighttime coughing. Indirect laryngoscopy may reveal arytenoid erythema, pachydermia laryngis, and vocal process ulcerations or granulomas. Studies have shown that acid applied to the vocal processes of dogs will indeed cause ulceration and granuloma formation of these areas. It is theorized that a combination of vocal process trauma (e.g., vocal fold abuse or misuse behaviors, endotracheal tube trauma) and acid reflux initiate ulcerative changes. With chronic acid exposure of these raw areas, a chondritis develops, resulting in an inflammatory reaction and granuloma formation. Treatment for this condition includes institution of dietary and lifestyle changes to decrease gastro-esophageal-reflux events. In addition, med-

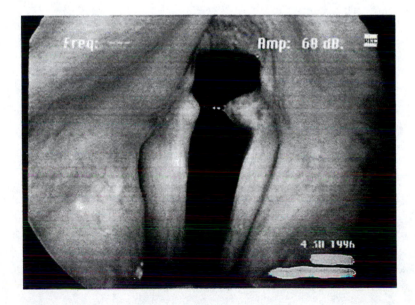

**FIGURE 6–33B.** This photograph was obtained roughly 4 weeks following the institution of an antireflux pharmacologic regimen. Note the response of the granuloma on the left side to this medication. The mass on the right side has changed only mildly.

ications to neutralize or inhibit acid secretion are prescribed. Voice therapy should be provided for those patients demonstrating vocal abuse behaviors. Using this regimen, resolution of granulomas may take up to 6 months. Surgical excision of these masses as a primary treatment modality results in a 50% recurrence rate, likely because of failure to treat the inciting reflux and voice abuse behaviors. However, if symptoms fail to resolve after prolonged medical therapy, biopsy or excision may be indicated.

# CASE 34
## *Reinke's Edema*

## HISTORY

This is a 30-year-old female who presented with the chief complaint of longstanding, intermittent dysphonia. The problem began following prolonged intubation after a serious horseback riding accident 7 years earlier. She admitted to daily voice abuse behaviors with worsening symptoms, which prompted her to seek a professional opinion.

## EXAMINATION FINDINGS

Perceptually, the patient's voice was moderately hoarse breathy with limited pitch and loudness controls. Maximum phonation time was less than 5 seconds. The next **voice sample** highlights these voice features.

**CD2
Track 1**

Acoustic analysis revealed the following: (1) fundamental frequency @ 175 Hz, (2) jitter @ 0.89%, (3) shimmer @ 0.50 dB, and (4) harmonic to noise ratio @ 2.3 dB. These results demonstrated significant pitch instability and noise characteristics in the voice signal.

Speech aerodynamic testing corroborated these findings.

Figure 6–34A illustrates the appearance of the vocal folds using videostroboscopy. Noted is a persistently small chink in the posterior glottis during phonatory efforts, due to bilateral polypoid degeneration of the vocal folds.

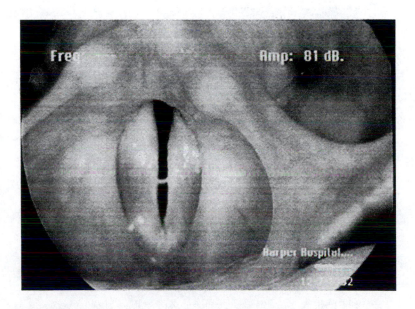

**FIGURE 6–34A.** This photograph illustrates bilateral Reinke's edema in a 30-year-old female who is a chronic voice abuser. In addition to the diffuse swelling, note the widespread erythema on the covers of both cords as well as in the interarytenoid regions.

The clinical diagnosis: Reinke's edema of the vocal folds. The condition was likely caused by chronic voice abuse behaviors. The treatment included bilateral vocal fold strippings, followed by speech therapy.

## TREATMENT RESULTS AFTER SURGERY

The patient returned for a full-scale voice evaluation after undergoing staged bilateral vocal fold stripping procedures.

**CD2
Track 1**

Perceptually, the patient's voice was mildly to moderately hoarse breathy in quality with difficulty in pitch and loudness control. The next **voice sample** highlights the postoperative voice characteristics.

Acoustic analysis revealed the following: (1) fundamental frequency @ 229 Hz, (2) jitter @ 1.06%, (3) shimmer @ 0.44 dB, and (4) harmonic/noise ratio @ 8.7 dB. These data point to a moderate improvement in pitch and reduced noise in the voice signal. Cycle-to-cycle vibratory instability had not improved, however.

Speech aerodynamic testing yielded the following: (1) mean airflow rate @ 198 cc/sec, and (2) glottal resistance @ 8.5 cmH$_2$O/lps. These data point to mild glottal leakage and moderately reduced laryngeal resistance.

Videostroboscopic examination (Figure 6–34B) illustrated the following: (1) mild edema and erythema of the left vocal fold, (2) fullness and erythema of the right vocal fold with associated irregularity along the medial surface, (3) persistent posterior glottic chink during phonation, and (4) mild irregularity of the mucosal wave characteristics, due to the associated fullness of the right vocal fold.

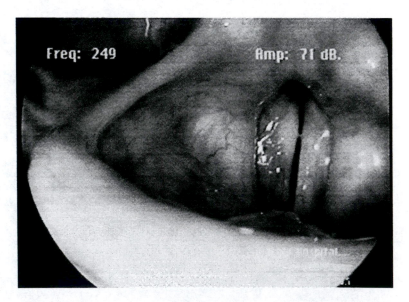

**FIGURE 6–34B.** This photograph was obtained after bilateral strippings of the true vocal folds. Note the diffuse edema and erythema of both true vocal folds. No appreciable difference in the swelling is noted in comparison to the preoperative state.

## TREATMENT RESULTS FOLLOWING SPEECH THERAPY

Following bilateral vocal fold strippings the patient underwent several months of speech therapy designed to introduce and implement appropriate vocal hygiene behaviors. Efforts were concentrated on eliminating vocal abuse behaviors, and improving vocal quality, loudness control, and breath support. Despite an understanding of the various concepts of good vocal hygiene, the patient was unable to adopt these new skills during ongoing speech. Her voice did not significantly improve during therapy, due to her persistent voice abuse behaviors. However, she felt her voice had improved as a result of this program.

## DISCUSSION

Reinke's edema results from chronic irritation of the vocal folds, which causes fluid collection in the superficial layer of the lamina propria (Reinke's space). It is a condition seen most frequently in voice abusers, and is nearly always associated with cigarette smoking. Other conditions, such as hypothyroidism, may be contributory.

Treatment for Reinke's edema includes elimination of the behaviors or conditions causing this disease process. Speech therapy plays a vital role in controlling voice abuse behaviors. If the diffuse polypoidal changes do not resolve after all irritants have been removed and vocal hygiene modified, surgery may be necessary. The once standard technique of vocal fold stripping has now been replaced by a more conservative, mucosa sparing procedure. This technique requires (1) an incision over the superior surface of the vocal fold, (2) elevation of a microflap of mucosa in the superficial layer of the lamina propria, (3) fine suctioning of the gelatinous material filling Reinke's space, (4) trimming of any redundant mucosa, and (5) replacement of the microflap of mucosa. The method may be performed bilaterally in one sitting, or as staged procedures. Most laryngologists have adopted this mucosa sparing approach because postoperative voice results have been significantly improved, compared with those following vocal fold stripping techniques.

# CASE 35
## *Recurrent Laryngeal Papillomas*

## HISTORY

This is a 28-year-old female who presented with a long history of recurrent laryngeal papillomas dating back more than 7 years. She underwent six previous procedures for removal of these lesions and at the time of examination was experiencing progressive dysphonia.

## EXAMINATION FINDINGS

**CD2
Track 2**

Perceptually, the patient's voice was severely breathy hoarse in quality with occasional high-pitched breaks. Maximum phonation time was less than 5 seconds. The next **voice sample** highlights the dysphonia.

Acoustic analysis revealed the following: (1) fundamental frequency @ 180 Hz, (2) jitter @ 3.4%, (3) shimmer @ 0.56 dB, and (4) harmonic to noise ratio @ 1.0 dB. These data are markedly abnormal, suggestive of a high degree of instability in the cycle-to-cycle vibratory characteristics of the vocal folds during phonation and a substantial amount of noise in the voice signal.

Figure 6–35A illustrates the appearance of the vocal folds using videostroboscopy. Note the exuberant amount of papillomatous tissue distributed over the left true vocal fold, virtually obscuring the entire fold from direct view. It does not appear that the right true fold is involved with disease. During phonatory efforts a persistent glottic chink exists, due to the papillomatous growths inhibiting complete glottic closure. The false folds adduct during phonation, likely as a compensatory mechanism for true fold disability.

The clinical diagnosis: recurrent laryngeal papillomas. The therapy of choice for such lesions is $CO_2$ laser ablation of the papillomatous growths without disruption of normal, uninvolved laryngeal mucosa. Postoperative speech therapy is often beneficial.

## TREATMENT RESULTS

**CD2
Track 2**

The patient underwent $CO_2$ laser excision of the laryngeal papillomas. She returned for speech therapy 2 weeks following the procedure. Perceptually, the patient's voice was markedly improved compared to the presurgical vocal status. She had only mild dysphonia characterized by episodic hoarse vocal quality and shrill-like outbursts. The next **voice sample** illustrates the voice gains postoperatively.

Videostroboscopic examination showed a remarkably improved appearance from that observed in the preoperative evaluation. Figure 6–35B reveals the postoperative appearance of the laryngeal inlet. There were persistent tags of papilloma tissue present in the anterior and posterior one-third of the undersurface of the true vocal fold on the left side.

## DISCUSSION

Laryngeal papillomas are cauliflower-like lesions caused by infection with the human papilloma virus (HPV). This lesion is the most common benign neoplasm of the larynx. During infancy or adulthood its presenting symptoms are hoarse vocal quality or

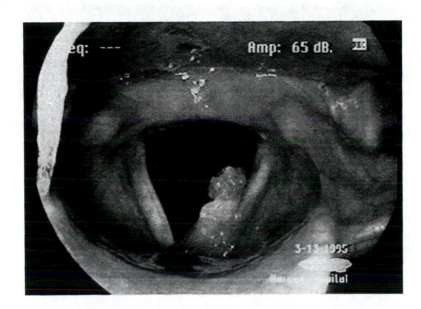

**FIGURE 6–35A.** This photograph was obtained from a 28-year-old female with recurrent laryngeal papilloma. Note the massive papilloma outgrowth off of the left true vocal fold. The right vocal fold is involved only at the anterior commissure level.

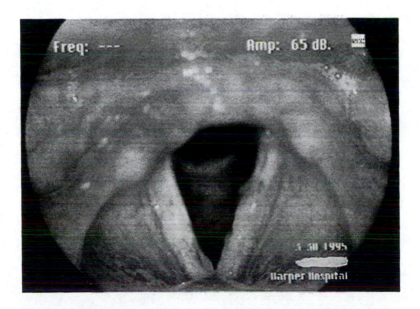

**FIGURE 6–35B.** This photograph was obtained following laser excision of the papilloma. Note that there are still tags of papilloma tissue on the left vocal fold.

airway obstruction. The natural history of this disease is one of multiple recurrences, especially with the juvenile onset type. Therefore, $CO_2$ laser vaporization of these lesions, although the accepted procedure of choice today, is only palliative in most cases. Multiple recurrences are believed to be caused by persistent growth of HPV in subclinically infected normal appearing tissue bordering the area of treatment. The goal of laser vaporization is to eradicate this lesion, establish an adequate airway, and facilitate functional voice without causing submucosal damage, scarring, and fibrosis of the vocal fold. Simultaneous removal of papillomas from both sides of the anterior or posterior commissure should be avoided, as this maneuver often results in web formation.

# CASE 36
## *Medialization Thyroplasty*

## HISTORY

The patient is a 40-year-old female who presented with the chief complaint of breathy voice quality for 18 months. When symptoms first occurred, diagnostic workup by an outside otolaryngologist revealed a left vocal fold paralysis. CAT scans of the neck and chest failed to provide an etiology for this disorder. The patient was a practicing physician who was unable to communicate effectively with patients due to the weak quality of her voice. She denied any swallowing difficulties with liquid or solid food substances; however, she struggled occasionally with aspiration of her own secretions.

## EXAMINATION FINDINGS

Perceptually, the patient's voice was mildly to moderately hoarse-breathy in quality with intermittent pitch breaks and aphonia. Maximum phonation time was within normal limits. The next **voice sample** highlights the patient's voice characteristics.

Acoustic analysis revealed the following: (1) fundamental frequency @ 237 Hz, (2) jitter @ 1.0%, (3) shimmer @ 0.20 dB, and (4) harmonic to noise ratio @ 2.8 dB. These acoustic findings are moderately abnormal. The jitter and shimmer data point to a mild to moderate degree of instability in the cycle-to-cycle vibratory characteristics of the true vocal folds associated with voice. The harmonics data point to a moderate to severe degree of noise in the voice signal.

**CD2**
**Track 3**

Figure 6–36A demonstrates the appearance of the larynx at the time of videostroboscopy. Note the paralyzed left vocal fold in the paramedian position. Also note that the arytenoid and aryepiglottic fold are collapsed into the inlet of the larynx and the ipsilateral fold has a slightly bowed appearance. During the closed phases of vibration associated with voice efforts a persistent chink exists along the length of the glottis. On occasion, only minimal contact occurs between the two folds.

The clinical diagnosis: vocal fold paralysis with glottal incompetence. This allows for excessive air escape through the glottis during phonation and a perceived breathy voice quality. The patient underwent a speech therapy session which provided exercises to be performed to help restimulate vocal fold functioning. These exercises were utilized both before and after performing a medialization thyroplasty procedure.

## TREATMENT RESULTS

A left medialization thyroplasty was performed with good voice quality obtained at the time of the operation. Postoperatively, the patient claimed her voice was significantly improved compared with preoperative vocal quality. Perceptually, the patient's voice had a slight hoarse vocal quality. This, however, is significantly improved over the preoperative status. The next **voice sample** illustrates this improvement.

**CD2**
**Track 3**

Acoustic analysis revealed the following: (1) maximum phonation time within normal limits, (2) fundamental frequency @ 230 Hz, (3) jitter @ 0.96%, (4) shimmer @ 0.16 dB, and (5) harmonic to noise ratio @ 9.0 dB. The jitter data are mildly elevated, suggestive of a mild degree of instability in the cycle-to-cycle vibratory characteristics of the true vocal folds associated with voice. The harmonics data point to a mild degree of noise in the voice signal.

Videostroboscopic examination (Figure 6–36B) illustrated no movement of the left vocal fold. She did achieve excellent glottal competency across the entire length of the glottis, with the exception of the most posterior portion.

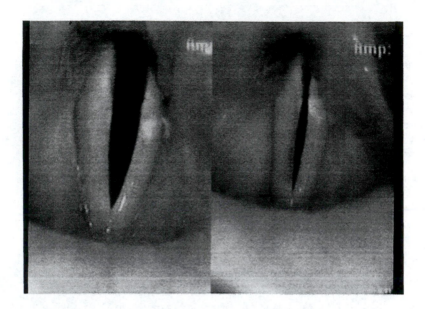

**FIGURE 6–36A.** This is the larynx of a 40-year-old female who presented with bowing of the left true vocal fold, of unknown origin. Note the pronounced degree of bowing of the left vocal fold and the glottal incompetency that results during phonation.

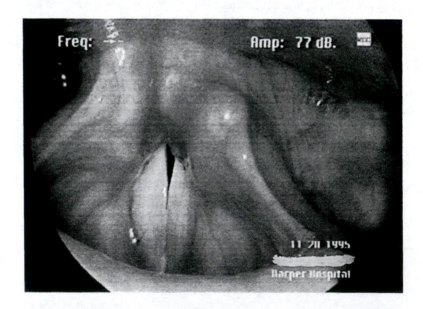

**FIGURE 6–36B.** This photograph was obtained after the patient underwent a left Isshiki thyroplasty to medialize the vocal fold. Note the improvement in glottal competency across two-thirds of the mechanism. A persistent chink still exists in the posterior glottis during phonation.

## DISCUSSION

Patients suffering glottal incompetency due to recurrent laryngeal nerve injury or presbylaryngis may benefit from a procedure that moves the affected vocal fold(s) toward the midline to allow better vibration during phonatory effort. The medialization thyroplasty is an external approach performed through an incision made in the neck over the thyroid ala. A rectangular window is carved from the thyroid ala at the level of the true vocal fold. A silastic wedge is then placed through the window to force the true fold toward the midline. The procedure is performed under a local anesthetic so that the patient can phonate, thus assuring proper vocal fold repositioning and better vocal quality. Other phonosurgical procedures designed to medialize the vocal fold include arytenoid adduction and injection of the true fold with substances such as gelfoam, Teflon, fat, or collagen. Indications and techniques for these procedures are described in Chapter 4.

# CASE 37
## *Verrucous Carcinoma of the Larynx*

## HISTORY

This is a 40-year-old male with a history of heavy smoking who presented with the chief complaint of progressive hoarseness, which had worsened over the previous several months. He experienced mild swallowing difficulties, with occasional aspiration on thin liquids. A recent endoscopy with biopsy revealed a verrucous carcinoma involving the left true vocal fold and extending across the anterior commissure. The patient presented for a full-scale voice evaluation prior to beginning radiation therapy.

## EXAMINATION FINDINGS

**CD2
Track 4**

Perceptually, the patient's voice was profoundly breathy-hoarse in quality. Maximum phonation time was less than 10 seconds. The next **voice sample** highlights the disturbed voice features.

Figure 6–37A illustrates the appearance of the vocal folds using videostroboscopy. An exophytic lesion involving the entire left true vocal fold with extension across the anterior commissure was noted. The vocal folds were hypomobile, and the vibratory wave was severely diminished, bilaterally. Because of the profound voice signal aperiodicity, neither acoustic nor aerodynamic measures were considered valuable.

The clinical diagnosis: verrucous carcinoma of the larynx. Surgical resection would include a near total or total laryngectomy. The patient did not want to lose his larynx,

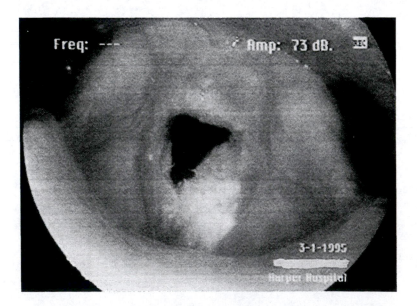

**FIGURE 6–37A.** This photograph was obtained from a 40-year-old male with the diagnosis of verrucous carcinoma of the larynx. Note the large exophytic lesion occupying most of the left true vocal fold and a portion of the right one as well.

therefore radiation therapy was recommended as primary treatment. Following radiation, he would undergo speech therapy.

## TREATMENT RESULTS DURING RADIATION THERAPY

The patient returned for a full-scale voice evaluation after undergoing 25 radiation therapy sessions. Perceptually, the patient's voice was moderately hoarse-breathy in quality with reduced pitch and volume dimensions. Maximum phonation time was less than 10 seconds.

Acoustic analysis revealed the following: (1) fundamental frequency @ 130 Hz, (2) jitter @ 2.4%, (3) shimmer @ 0.93 dB, and (4) harmonic to noise ratio @ 0.1 dB. These findings are moderately to severely abnormal.

The following **voice sample** demonstrates the patient's voice characteristics, which have improved slightly.

**CD2**
**Track 4**

Speech aerodynamic testing yielded the following: (1) mean airflow rate @ 1652 cc/sec, (2) subglottal pressure @ 19.8 cm $H_2O$, and (3) glottal resistance @ 17.0 cm $H_2O$/lps. These findings are markedly abnormal. They point to a hypofunctioning laryngeal valve with excessive airflow and reduced compression forces of the true vocal folds during phonation efforts.

Videostroboscopic examination (Figure 6–37B) illustrated the following: (1) yellowish, white patchy changes are noted along the arytenoid apices, piriform sinus, ventricular vocal folds, and interarytenoid zone; these changes are consistent with radiation induced mucositis; (2) the vocal folds appear bulky; (3) the patient now recruits the ventricular folds during phonatory efforts; and (4) the airway is not compromised.

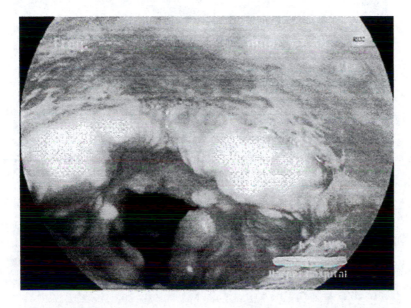

**FIGURE 6–37B.** This photograph was obtained at the conclusion of radiation therapy for the verrucous carcinoma. Note the widespread mucositis changes throughout the laryngeal inlet, including the vocal folds.

# TREATMENT RESULTS AT THE CONCLUSION OF RADIATION THERAPY

The patient returned for a full-scale voice evaluation roughly 2 months after undergoing radiation therapy. He admitted to persistent smoking abuse behaviors.

**CD2
Track 4**

Perceptually, the patient's voice was moderately to severely hoarse-harsh-breathy in quality. Maximum phonation time was 6 seconds. The next **voice sample** demonstrates these changes.

Acoustic analysis revealed the following: (1) fundamental frequency @ 93 Hz, (2) jitter @ 0.71%, (3) shimmer @ 0.61 dB, and (4) harmonic to noise ratio @ 4.0 dB. These numbers are moderately to severely abnormal. The jitter and shimmer data point to a moderate degree of instability in the cycle-to-cycle vibratory characteristics of the true vocal folds associated with voice. The harmonics data point to a substantial amount of noise in the voice signal.

Videostroboscopic examination (Figure 6–37C) illustrates the following: (1) the left true vocal fold is edematous and has an irregular free mucosal margin; (2) the right true vocal fold also has an irregular free mucosal margin and is partially obscured from full view by the overhanging right false vocal fold; (3) during the closed phases of vibration associated with voice the entire laryngeal inlet squeezes down, obstructing a view of the true vocal fold mechanism; and (4) significant interarytenoid hyperplastic mucosal changes are noted.

# SPEECH THERAPY

The patient was encouraged to stop smoking and warned about the dangers of continuing this destructive behavior. He was placed in a speech therapy program. To date,

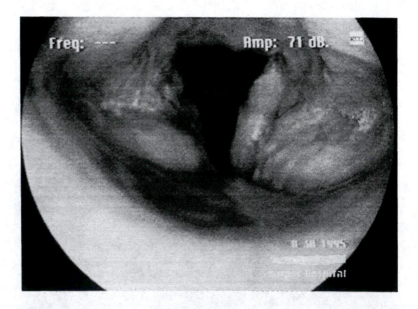

**FIGURE 6–37C.** This laryngeal photograph was obtained 2 months after radiation therapy. Note the mild to moderate improvement in the mucositis changes of the laryngeal inlet. However, there is still gross abnormality in the anatomy of the entire mechanism. These disturbances correlate significantly with the patient's pronounced dysphonia.

vocal quality has not improved, and monthly follow-up evaluations have demonstrated no evidence of persistent or recurrent disease.

## DISCUSSION

Verrucous carcinoma accounts for approximately 4% of all laryngeal cancers, with squamous cell carcinoma being the most common laryngeal malignancy by far, accounting for 90–95% of all cases. Verrucous lesions of the larynx typically involve the glottis or supraglottis. They tend to be well differentiated and demonstrate a superficial, noninvasive, exophytic, "pushing border" type growth pattern. Thus, these cancers are rarely found to be deeply invasive or metastatic.

Treatment for verrucous carcinoma includes surgery or radiation therapy. Surgical excision of this tumor results in local control and survival rates around 95%. The literature is controversial regarding use of radiation therapy to treat such lesions. Some researchers claim verrucous cancers are radioinsensitive, or that these lesions may be transformed into more aggressive tumors by radiation therapy. To date, both therapeutic modalities are utilized, but no overwhelming evidence supports one form of treatment over the other.

# CASE 38
## *Vocal Fold Cyst*

## HISTORY

This is a 38-year-old male who presented with a chief complaint of persistent hoarse vocal quality for the past 6 months. He was a nonsmoker who complained of excessive postnasal mucous secretions, chronic coughing, throat clearing, and gastric reflux. He admitted to voice abuse patterns both at work and as a singer in a local band.

## EXAMINATION FINDINGS

**CD2
Track 5**

Perceptually, the patient's voice was moderately hoarse-breathy in quality with limitations in pitch and volume range. Maximum phonation time was within normal limits. The next brief **voice sample** highlights these voice features.

Acoustic analysis revealed the following: (1) fundamental frequency @ 165 Hz, (2) jitter @ 0.63%, (3) shimmer @ 0.13 dB, and (4) harmonic to noise ratio @ 16.0 dB. These data are mildly abnormal, suggestive of instability in the cycle-to-cycle vibratory characteristics of the vocal folds, and a mildly elevated pitch level.

Figure 6–38A illustrates the appearance of the vocal folds using videostroboscopy. Note the presence of a large submucosal cyst-like structure over the middle one-third of the left true vocal fold. During phonatory efforts this mass hampers the vibratory activities of the involved fold and compresses the opposing fold during the closed phase of vibration. The cyst inhibits full glottic closure, resulting in a persistent glottic gap both anterior and posterior to the mass. At no time during phonation is full glottic competency observed.

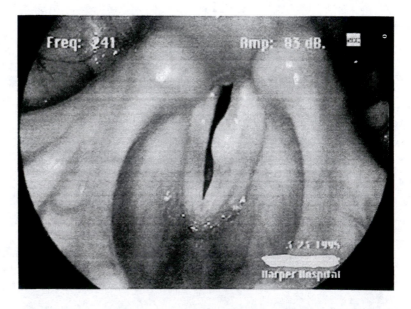

**FIGURE 6–38.** This photograph illustrates a cyst on the middle one-third of the left true vocal fold. Note the pronounced outgrowth of this mass and its effect on glottal competency.

The clinical diagnosis: left vocal fold submucosal cyst. The relatively large size of this lesion would likely preclude its complete resolution with speech therapy alone. Microflap excision of the vocal fold cyst with postoperative speech therapy was the recommended treatment plan.

## TREATMENT RESULTS

The patient underwent microflap excision of the left vocal fold cyst. Postoperatively, he was placed on an H2 blocker to lessen the likelihood of acid regurgitation onto the healing vocal fold. He was instructed to refrain from voice use for 2 weeks and he was then slowly rehabilitated through a voice therapy program.

A laryngeal study and vocal assessment were obtained 2 weeks postoperatively. Perceptually, the patient's voice was only mildly hoarse during connected speech. The next brief **voice sample** highlights the voice improvement.

Acoustic analysis revealed the following: (1) maximum phonation time within normal limits, (2) fundamental frequency @ 148 Hz, (3) jitter @ 0.53%, (4) shimmer @ 0.22 dB, and (5) harmonic to noise ratio @ 8.0 dB. These data were relatively normal, with perhaps only a trace of noise in the signal

Videostroboscopic examination (Figures 6–38B & 6–38C) illustrated mild erythema on the left true vocal fold surgical site. The free margins of both folds were clean. A small amount of mucous beading was noted to collect on the surfaces of the folds throughout the exam, causing the patient to occasionally clear his throat. These findings were considered normal postoperative changes. The patient was instructed on the importance of hydration to thin secretions and to provide a better vibratory environment during phonation. Overall, he was very pleased with the postoperative results, as voice was significantly improved compared with the preoperative status.

**CD2**
**Track 5**

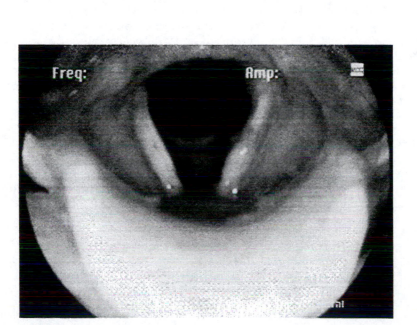

**FIGURE 6–38B.** This photograph was obtained following microexcision of the vocal fold cyst. Note there is still a residual degree of swelling in the middle one-third of the left true vocal fold.

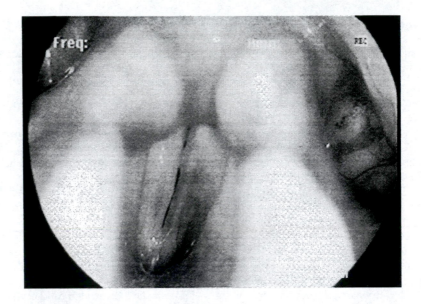

**FIGURE 6–38C.** This photograph illustrates closure at the midline during voice effort postsurgically. Note that there is a mild degree of glottal incompetency but a significant improvement over the preoperative condition.

## DISCUSSION

Vocal fold cysts are most often mucous retention cysts and occasionally are of epidermoid origin. Cysts are usually unilateral submucosal masses involving the membranous true vocal fold. They typically cause hoarse vocal quality and are diagnosed using indirect laryngoscopy. However, if small, the only physical finding may be an asymmetric and retarded mucosal wave of the involved side, seen only with stroboscopy.

Voice therapy is usually the treatment option of choice for such lesions. However, if nonsurgical therapy fails to resolve symptoms, microflap excision of the cyst under microscopic vision can be performed. A description of this procedure was outlined in Chapter 4. Briefly, the technique includes incision of mucosa over the superior surface of the vocal fold, just lateral to the cyst. A small mucosal flap is elevated directly over the cyst and the mass is then gently dissected from surrounding tissues. After removal of the cyst, the mucosal flap is redraped over the superior surface of the fold and excess mucosa is trimmed. Voice therapy after excision should be directed at controlling vocal abuse behaviors.

# CASE 39
## *Hemorrhagic Polyp of the True Vocal Fold*

### HISTORY

The patient is a 65-year-old female who presented with the chief complaint of mild dysphonia, characterized as a low pitched voice developing over a prolonged period of time. She was a high school gym teacher for more than 20 years and admitted to a strong history of vocal abuse behaviors during class. She was a nonsmoker and denied any other voice abnormalities

### EXAMINATION FINDINGS

Perceptually, the patient's voice was within normal limits but of low pitch dimensions. Maximum phonation time was also within normal limits. The next **voice sample** highlights the patient's voice.

Acoustic analysis revealed the following: (1) fundamental frequency @ 146 Hz, (2) jitter @ 0.55%, (3) shimmer @ 0.10 dB, and (4) harmonic to noise ratio @ 12.3 dB. With the exception of the pitch findings, which indicate a lower than average pitch for the patient's age and sex, all of these acoustic data are within normal limits.

Figure 6–39A illustrates the appearance of the vocal folds using videostroboscopy. Note the presence of a large hemorrhagic polyp occupying the middle one-third of the right true vocal fold. During phonation only a mild chink in the glottis is evident during the closed phases of vibration. Stroboscopy reveals a mildly retarded mucosal

**CD2**
**Track 6**

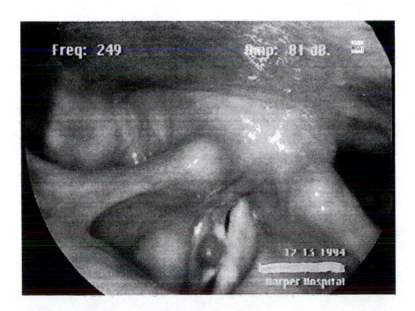

**FIGURE 6–39A.** This is a 65-year-old female with a hemorrhagic polyp occupying a large portion of the right true vocal fold. Note the deformation of the opposing fold during phonation, and the chink in the posterior and anterior glottis around this mass.

wave action on the affected side, especially over the superior surface of the true fold. Slight discoloration of the ipsilateral fold is evident. The polyp does not appear to interfere with the free margin vibratory characteristics of the involved vocal fold. This likely accounts for the relatively normal phonation features seen.

The clinical diagnosis: hemorrhagic polyp involving the middle one-third of the right true vocal fold. The relatively large polyp has caused mild retardation of the mucosal wave over the superior surface of the true vocal fold due to its mass effect. This likely inhibits the speed of vibration of the vocal folds and accounts for the abnormally low vocal pitch. However, the free margin of the fold is uninvolved, reflecting the normal perceptual and objective voice data.

The recommended treatment for this lesion was surgical excision, followed by speech therapy.

## TREATMENT RESULTS

The patient underwent uneventful surgical excision of the right hemorrhagic polyp, followed by speech therapy. Figure 6–39B demonstrates the vocal fold appearance 1 month postoperatively. Perceptually, she demonstrated normal voice, but persistent low pitch quality. She was placed on a voice program aimed at improving vocal pitch level and reducing vocal abuse patterns. The Visi-Pitch apparatus was utilized to raise her habitual speech frequency from 150 Hz to approximately 190 Hz. At this new fundamental frequency she demonstrated excellent vocal quality. She is currently undergoing further voice therapy.

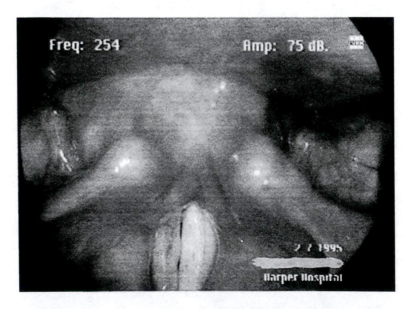

**FIGURE 6–39B.** This photograph was obtained following surgical excision of the hemorrhagic polyp. Note the marked improvement in the appearance of the larynx overall.

## DISCUSSION

Vocal fold polyps develop secondary to vocal abuse behaviors. They may occur abruptly with a submucosal hemorrhage, usually accompanied with acute dysphonia. The polyp may progressively enlarge due to repeated vocal trauma. Likewise, polyps may develop insidiously, owing to chronic abusive voice patterns. Vocal quality is usually altered when a polyp develops over the free margin of the true vocal fold, owing to mucosal wave disruption secondary to a mass effect. If the polyp is located distant from the vibratory margin of the true vocal fold, voice may be unaffected. Treatment for vocal fold polyps includes voice therapy, with or without surgical excision. Generally, therapy aimed at stopping vocal abuse behaviors will result in resolution of small and immature polyps. Large or mature polyps are better treated with surgical excision followed by therapy.

It is interesting to note that females are generally more apt to seek help for this condition than males. The low-pitch side effects are not usually of concern to males. In fact, we have discovered surface level vocal fold polyps on routine laryngeal examinations that did not result in clinically significant dysphonia in both males and females. With this fact in mind and strictly from a pathologic viewpoint, laryngologists and speech pathologists should not always believe what they hear in the voices of their patients. Conversely, when treating patients and analyzing the results of intervention, practitioners should be equally careful not to hear what they believe.

The current patient did not need to undergo phonosurgery. She elected to have the polyp excised for two reasons. First, she was uncomfortable with the low pitch feature. Second, she preferred to have the lesion removed for fear that it might cause more difficulty at a later time. Other patients may choose to wait and see, or try voice therapy alone.

# CASE 40
## *Early Vocal Fold Granuloma*

## HISTORY

The patient is a 46-year-old male college professor who presented with the chief complaint of progressive voice difficulty for the prior 2 months, as well as generalized vocal and cervical muscle fatigue. He admitted to occasional voice abuse and a high level of occupation-related stress. He denied reflux symptoms, smoking, throat clearing, or coughing behaviors.

## EXAMINATION FINDINGS

Perceptually, the patient's voice was moderately harsh-hoarse in quality with episodes of high pitch outbursts. Maximum phonation time was within normal limits. The next **voice sample** highlights this patient's dysphonic features.

**CD2
Track 7**

Acoustic analysis revealed the following: (1) fundamental frequency @ 118 Hz, (2) jitter @ 0.41%, (3) shimmer @ 0.12 dB, and (4) harmonic to noise ratio @ 10.1 dB. These acoustic findings are within normal limits.

Speech aerodynamic testing revealed the following: (1) mean transglottal airflow rate during phonation @ 707 cc/sec, (2) subglottal pressure estimate @ 5.3 cm $H_2O$, and (3) glottal resistance @ 83 cm $H_2O$/lps. The transglottal airflow findings were roughly seven times normal during phonation. The resistance data are roughly two times the normal degree of compression forces between the true vocal folds during phonation efforts. Whereas the flow findings suggest a hypofunctioning laryngeal mechanism, the resistance findings suggest glottal hyperfunctioning during voice efforts. These contradictory observations are not uncommon and are often associated with laryngeal muscle tension disorders.

Figure 6–40A demonstrates the appearance of the larynx at the time of videostroboscopy. Note the area of swelling on the posterior one-third of the superior surface and free margin of the right true vocal fold. Mucous tends to adhere to this irregular region. There is mild mucosal irregularity of the free edge of the right true fold as well. Diffuse arytenoid erythema and hyperplastic posterior commissure mucosa is evident. With phonatory efforts there is a generalized squeezing together of the supraglottic and glottic vocal tract, with a persistent posterior glottic chink. The mucosal wave dynamics remain unaffected.

The clinical diagnosis: mucosal edema and early granuloma formation of the posterior right true vocal fold, likely resulting from a muscle misuse voice disorder. Although the patient is asymptomatic, the mucosal changes are suggestive of reflux laryngitis. The aerodynamic findings suggest a mixture of excessive transglottic airflow during phonation and increased glottal resistance. These findings are not uncommon in patients suffering from muscle tension dysphonia. Treatment recommendations included voice therapy aimed at correcting abusive vocal behaviors and antireflux measures.

## TREATMENT RESULTS

The patient underwent several voice therapy sessions with focus on various aspects of proper breath support and easier onset of phonation behaviors. Although the acoustic analysis revealed a fundamental frequency of 118 Hz, the patient continually demonstrated an abnormally low habitual speech frequency in the 80–90 Hz range. Therefore,

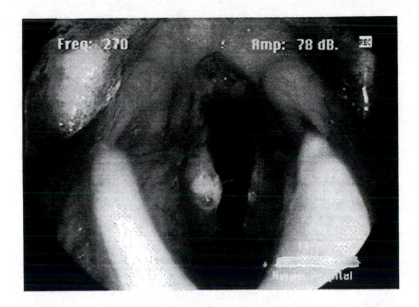

**FIGURE 6–40A.** Note the presence of early vocal fold granuloma on the posterior one-third of the right true vocal fold in a 46-year-old male patient. Pachydermal growth is also seen in the interarytenoid region.

emphasis was placed on raising the patient's habitual speech frequency to a slightly higher normal range.

The patient was discharged from the speech therapy program after demonstrating significant improvements in phonation. His voice was subjectively normal and the nodule had completely resolved. Figure 6–40B illustrates these results. The next brief **voice sample** highlights this gain.

**CD2**
**Track 7**

## DISCUSSION

Voice disorders may result from misuse of voluntary muscles of the supraglottic, glottic, and infraglottic vocal tract. These conditions have been referred to as muscle misuse voice disorders. Generalized isometric tension of all the laryngeal muscles is often associated with a posterior glottic chink due to the overpowering pull of the posterior cricoarytenoid muscles during phonation. This disorder may result in mucosal changes of the vocal folds, including nodules, chronic laryngitis, and polypoid degeneration. Acoustic analysis of such patients may reveal a mixed hypo-/hyperfunctional laryngeal mechanism. Treatment is aimed at correcting the muscle misuse behaviors. Surgery can often be avoided in most patients who comply with the voice therapy requirements.

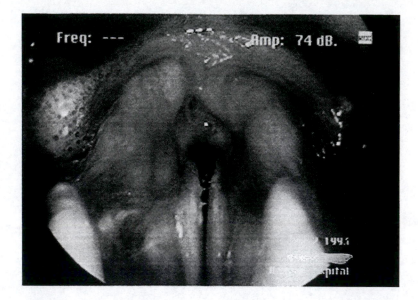

**FIGURE 6–40B.** This photograph was obtained following a voice therapy program. Note the resolution of the granulation change on the posterior one-third of the right true vocal fold. There is still some degree of mild pachydermia laryngis.

# CASE 41
## *T1 Glottic Carcinoma*

## HISTORY

This is a 52-year-old male who presented with the chief complaint of progressive hoarseness for the prior 4 months. He admitted to smoking one-half pack of cigarettes per day for the past 30 years and occasional alcohol use. He denied vocal abuse behaviors, reflux symptoms, hemoptysis, dyspnea, or weight loss. A recent biopsy of both vocal folds revealed squamous cell carcinoma, staged as T1b.

## EXAMINATION FINDINGS

Perceptually, the patient's voice was moderately hoarse-breathy with limited pitch and loudness controls. Maximum phonation time was 20 seconds. The next **voice sample** highlights these dysphonic features.

**CD2**
**Track 8**

Acoustic analysis revealed the following: (1) fundamental frequency @ 126 Hz, (2) jitter @ 0.69%, (3) shimmer @ 0.57 dB, and (4) harmonic to noise ratio @ 6.3 dB. These data point to a moderately unstable laryngeal mechanism, with excessive noise in the voice signal and abnormal variability in the frequency and amplitude vibratory activities of the vocal folds.

Speech aerodynamic testing revealed the following results: (1) mean transglottal airflow rate during phonation @ 20 cc/sec, (2) subglottal pressure estimate @ 9.6 cm $H_2O$, and (3) glottal resistance @ 280 cm $H_2O$/lps. These findings point to a significantly hyperfunctioning vocal fold mechanism, which disrupts airflow rate and increases vocal fold contact tension.

Figure 6–41A illustrates the appearance of the vocal folds using videostroboscopy. Note the following: (1) irregular anatomy of the vocal fold covers bilaterally, which may be the result of the recent biopsies, (2) absence of mucosal wave characteristics bilaterally, (3) complete closure at the midline during phonation efforts, and (4) mild hyperactivity of the ventricular folds during phonatory efforts.

The clinical diagnosis: bilateral squamous cell carcinoma of the true vocal folds with unimpaired vocal fold mobility, staged as T1b. Treatment for this lesion included full-course radiation therapy, followed by speech therapy.

## TREATMENT RESULTS: HALFWAY THROUGH RADIATION THERAPY

The patient returned for a full-scale voice evaluation halfway through radiation treatment. He reported frequent throat clearing behaviors, as well as mild dysphagia and odynophagia.

Perceptually, the patient's voice was mildly hoarse with occasional pitch breaks. The following **voice sample** demonstrates the patient's voice at this point in time.

**CD2**
**Track 8**

Acoustic analysis revealed the following: (1) fundamental frequency @ 137 Hz, (2) jitter @ 0.65%, (3) shimmer @ 0.52 dB, and (4) harmonic to noise ratio @ 4.5 dB. These data are not significantly different from that collected before treatment.

Speech aerodynamic testing yielded the following: (1) mean airflow rate @ 86 cc/sec, (2) subglottal pressure estimate @ 9.0 cm $H_2O$, (3) glottal resistance @ 30.0 cm $H_2O$/lps. The glottal resistance data are significantly improved over previous findings. In the previous evaluation the patient was generating hyperfunctional, compensatory vocal fold behavior. At this sitting glottal resistance measures were near normal.

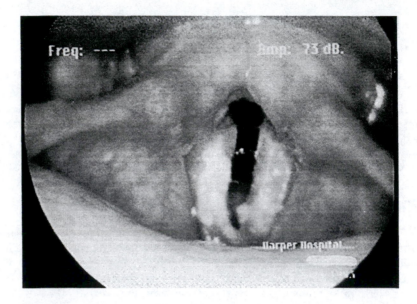

**FIGURE 6–41A.** This laryngeal photograph was obtained from a 52-year-old male with the diagnosis of T1b glottic squamous cell carcinoma. Note the diffuse erythema and cancerous growths along the covers and free edges of both true vocal folds.

Videostroboscopic examination (Figure 6–41B) illustrated the following: (1) bilateral erythema of the vocal folds and surrounding soft tissue, (2) a persistent chink in the middle third of the membranous glottis during phonation efforts, and (3) irregular vibratory mucosal wave characteristics during phonation. The patient's mildly hoarse dysphonia results from the overall edema and free edge irregularity of the vocal folds.

## TREATMENT RESULTS AFTER COMPLETION OF RADIATION THERAPY

After completion of radiation therapy the patient returned for a full-scale voice evaluation. He continued to experience dysphagia and odynophagia, with progressively worsening voice quality.

Perceptually, the patient's voice was mildly hoarse-harsh in quality, although pitch and loudness controls did not seem significantly altered. The following **voice sample** demonstrates the patient's voice.

**CD2
Track 8**

Acoustic analysis revealed the following: (1) fundamental frequency @ 128 Hz, (2) jitter @ 0.48%, (3) shimmer @ 0.70 dB, and (4) harmonic to noise ratio @ 13.1 dB. The harmonic to noise data are significantly improved over the previous session, indicating less noise in the voice signal. All other data are not significantly different from that collected previously.

Speech aerodynamic testing yielded the following: (1) mean airflow rate during phonation @ 277 cc/sec, and (2) subglottal pressure estimate @ 8.9 cm $H_2O$. These data point to a slightly greater airflow rate through the glottis during phonation than was obtained during previous sessions. This was likely due to the increased loudness used during this session.

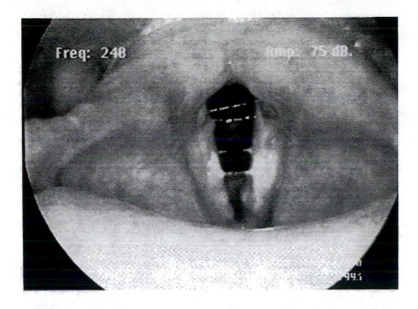

**FIGURE 6–41B.** This photograph was obtained from the same patient roughly halfway through radiation therapy. Note the moderate improvements in the appearance of the vocal folds.

Videostroboscopic examination (Figure 6–41C) illustrates the following: (1) mild erythema of the false vocal folds, (2) a small, persistent glottic chink in the middle third of the vocal folds during phonation efforts, and (3) irregular vibratory mucosal wave characteristics during phonation. These findings are not significantly different from previous exams, except that the true vocal folds themselves are less edematous and erythematous.

## TREATMENT RESULTS FOLLOWING SPEECH THERAPY

Two weeks following completion of radiation the patient began voice therapy aimed at adjusting the fundamental frequency and average loudness levels during conversational speech. Using the VisiPitch apparatus he was able to raise his fundamental frequency, measured at 100 Hz, to a more optimal level of 135 Hz. Using exercises to provide better breath support, conversational volume was raised from 30 dB to 45 dB. After three treatment sessions the patient demonstrated significant improvement in vocal quality.

## DISCUSSION

Squamous cell carcinoma of the larynx usually results from repeated exposure of the laryngeal mucosa to cigarette smoke. If the carcinoma is confined to the true vocal folds, patients will generally present with persistent hoarseness. Therefore, hoarseness lasting greater than 3 weeks in any patient with a smoke exposure history should be intensively evaluated. Unlike other head and neck malignancies, glottic carcinoma presents with symptoms (i.e., hoarseness, sore throat, ear pain) early in the course of disease, therefore allowing for diagnosis of earlier stage cancers. The standard treat-

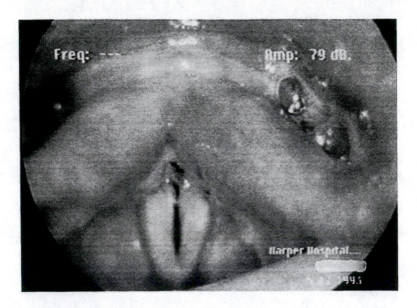

**FIGURE 6–41C.** This photograph was obtained at the completion of radiation therapy. Note the marked improvement in comparison to Figure 6–41A. The patient still struggles with a mild degree of glottal incompetency and this correlates with his persistent mild degree of hoarse vocal quality.

ment of T1 glottic carcinomas is radiation therapy, with surgical intervention utilized for radiation treatment failures. A subset of patients with superficial mid vocal fold lesions can be effectively treated by $CO_2$ laser excision, instead of radiation therapy, with comparable local control, survival, and vocal quality. Radiation therapy for T1 glottic carcinomas results in a 90% local control and 5 year disease-free survival rate. Vocal quality, however, rarely returns to normal.

# CASE 42
## *Bilateral Vocal Fold Nodules*

## HISTORY

This is a 39-year-old female who presented with a chief complaint of progressive hoarseness occurring over a 3-month period. Her history was significant for increased voice use due to choir activities in her local church during the past few months. She also admitted to chronic throat clearing behaviors and a 16 pack per year smoking history.

## EXAMINATION FINDINGS

Perceptually, the patient's voice was moderately hoarse-breathy in quality with low pitch characteristics. Maximum phonation time was within normal limits. The next **voice sample** highlights these dysphonic features.

**CD2**
**Track 9**

Acoustic analysis revealed the following: (1) fundamental frequency @ 173 Hz, (2) jitter @ 0.77%, (3) shimmer @ 0.23 dB, and (4) harmonic to noise ratio @ 12.5 dB. The pitch findings are lower than normal for the patient's age and sex. The other acoustic data collected fall within normal limits.

Speech aerodynamic testing revealed the following results: (1) mean transglottal airflow rate during phonation @ 282 cc/sec, (2) subglottal pressure estimate @ 6.5 cm $H_2O$, and (3) glottal resistance @ 17.7 cm $H_2O$/lps. The flow data are roughly three times the normal degree of transglottal airflow during voice efforts. The airflow resistance at the glottal inlet is roughly one-half the normal value measured during phonation. These findings are suggestive of a hypofunctioning laryngeal mechanism.

Figure 6–42A illustrates the appearance of the vocal folds using videostroboscopy. Multiple nodule formations are noted bilaterally on the free margins of the true vocal folds. During the closed phase of vibration the glottis assumes an hourglass configuration caused by interruption of complete vocal fold closure by these nodular masses. Under stroboscopic visualization mild irregularities of the mucosal waves are noted, more pronounced on the left, secondary to the load effects from these multiple nodules.

The clinical diagnosis: multiple bilateral vocal fold nodules, more pronounced on the left free margin of the vocal fold. Complete resolution of these nodules with voice therapy alone was thought unlikely due to the multiplicity of these masses. Therefore, surgical removal followed by speech therapy was recommended.

## TREATMENT RESULTS

The patient underwent surgical excision of bilateral vocal fold nodules. This was performed as staged procedures to lessen the likelihood of anterior commissure webbing. The excisions were performed uneventfully and, following recovery, the patient was started on a voice therapy program. Treatment focused on teaching vocal hygiene through pitch, loudness, and breath support regulation exercises using the VisiPitch device. The patient was extremely motivated to improve vocal behaviors and she worked diligently during this 8-week treatment program.

**CD2**
**Track 9**

Laryngeal study and vocal assessment were obtained just prior to discharging the patient from voice therapy. Perceptually, her voice was significantly improved, with only mild dysphonia and a higher pitch level compared to her pretreatment fundamental frequency. The following **voice sample** demonstrates the patient's posttherapy voice. Acoustic analysis revealed the following: (1) maximum phonation time within

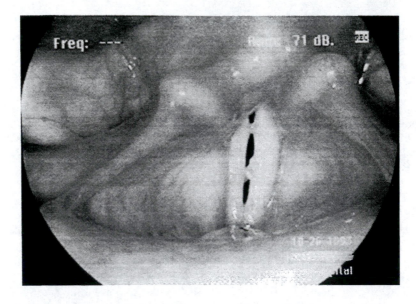

**FIGURE 6–42A.** This photograph demonstrates the presence of multiple bilateral vocal fold nodules, which interfere with glottal competency.

normal limits, (2) fundamental frequency @ 238 Hz, (3) jitter @ 1.72%, (4) shimmer @ 0.12 dB, (5) harmonic to noise ratio @ 15.7 dB.

Speech aerodynamic testing yielded the following: (1) mean airflow rate @ 469 cc/sec, (2) subglottal pressure estimate @ 5.3 cm $H_2O$, (3) glottal resistance @ 12 cm $H_2O$/lps. These data are mildly abnormal, suggestive of four times the normal degree of transglottal air flow during phonation and one-half the normal degree of compression forces between the true vocal folds during phonation.

Videostroboscopic examination (Figure 6–42B) illustrated mild irregularity of the true vocal fold free margins, which represents substantial improvement over the multinodular appearance presurgically. During phonation efforts the true vocal folds display a persistent chink across the entire length of the glottis, which may account for the increased airflow and reduced resistance findings.

Overall, the patient demonstrated significant subjective improvement in voice quality and resolution of multiple vocal fold nodules, as seen with videostroboscopy.

## DISCUSSION

Vocal fold nodules develop secondary to vocal abuse behaviors. Nodules are usually single, bilateral, small masses that involve the anteroposterior midpoint of the membranous true vocal fold. Multiple nodules may uncommonly occur over the free margins of the true vocal folds. These lesions may disrupt mucosal wave characteristics, owing to their load effect on the superficial layer of the lamina propria. Incomplete glottic closure may occur due to the mass effect of these lesions. These findings explain the perceptual hoarse-breathy quality heard in this patient. Surgical excision is often recommended followed by speech therapy for multiple mature nodules. Certainly, if the patient fails to practice proper vocal hygiene postoperatively, the pathology is likely to recur.

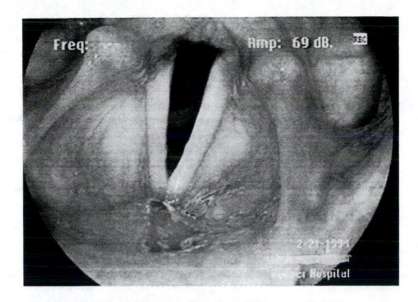

**FIGURE 6–42B.** This photograph was obtained from the same 39-year-old female following surgical excision of the nodules. Note that with the exception of a mild degree of irregularity on the free margins of the vocal folds there is substantial improvement in the overall appearance of this mechanism.

# CASE 43
## *Recurrent Vocal Fold Papillomas*

## HISTORY

This is a 27-year-old female who presented with a 2-year history of papillomas involving the true vocal folds. She underwent $CO_2$ laser excision of right-sided vocal fold papillomas approximately 2 years previously. Postoperatively, her voice was subjectively normal. However, 1 month following this procedure voice difficulties returned. She presented at this point in time with the chief complaint of hoarseness, vocal fatigue, and mild shortness of breath.

## EXAMINATION FINDINGS

**CD2**
**Track 10**

Perceptually, the patient's voice was moderately hoarse-breathy. Maximum phonation time was less than 7 seconds. The next **voice sample** highlights these voice abnormalities.

Acoustic analysis revealed the following: (1) fundamental frequency @ 232 Hz, (2) jitter @ 4.6%, (3) shimmer @ 0.61 dB, and (4) harmonic to noise ratio @ 0.60 dB. These data are moderately to severely abnormal. The jitter findings point to a marked degree of instability in the cycle-to-cycle vibratory characteristics of the true vocal folds. The harmonics data point to a substantial amount of noise in the voice signal.

Figure 6–43A illustrates the appearance of the laryngeal inlet using videostroboscopy. Note the appearance of bilateral papillary growths emanating from the free margins of the vocal folds. The right fold has two focal areas of involvement, whereas the left fold is less severely involved. At no time during vocal efforts is complete glottal competency observed due to these lesions. Mucosal waves are diminished in response to the load effects of these masses. The patient demonstrates normal vocal fold mobility and the airway is not compromised.

The clinical diagnosis: bilateral recurrent vocal fold papillomas. Recommended treatment included surgical excision of these lesions, followed by voice therapy. The technique of microflap excision of diseased mucosa, with the hope of completely eradicating the papilloma, versus a more standard technique of $CO_2$ laser ablation, without complete elimination and probable recurrence of disease, was discussed with the patient. She elected for microflap excision of these lesions.

## TREATMENT RESULTS AFTER THERAPY

Microflap excisions of bilateral vocal fold papillomas were performed in a one-stage procedure. Under high magnification intraoperatively, papillomatous growths were noted to involve the anterior commissure region. These particular lesions were carefully ablated using a $CO_2$ laser in an attempt to avoid web formation. Postoperatively the patient was placed on antibiotics for 7 days, H2 blockers for 6 weeks, and absolute voice rest for 2 weeks.

**CD2**
**Track 10**

The patient returned 17 days postoperatively for evaluation and institution of a voice therapy program. Perceptually, the voice was moderately to severely hoarsebreathy in quality. Acoustic analysis data corroborated these findings. Figure 6–43B demonstrates the videostroboscopic examination. The free edges of the true vocal folds look smooth and clean. During phonation there is a persistent chink in the glottis across the entire length, and mucosal waves are retarded. These findings likely account for the aforementioned dysphonia. The next **voice sample** illustrates the postoperative voice.

At the outset of voice therapy the primary objective was to improve valving capabilities of the true vocal folds. Several valving techniques were introduced, including

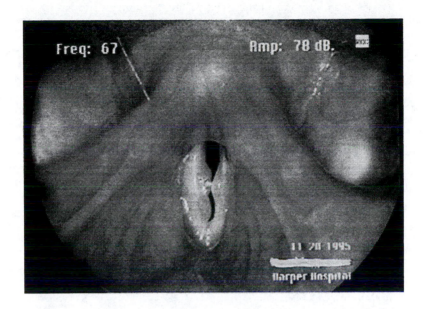

**FIGURE 6–43A.** This photograph was obtained from a 27-year-old female with recurring laryngeal papillomas. Note the growths on the free margin of both vocal folds, more pronounced on the right side.

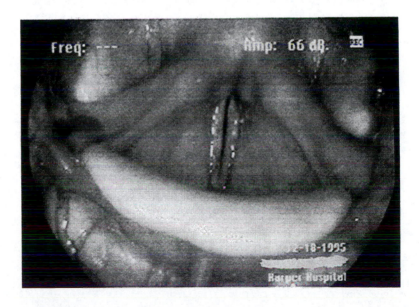

**FIGURE 6–43B.** This illustration was obtained from the patient roughly 2 weeks following surgical excision of the papillomas. Note the improved appearance of both vocal folds.

the use of a neck band, pushing and pulling techniques, and head turning, especially to the left. These methods proved beneficial to improving voice output in terms of vocal quality and intensity measures. However, without these valving maneuvers voice quality diminished during contextual speech. In addition, breath support exercises were prescribed as homework assignments between sessions.

One month postoperatively the patient demonstrated a harsh-strained vocal quality. The muscle tension dysphonia was likely a compensatory reaction to the inability to effectively vibrate the vocal folds. In addition, during contextual speech there was a tendency to drift significantly higher in pitch, thus causing shrill vocal quality and poor overall speech. Using the Visi-Pitch apparatus, the patient decreased her habitual speech frequency from 290 Hz to 256 Hz. At this level she generated reasonably good voice quality, both in isolated vowel production and in running speech.

After eight sessions she continued to have a harsh-strained vocal quality. Stroboscopic examination revealed the vocal folds to be free of papillomas. However, mucosal waves were virtually absent during phonation and she was heavily recruiting the false vocal folds during most vocalizations. With no demonstrable voice improvement 2½ months postoperatively, the patient elected to seek further treatment elsewhere.

## DISCUSSION

Laryngeal papillomas are cauliflower-like lesions caused by infection with the human papilloma virus (HPV). This lesion is the most common benign neoplasm of the larynx. During infancy or adulthood its presenting symptoms are hoarseness or airway obstruction. The natural history of this disease is one of multiple recurrences, especially with the juvenile onset type. Therefore, $CO_2$ laser vaporization of these lesions, although the accepted procedure of choice today, is thought to be only palliative in most cases. Multiple recurrences are thought to be caused by persistent growth of HPV in subclinically infected normal appearing tissue bordering the area of treatment. The goals of laser vaporization are to eradicate this lesion, establish an adequate airway, and improve voice without causing submucosal damage, which may result in vocal fold scarring and fibrosis. Simultaneous removal of papillomas from both sides of the anterior or posterior commissure should be avoided, as this maneuver often results in commissure web formation.

Microflap excision of vocal fold papillomas is a technique whereby diseased mucosa from the vocal fold is microscopically elevated and removed. In contrast to $CO_2$ laser ablation of only the surface of such lesions, this procedure is designed to fully eradicate HPV-containing tissues without disrupting the vocal ligament. Thus, lesions are removed in one stage with hopes of reducing the likelihood of recurrence and vocal fold scarring. The current patient remained disease-free nearly 3 months after her original operation. However, her voice remained moderately to severely harsh-strained, due to submucosal scarring.

# CASE 44
## *Closed Head Injury with Vocal Fold Paralysis*

## HISTORY

This is a 46-year-old male who suffered a closed head injury 10 months prior to this evaluation. The injury resulted in cognitive deficits, breathy dysphonia, hypernasal speech, and dysphagia for both liquids and solids, necessitating placement of a gastrostomy feeding tube. The patient complained of inability to handle his own secretions, with frequent coughing and throat clearing behaviors.

## EXAMINATION FINDINGS

Perceptually, the patient's voice had a moderate to severe wet-gurgly, hoarse-breathy quality with mild hypernasality. Maximum phonation time was less than 5 seconds. The next **voice sample** highlights the patient's speech and voice behaviors.

Acoustic analysis revealed the following: (1) fundamental frequency @ 183 Hz, (2) jitter @ 1.64%, (3) shimmer @ 0.52 dB, and (4) harmonic to noise ratio @ 6.8 dB. These results demonstrate significant pitch instability and features of excessive noise in the voice signal.

**CD2**
**Track 11**

Figure 6–44A illustrates the appearance of the vocal folds using videostroboscopy. The following salient characteristics are noted: (1) the left true vocal fold is paralyzed in a lateral position with incomplete closure of the folds at the midline during phonatory efforts, thus explaining the breathy dysphonia, and (2) there is profound pooling of secretions in the vallecula, piriform sinuses, and postcricoid regions, with spillage of saliva into the glottic inlet. This results in the wet-gurgly voice quality and episod-

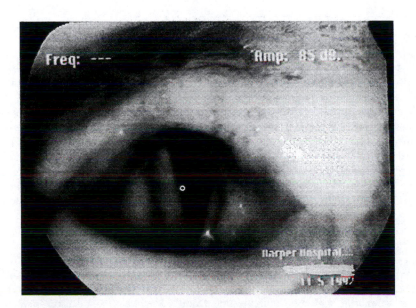

**FIGURE 6–44A.** This photograph demonstrates left vocal fold paralysis in a 46-year-old male who suffered a closed head injury. Note the profound glottal incompetency during phonation effort as well as the marked degree of secretion pooling in the piriform sinuses.

ic coughing and choking events. Oral cavity examination revealed left soft palate paralysis causing velopharyngeal insufficiency and hypernasality of speech.

The clinical diagnosis: left vagal nerve injury at the brainstem level resulting in: (1) vocal fold paralysis with breathy dysphonia, (2) velopharyngeal incompetency with hypernasal speech quality, and (3) dysphagia with aspiration, likely resulting from a combination of glottal and palatal incompetence, and left-sided pharyngeal weakness. Treatment for this constellation of flaccid dysarthric symptoms involved rendering glottal and velopharyngeal competency by performing a medialization thyroplasty and fitting a palatal lift appliance, respectively. The patient was immediately started on a speech and swallowing therapy program.

## TREATMENT RESULTS AFTER SURGERY

The patient returned for a full-scale voice evaluation after undergoing a left-sided medialization thyroplasty. He continued to display hypernasality of speech due to the aforementioned palatal incompetence. A modified barium swallow showed persistent aspiration of both liquid and paste substances due to oral and pharyngeal musculature dysmotility.

**CD2**
**Track 11**

Perceptually, the patient's voice was mildly improved. Maximum phonation time was 5 seconds. The next **voice sample** highlights the patient's persistent speech and voice difficulties.

Acoustic analysis revealed the following: (1) fundamental frequency @ 141 Hz, (2) jitter @ 1.2%, (3) shimmer @ 0.37 dB, and (4) harmonic to noise ratio @ 5.8 dB. These data suggest a more natural "male" pitch and less instability of vibration of the vocal folds during phonation.

Videostroboscopic examination (Figure 6–44B) illustrates the medialized left vocal fold. There remains a persistent posterior glottic chink during phonatory efforts. Pooled secretions persist in the vallecula and piriform sinuses.

## TREATMENT RESULTS AFTER PALATAL PROSTHESIS FITTING

The patient was lost to follow-up for 10 months, but returned for a full-scale voice evaluation after being fit with a palatal lift prosthesis. The patient now claimed to be tolerating regular diet without symptoms of aspiration.

Perceptually, phonation was hoarse-breathy in quality with a wet-gurgly overlay. Resonation was moderately hypernasal with marked degrees of nasal air emissions during ongoing speech. Maximum phonation time was approximately 5 seconds.

**CD2**
**Track 11**

Acoustic analysis with the lift in place revealed the following: (1) fundamental frequency @ 169 Hz, (2) jitter @ 1.5%, (3) shimmer @ 0.50 dB, and (4) harmonic to noise ratio @ 12.0 dB. Pitch jitter data point to instability of vibration of the vocal folds and a higher than normal fundamental frequency. The following **voice sample** demonstrates the patient's voice and speech characteristics.

Speech aerodynamic testing with the lift in place yielded the following: (1) mean airflow rate @ 3,465 cc/sec, (2) subglottal pressure @ 9 cm $H_2O$, and (3) glottal resistance @ 2.2 cm $H_2O$/lps. These data were similar to that obtained without the lift. They indicate transglottal airflow to be roughly 30 times normal and glottal resistance roughly 1/25 the normal amount of compression forces between the vocal folds during phonation efforts. Maximum volume produced by the patient during speaking efforts was approximately one-third the normal level expected.

Nasal airflow velocities with and without the prosthesis in place were approximately 250 cc/sec, which is moderately excessive.

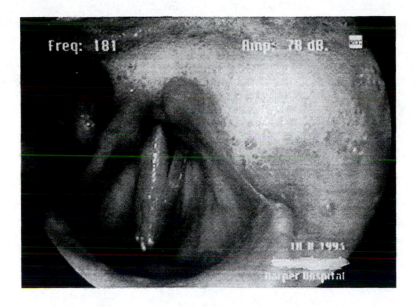

**FIGURE 6–44B.** This photograph was collected following a left Isshiki medialization thyroplasty. Note the improvement in glottal competency. Salivary secretions continue to pool in the piriform sinuses. This difficulty correlates with the patient's coexistent dysphagia and velopharyngeal paralysis.

Videostroboscopic examination illustrates the following: (1) the left true vocal fold is atrophic and hanging in a paramedian position, (2) closure at the midline is incomplete, as there remains a persistent posterior glottic chink during phonatory efforts, (3) there is pooling of secretions in the piriform sinuses and vallecula, and (4) mucosal wave characteristics are irregular due to the vocal fold paralysis.

Clinical impression: persistent incompetency of the glottis and palate resulting in breathy dysphonia and hypernasality of speech, respectively. The patient was referred back to his prosthodontist for palatal lift augmentation. He was encouraged to continue voice therapy sessions focused on voice building exercises, as well as a swallowing program designed to gradually advance oral feedings. Shortly thereafter the patient was lost again to follow-up and has not been seen in the voice and swallowing center to date.

## DISCUSSION

The patient described suffered a vagal nerve injury at the level of the brainstem. This resulted in glottic and palatal incompetence, as well as pharyngeal weakness. The clinical diagnosis was flaccid dysarthria. Primary treatment for this condition usually includes speech and swallowing therapy to facilitate glottic and velopharyngeal competency and to reduce the risk of aspiration pneumonia. Ancillary procedures, including medialization thyroplasty or vocal fold injections, often result in immediate glottic competency, improved phonation, and better airway protection because of a stronger cough mechanism. A palatal adhesion technique or palatal lift appliance usually reduces velopharyngeal incompetency and augments both speech and swallowing activities.

In the present case history, hypernasality and associated articulatory imprecision were not corrected with the palatal lift appliance. This was probably due to a suboptimal prosthetic fit. Although the patient experienced mild voice improvement after the medialization thyroplasty procedure, he continued to suffer from a posterior glottic chink, which likely accounted for his persistent breathy voice. Adding an arytenoid adduction procedure to the medialization thyroplasty may have reduced this chink, improved vocal quality, increased phonation time, and lessened symptoms of vocal fatigue. This secondary procedure was mentioned to the patient, but he refused to submit to further surgery.

# CASE 45
## *Supraglottic Laryngectomy*

## HISTORY

This is a 57-year-old male with a significant drinking and smoking history who presented 8 months prior with a T1 squamous cell carcinoma of the left piriform sinus. The lesion was treated with full course radiation therapy, but a repeat triple endoscopy with biopsy of the original cancer site revealed persistent disease. A salvage operation was performed, which included an extended supraglottic laryngectomy (supraglottic laryngectomy, partial pharyngectomy) and left modified radical neck dissection. Postoperatively, the patient was tracheotomy and nasogastric tube dependent due to supraglottic and hypopharyngeal edema. He presented at this time for postoperative speech and swallowing therapy.

## TREATMENT RESULTS AFTER SWALLOWING THERAPY

The patient had an uneventful postoperative recovery and was started on a swallowing therapy program 12 days after surgery. He was initially taught a supraglottic swallow technique using thickened nectar and pudding food substances. Briefly, the technique included: (1) tucking the chin to chest, (2) swallowing against a closed glottis (i.e., holding the breath), and (3) coughing to clear the glottis of any residue before inhaling. Although he understood and was able to perform the maneuver, first attempts at swallowing resulted in aspiration of approximately 50% of all food substances. He made moderate gains over the next 2 weeks, demonstrating improved success with strained peaches and thickened juices, only aspirating approximately 10–20% of the bolus. Nasogastric tube feedings were continued to provide supplemental nourishment. He was instructed on a home oral feeding diet which included such foods as strained vegetables, pureed foods, oatmeal, milkshakes, and small curd cottage cheese. The next **voice sample** demonstrates the patient's voice characteristics.

Videostroboscopic exam (Figure 6–45A) reveals the postoperative larynx and hypopharynx. Note erythema and edema of the arytenoids, obliteration of the left piriform sinus, and pooling of secretions around the operative site.

After a 6-week absence from the swallowing and voice center due to complications from chemotherapy, the patient returned for further swallowing therapy. Using the supraglottic swallow technique and valving maneuvers designed to enhance glottic closure, he demonstrated minimal signs of aspiration with thickened juices, soups, and shakes. Within 1 week the nasogastric feeding tube was removed. Thereafter, he continued to show improvement, steadily gained weight, and was soon tolerating a variety of food substances. Videostroboscopic exam (Figure 6–45B) demonstrates a slightly bowed and weakened right true vocal fold, due to a right-sided superior laryngeal nerve injury following surgery. However, adequate glottic closure occurs during phonatory and swallowing efforts. There is mild pooling of secretions in the postcricoid region that is readily cleared with coughing or swallowing maneuvers.

**CD2**
**Track 12**

## TREATMENT RESULTS AFTER SPEECH THERAPY

After achieving adequate oral intake following several swallowing therapy sessions, attention was turned to the voice. Perceptually, the patient had a hoarse-breathy vocal

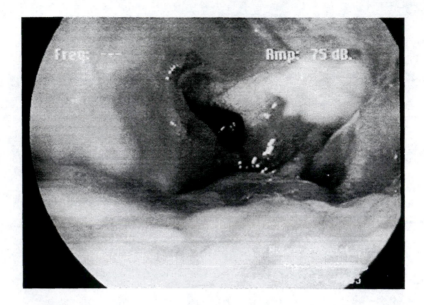

**FIGURE 6–45A.** This photograph was obtained from a 57-year-old male who had undergone a supraglottic laryngectomy within a week of this examination. Note the profound degree of erythema and thick secretion accumulation in the surgical field.

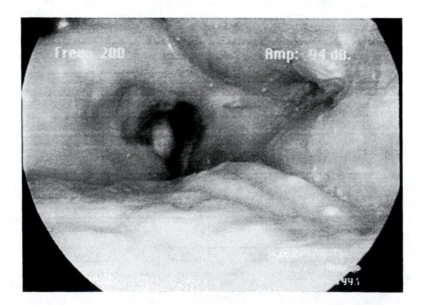

**FIGURE 6–45B.** This photograph was obtained roughly 6 weeks following surgery. Note the significant resolution of the erythema in the surgical field. Glottal functioning has become easier as a result of these changes. Note the persistent chink in the posterior one-half of the glottis during the closed phases of vibration of the vocal folds associated with voice activity.

quality due to the aforementioned superior laryngeal nerve injury. The next **voice sample** demonstrates the voice quality. Periodically, secretions penetrated the laryngeal inlet causing a wet-gurgly voice. Using the Visi-Pitch apparatus, vocal exercises were aimed at reproducing his optimal fundamental frequency of 140 Hz during conversational speech. Vocal intensity was targeted between 40–50 dB. He was given homework assignments using vowel sounds to practice pitch and intensity control. During this time period the patient made some gains, but the voice remained hoarse-breathy in quality. Despite these difficulties the patient did quite well and no longer needed formal voice or swallowing therapy. Upon discharge from the treatment center, he was delighted with the progress he had made, and was referred back to his treating physician.

**CD2
Track 12**

## DISCUSSION

Treatment for piriform sinus cancers has traditionally included surgery followed by radiation therapy, with dismal overall 5-year disease-free survival rates ranging between 10 and 35%. Surgical options include partial laryngopharyngectomy or, if there is high suspicion for swallowing difficulties and/or aspiration after surgery, total laryngectomy and partial pharyngectomy.

Recently, organ preservation using induction chemotherapy (ci-platinum plus 5-fluorouracil) followed by radiation if a complete response is achieved, or surgery if less than a complete response occurs (arm 1), has been compared to standard surgery following by radiation therapy (arm 2) in a European Organization of Research Therapy in Cancer (EORTC) study reported in 1994. The study included 197 patients with piriform sinus carcinomas, all of whom were considered resectable. A comparison of 3year disease-free survival rates between the two arms showed no statistically significant differences. However, it was possible to save the larynx of approximately 1 out of 3 patients using the organ preservation protocol. To date, 5-year disease-free survival rates have not been reported.

There are significant indications suggesting that piriform sinus carcinoma is a less than ideal site for organ preservation. Of primary concern is the realization that over two-thirds of patients receiving the organ preservation regimen will fail treatment and need salvage surgery. Performing a laryngopharyngectomy in irradiated tissues is problematic because of increased morbidity and mortality rates. In addition, detecting recurrent or persistent disease is difficult because of the relative inaccessibility of the piriforms during office examinations.

Induction chemotherapy may play an important role in determining which tumors will respond to radiation therapy and which ones should undergo early surgical resection. However, until more definitive data are collected to compare the two treatment arms, controversy will exist regarding the best treatment plan for this lethal cancer.

# CASE 46
## *Fungal Involvement of the Vocal Fold*

### HISTORY

This is a 71-year-old male who presented to the voice center 9 months after undergoing resection of an extensive right submandibular gland adenoid cystic carcinoma, followed by combination photon and neutron therapy to the primary site and cervical region. His postradiation course was complicated by wound breakdown and severe oral and laryngeal mucositis. He returned with complaints of progressive breathy dysphonia and symptoms of aspiration on liquids.

### EXAMINATION FINDINGS

**CD2
Track 13**

Perceptually, the patient's voice was profoundly breathy in quality. Maximum phonation time was less than 3 seconds, which was significantly abnormal. The next brief **voice sample** highlights this voice disturbance.

Figure 6–46A illustrates the appearance of the vocal folds using videostroboscopy. The patient exhibits a large, exophytic plaque emanating from the left true vocal fold. The lesion fixes the fold in a paramedian position, inhibiting any movements during phonatory efforts. The right side of the larynx looks inflamed, and the true fold is hypomobile and poorly visualized.

Clinical diagnosis: The patient was taken to the operating room for direct laryngoscopy and biopsy of the left vocal fold growth. Histopathological analysis confirmed the characteristic fungal hyphae of candida. The patient was started on oral antifungal medication.

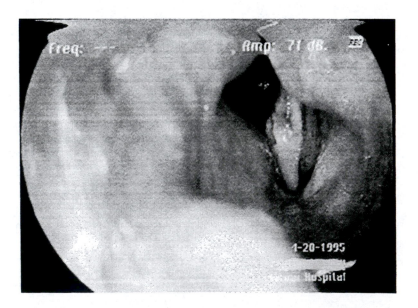

**FIGURE 6–46A.** This illustration demonstrates a fungal lesion of the left true vocal fold and surrounding soft tissue in a 71-year-old male who had recently received a combination of photon and neutron therapy for adenoid cystic carcinoma of the submandibular gland on the right side.

## TREATMENT RESULTS

After receiving 6 weeks of oral ketoconazole the patient returned for a repeat laryngeal evaluation.

Perceptually, the patient's voice remained profoundly breathy during all conversational efforts. Maximum phonation time was less than 5 seconds.

Videostroboscopic examination (Figure 6–46B) shows resolution of the left-sided fungal lesion. Movement of the left fold has returned; however, both folds remain paretic. During the entire examination, glottal incompetency was evident.

## DISCUSSION

The pathology presented in this case is unusual. The differential diagnosis for such a lesion includes carcinoma, chondritis with exuberant granulation formation, or an infectious etiology. The severe laryngeal mucositis induced by radiation therapy, combined with the patient's debilitating illness, likely accounted for his fungal superinfection. Other fungal organisms known to infect the larynx include histoplasmosis, blastomycosis, coccidiomycosis, actinomycosis, cryptococcosis, sporotrichosis, and aspergillosis. These organisms typically affect immunocompromised or debilitated patients and histology will show multinucleated giant cells associated with an inflammatory reaction. Not uncommonly, the inflammatory reaction may stimulate hyperplasia of the overlying squamous epithelium, resembling invasive carcinoma. Histologic confirmation of giant cells will suggest the diagnosis of fungal disease, rather than carcinoma. Treatment for this condition includes use of IV or oral antifungal medications, such as ketoconazole, nystatin, flucytosine, fluconazole, itraconazole, or amphotericin B.

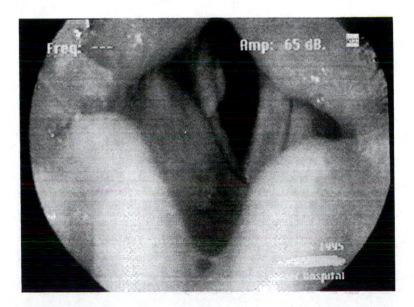

**FIGURE 6–46B.** This laryngeal photograph was obtained 6 weeks following pharmacologic treatment for the fungal lesions. Note the marked improvement in the appearance of the laryngeal inlet. There is still a tag of hyperplastic tissue on the posterior one-half of the right true vocal fold. Also note the bowing of the left true vocal fold.

# CASE 47
## Gelfoam Injection for Vocal Fold Paralysis

## HISTORY

This is a 65-year-old male who presented with a chief complaint of breathiness after undergoing a left-sided carotid endarterectomy. He was extubated uneventfully immediately after the operation with no voice difficulties, but became progressively dysphonic 72 hours after the operation. Upon further questioning he admitted to becoming "winded" when attempting to carry on a conversation, and suffered from aspiration with administration of liquids.

## EXAMINATION FINDINGS

Perceptually, the patient's voice was moderately to severely breathy-hoarse in quality. Maximum phonation time was less than 5 seconds, which was significantly abnormal. The next **voice sample** highlights these voice features.

**CD2**
**Track 14**

Acoustic analysis revealed the following: (1) fundamental frequency @ 151 Hz, (2) jitter @ 4.7%, (3) shimmer @ 1.4 dB, and (4) harmonic to noise ratio @ 0.91 dB. These data are markedly abnormal. The jitter and shimmer findings point to a substantial amount of instability in the vibratory cycles of the true vocal folds. The harmonics data indicate a significant amount of noise in the voice signal.

Figure 6–47A illustrates the appearance of the vocal folds using videostroboscopy. The left vocal fold is in a paramedian position and remains relatively motionless dur-

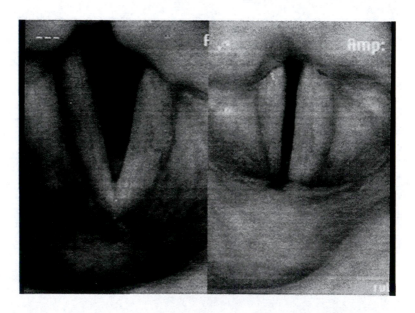

**FIGURE 6–47A.** This photograph illustrates the appearance of the vocal folds at rest as well as during phonatory effort in a 65-year-old male with left vocal fold paresis following an endarterectomy. Note the bowing of the involved side and the glottal incompetency that results.

ing all phonatory maneuvers. There is mild bowing of the left fold as a result of its inherent muscle weakness. The right true fold crosses the midline to provide near complete posterior glottic seal at the level of the vocal processes of the arytenoids. However, there is inadequate closure of the membranous vocal folds, thus creating an "elliptical" shaped anterior glottic defect during phonatory efforts. This defect accounts for the aforementioned perceptual and acoustic disturbances.

The clinical diagnosis: left-sided vocal fold paralysis after a carotid endarterectomy procedure. The history of normal voice after extubation, with progressive hoarseness beginning 72 hours later, points toward a neurapraxic (temporary) injury of the left recurrent laryngeal nerve. Treatment for this condition included gelfoam injection of the left vocal fold, followed by stimulative voice therapy to help provide greater valving at the level of the glottis.

## TREATMENT RESULTS AFTER SURGERY

The patient returned for a full-scale voice evaluation after undergoing gelfoam injection of the left true vocal fold. Immediately after the injection the patient had improved voice quality and swallowing, better cough, and less shortness of breath during conversational speech.

Perceptually, the patient's voice was mildly to moderately hoarse-breathy in quality with occasional coughing and throat clearing behaviors. The next **voice sample** highlights the postoperative voice characteristics.

**CD2**
**Track 14**

Acoustic analysis revealed the following: (1) fundamental frequency @ 152 Hz, (2) jitter @ 0.63%, (3) shimmer @ 0.26 dB, and (4) harmonic to noise ratio @ 10.8 dB. These data are considered normal.

Videostroboscopic examination (Figure 6–47B) illustrates the left vocal fold to be full and resting in a near median position. During phonatory efforts adequate glottic seal is obtained over the entire free margin. No motion of the involved cord was observed.

## TREATMENT RESULTS AFTER VOICE THERAPY

Postoperatively the patient was placed in a voice therapy program designed to stimulate return of true vocal fold function through valving exercises. To date, he continues therapy and is making nice progress.

## DISCUSSION

Not infrequently, a patient will suffer a neurapraxic or sometimes permanent injury of the recurrent laryngeal nerve after a carotid endarterectomy or other type neck procedure. The patient will typically complain of the following: (1) breathy dysphonia, due to weakness of the thyroarytenoid muscle complex, (2) coughing spells from aspiration of saliva or liquids due to inadequate glottic seal during swallowing, and (3) shortness of breath during attempts at conversational speech because of excess glottal air escape while phonating. Voice therapy, designed to stimulate return of vocal fold function or to help provide better compensation from the normal functioning fold, can yield encouraging results. However, improvement may not be seen for days, or even months. For those symptomatic patients with presumed neurapraxia of the recurrent laryngeal nerve and "elliptical" glottal defects, gelfoam injection can provide immediate improvement of swallowing function and voice quality. Gelfoam is nearly completely reabsorbed by the tissues within 10 weeks of injection, thus giving symptomatic relief while waiting for return of function. If vocal fold compensation or normal movement fails to occur, and voice quality deteriorates after 10 weeks, repeat gelfoam injection can

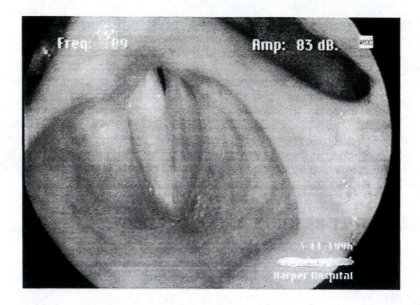

**FIGURE 6–47B.** This photograph was obtained following gelfoam injection into the left true vocal fold to augment glottal competency. Note the improvement in closure at the midline during phonatory effort. Also note the overall discoloration of the treated vocal fold.

be performed. For protracted paralysis, that which lasts more than 9 months, more definitive phonosurgical intervention may be indicated. Use of Teflon, fat, collagen, or medialization thyroplasty techniques will usually produce good results.

# CASE 48
## *Vocal Process Contact Ulcerations*

## HISTORY

This is a 58-year-old male with a smoking history who presented to his local otolaryngologist with a chief complaint of progressive hoarseness occurring over a 12-month period. The patient admitted to chronic voice abuse patterns, both at work and at home. He also described reflux symptoms, including heartburn, acid regurgitation, chronic throat clearing, morning sore throat, and nocturnal coughing. The patient was placed on an H2 blocker and instructed on dietary and lifestyle changes to help prevent acid reflux. When symptoms failed to resolve after 6 weeks of therapy, a biopsy was obtained revealing chronic inflammation. The patient was subsequently referred to the voice center for further recommendations.

## EXAMINATION FINDINGS

Perceptually, the patient's voice was moderately hoarse-harsh in quality with low pitch characteristics. The next **voice sample** demonstrates these dysphonic features.

Figure 6–48A illustrates the appearance of the vocal folds using videostroboscopy. Note the presence of mucosal erythema and ulcerative changes located over the vocal processes of the arytenoids, most notably on the right side. The right-sided lesion appears to partly inhibit vocal fold competency of the posterior cartilaginous glottis. The posterior commissure mucosa is thickened, redundant, and keratinized; these physical findings are referred to as pachydermia laryngis.

**CD2**
**Track 15**

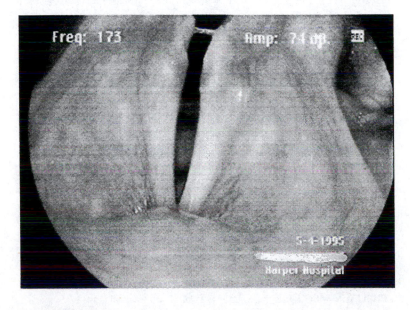

**FIGURE 6–48A.** This is the larynx of a 58-year-old male with the diagnosis of contact ulcerations on the vocal processes of the true vocal folds. Note the erythema and edema of the medial surfaces of the structures.

The clinical diagnosis: contact ulcers and laryngeal mucosal changes resulting from chronic voice abuse behaviors and gastro-esophageal-reflux disease. The patient was started on a speech therapy program designed to reduce voice abuse behaviors. He was again instructed on dietary and lifestyle changes that would reduce the number of reflux events, and Prilosec (Omeprazole) was substituted for the H2 blocker.

## TREATMENT RESULTS

At the outset of speech therapy the patient was noted to use hard glottal attacks and frequent throat clearing during contextual speech. This was largely attributed to his aggressive personality. He was encouraged to recognize and avoid these behaviors at work and at home. The Visi-Pitch apparatus was utilized to help identify his optimal and habitual pitch levels, as well as to provide instant feedback during exercises of easy onset of phonation and to regulate breathing and vocal intensity output.

After 2 months of therapy the patient denied further reflux symptoms, although he complained of occasional sore throats. Perceptually, his voice was significantly improved, but he continued occasionally to attack phonation with a hard and abrupt onset of voice. The next **voice sample** demonstrates improved voice characteristics. Acoustic analysis revealed voice to be within normal limits with respect to parameters of pitch, jitter, shimmer, and harmonic to noise ratio.

**CD2**
**Track 15**

Videostroboscopic examination (Figure 6–48B) illustrates significant resolution of the contact ulcerations over the vocal processes. Although a mild amount of erythema is evident over the posterior glottis, these changes are dramatically improved when compared to original observations.

Overall, the patient demonstrated significant voice improvement and near complete resolution of his laryngeal pathology. He was discharged from the voice center

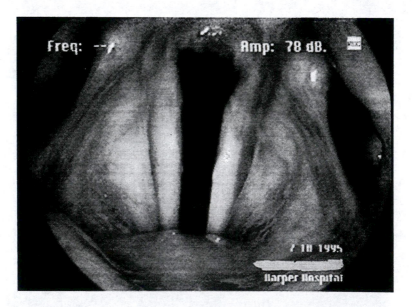

**FIGURE 6–48B.** This photograph was obtained following antireflux medication and voice therapy. Note the improvement in the appearance of the vocal folds bilaterally. Significant resolution of the erythema and edema has occurred in the affected sites. This correlates with the patient's improved phonatory skills.

with encouragement to continue proper vocal hygiene. He will continue antireflux therapy under the guidance of his primary care physician.

## DISCUSSION

Vocal process ulcerations are a common sequelae of chronic voice abuse behaviors. Hard glottal attacks and frequent throat clearing actions cause trauma to the mucosa overlying the vocal processes of the arytenoids, as they repeatedly and forcefully come into contact. Often, gastro-esophageal reflux disease compounds the laryngeal pathology, either because of symptoms evoked by acid reflux (i.e., chronic cough, throat clearing), or as a result of the direct inflammatory effect of acid contacting the laryngeal mucosa. Treatment for such a condition includes a combination of speech behavior modification and antireflux measures. Failure to control either voice abuse or acid reflux will likely result in persistent symptoms or recurrence of disease.

The patient described in this case history remained symptomatic, despite dietary and lifestyle changes and treatment with an H2 blocker to control acid reflux. Studies have shown that those failing treatment with some of the more commonly used H2 blockers (Zantac, Tagamet, Pepsid) may respond to Prilosec, a potent acid inhibitor. Resolution of symptoms may take 6 weeks to 3 months. Of equal importance regarding treatment outcome was the institution of voice therapy to initiate behavior modification guidelines.

# CASE 49
## *Psychogenic Dysphonia*

## HISTORY

This is a 35-year-old male who presented with a chief complaint of high pitched, squeal-like dysphonia that had persisted over a 3-month period. He claimed the voice difficulties occurred acutely, and that they worsened during stressful situations. After more in-depth questioning regarding the patient's psychosocial history, he admitted to having a very stressful lifestyle, rearing two children on his own.

## EXAMINATION FINDINGS

**CD2
Track 16**

Perceptually, the patient's voice was profoundly harsh, high pitched, and squeal-like in quality, with reduced volume dimensions. The next **voice sample** highlights these dysphonic features.

Figure 6–49A illustrates the appearance of the vocal folds using videostroboscopy. Note the profound degree of hyperactivity of the ventricular folds bilaterally, which obscure view of the true folds during phonatory efforts. At no time during phonation are the true fold behaviors identified for vibratory analysis. However, during inspiration, the false folds abduct, allowing view of normal appearing and symmetrically moving true vocal folds.

The clinical diagnosis: psychogenic dysphonia causing a muscle misuse voice disorder. The extreme hyperactivity of the ventricular folds (plica ventricularis) obscures

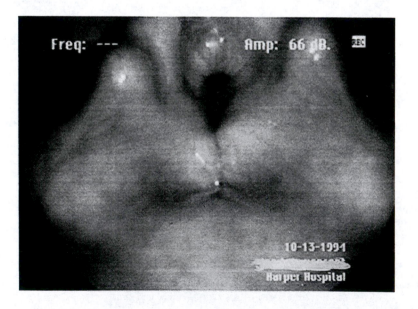

**FIGURE 6–49A.** This photograph demonstrates profound hyperactivity of the ventricular vocal folds in a patient diagnosed as having psychogenic dysphonia. Note that the examination of the true vocal folds is virtually impossible because of these supraglottal activities.

view of the tightly squeezed true folds during phonatory efforts. The hyperadducted true vocal folds actually produce the aforementioned dysphonic features. Treatment for this condition includes both behavior modification designed to "reeducate" the patient on proper vocal fold positioning during phonation and psychological counseling to help reduce emotional conflict.

## TREATMENT RESULTS

The patient was referred for psychologic counseling and underwent several speech therapy sessions, but remained profoundly dysphonic. An attempt to minimize supraglottic hyperactivity with lidocaine injection into the false folds bilaterally resulted in immediate return of normal voicing. This response is demonstrated with the next **voice sample.** The patient was encouraged to continue practicing his new vocal behaviors at home. One week later he returned to the voice center with recurrent severe dysphonia. Speech therapy failed to revert the voice to normal. Given the psychogenic nature of this condition and the dramatic response to the first injections, a transtracheal injection of topical lidocaine was performed to anesthetize the tracheal mucosa. This resulted in sudden return of normal voicing. Figure 6–49B demonstrates a normal glottis and supraglottis shortly after the injection procedure. Again, the patient was given encouragement to continue these normal vocal behaviors. In addition, he was prescribed a placebo pill to take daily for 1 week with the hope of providing a longer time period of symptom relief and further behavioral reinforcement. To date, he continues to vocalize normally.

**CD2**
**Track 16**

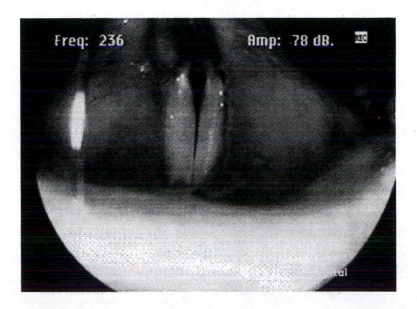

**FIGURE 6–49B.** This photograph was obtained immediately following transtracheal injection of topical lidocaine. The ventricular vocal folds are virtually motionless during phonatory activity, which correlates with significantly better voice output.

## DISCUSSION

Voice disorders may result from abnormal use of muscles associated with phonation, including the intrinsic and extrinsic laryngeal muscles, as well as muscles of the tongue, jaw, pharynx, and respiratory system. These conditions, referred to as muscle misuse disorders, may present with a variety of symptoms and physical findings. Depending on the posture of the larynx during phonation, patients may exhibit no audible voice, profound breathiness, or abnormally high or low pitched vocal quality. Muscle misuse voice disorders may present with no organic changes of the vocal folds, while others are associated with secondary pathologies, including nodules, polypoid degeneration, Reinke's edema, chronic laryngitis, vocal process ulcerations, or scarring. When psychologic conflict causes a muscle misuse voice disorder, the condition is referred to as "psychogenic dysphonia."

Lateral contraction, or hyperadduction, of the larynx is a type of muscle misuse disorder where the glottis and/or supraglottis is squeezed together during phonatory efforts. Isolated glottic hyperadduction will usually produce a tense sounding voice because of incorrect vocal technique. Occasionally, the condition is caused by emotional stress. Not uncommonly, it is triggered by an upper respiratory tract infection, but dysphonia persists weeks after the viral illness has resolved. Koufman has described this condition as "habituated" hoarseness.

The patient described in this case history suffered from hyperadduction of the false vocal folds, a condition referred to as plica ventricularis. The adducted ventricular folds obscured view of the tightly adducted true vocal folds. The true folds actually produced the patient's high-pitched squeaky voice quality. This is the most common muscle misuse type seen in patients suffering from psychogenic dysphonia. Treatment of this disorder relies on both correction of the specific muscle misuse pattern and management of psychological stressors triggering the condition.

# CASE 50
## *Sulcus Vergeture/Vocalis*

## HISTORY

This is a physician who presented with a longstanding history of dysphonia and vocal fatigue that became progressively worse upon joining and participating in a barbershop quartet. He complained that his voice quality deteriorated when attempting to ascend in pitch. He denied any reflux symptoms or voice abuse behaviors.

## EXAMINATION FINDINGS

Perceptually, the patient's voice was mildly hoarse-raspy in quality. Maximum phonation time was within normal limits. The next **voice sample** highlights these dysphonic voice features.

**CD2**
**Track 17**

Acoustic analysis revealed the following: (1) fundamental frequency @ 109 Hz, (2) jitter @ 0.63%, (3) shimmer @ 0.76 dB, and (4) harmonic to noise ratio @ 10.9 dB. The jitter and shimmer data are slightly elevated, pointing toward cycle-to-cycle voice signal variability. Speech aerodynamic testing was within normal limits.

Figures 6–50A and 6–50B illustrate the appearance of the vocal folds using videostroboscopy. Note the appearance of linear atrophic mucosal depressions or sulci, which parallel the free margins of both true vocal folds. During phonatory efforts the medial free margins of both vocal folds appear concave and slightly bowed, left greater than right; a persistent anterior glottal chink is produced. With ascending pitch the left false fold progressively medializes, partially obscuring the true cord beneath. Mucosal waves are slightly diminished and asymmetrical.

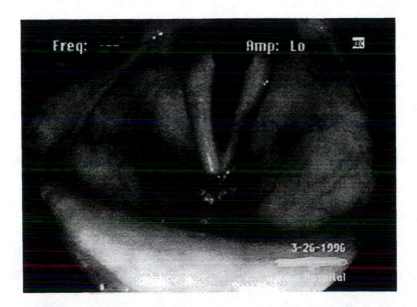

**FIGURE 6–50A.** This photograph was taken from a man with the diagnosis of sulcus vocalis. Note the vertical grooves parallel to the free margins of the true vocal cords.

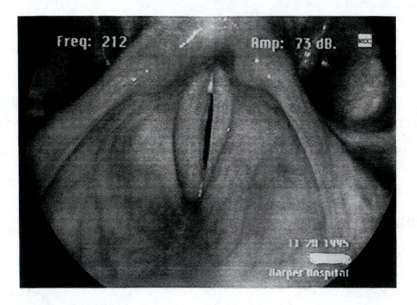

**FIGURE 6–50B.** This photograph was obtained from the same patient during the closed phases of vibration associated with voice. Note the persistent elliptical-shaped glottal chink caused by the bilateral sulcus formation that correlates with the patient's breathy-hoarse dysphonia.

The clinical diagnosis: sulci involving both vocal folds, resulting in bowing of the cords and glottal incompetence. Hyperadduction of the left vestibular fold is likely a compensatory movement to help overcome the persistent anterior glottic chink during phonatory efforts. The sulci result in mildly stiffened mucosal wave characteristics. These aforementioned vocal fold disturbances likely account for the patient's dysphonic features. The recommended treatment for this condition includes speech therapy and microsurgical excision of the sulci.

## DISCUSSION

Bouchayer and Cornut have described two types of vocal fold "sulci," sulcus vocalis and sulcus vergeture. Both lesions can be identified using videostroboscopy. However, definitive diagnosis is usually obtained at the time of intraoperative microlaryngoscopy. Sulcus vocalis is defined as an invagination of epithelium over the free margin of the true vocal fold, which extends through the superficial lamina propria and attaches to the vocal ligament. There may be an associated inflammatory reaction. The invaginated mucosa is stratified squamous epithelium, histologically resembling an open epidermal cyst. Therefore, it is believed that these lesions are derivatives of vocal fold epidermal cysts that have opened toward the free margin.

Sulcus vergeture is a linear atrophic mucosal depression that parallels the free margin of the true vocal fold, adhering to the underlying vocal ligament. This condition occurs more commonly in males, is bilateral, and thought to be of congenital origin. The mucosal tethering caused by the linear invagination results in bowing of the vocal fold and a concavity of the free margin.

Treatment for such conditions includes speech therapy and/or surgical intervention. There are no procedures available that replace the stiffened tissues surrounding the sulcus with normal tissue of the superficial lamina propria. Therefore, treatment will not likely revert vocal quality to a normal level. Surgery for sulcus vocalis includes microexcision of the invaginated mucosa with reapproximation of the free mucosal edges. Sulcus vergeture is surgically treated by carefully freeing the atrophic mucosa from the vocal ligament and injecting steroid submucosally to help prevent scarring of the ligament. Often, the mucosa cannot be effectively elevated, therefore microexcision of the mucosa with reapproximation of the free mucosal edges is performed. Although considered experimental, collagen injection into the true vocal folds may prove beneficial for such lesions.

The patient described in this case history likely suffers from bilateral sulcus vergeture. Although speech therapy and surgical excision of these lesions were recommended, he declined any intervention at this time.

# CASE 51
## *Subglottic Granular Cell Tumor*

## HISTORY

This is a 38-year-old male smoker who presented with a 1-year history of intermittent aphonia, lasting a few minutes at a time. He admitted to occasional voice abuse behaviors at home while helping to raise three children. He also described chronic gastro-esophageal-reflux symptoms, including heartburn, acid regurgitation, chronic throat clearing, and paroxysmal nighttime coughing. Flexible laryngoscopy revealed reflux changes of the mucosa and a large subglottic mass. The patient was referred to the voice center for full-scale laryngeal and videostroboscopic evaluation.

## EXAMINATION FINDINGS

**CD2**
**Track 18**

Perceptually, the patient's voice was mildly hoarse in quality. Maximum phonation time was within normal limits. The next **voice sample** highlights the mild dysphonic voice features.

Acoustic analysis revealed the following: (1) fundamental frequency @ 121 Hz, (2) jitter @ 0.7%, (3) shimmer @ 0.38 dB, and (4) harmonic to noise ratio @ 15.0 dB. These data are all within normal limits.

Speech aerodynamic testing revealed the following: (1) mean airflow rate through the glottis during phonation @ 540 cc/sec, (2) subglottic pressure estimates @ 9.0 cm $H_2O$, and (3) glottic resistance @ 24.1 cm $H_2O$/lps. The flow findings suggest over five times the expected degree of transglottal airflow during phonation efforts. The glottal resistance findings reveal one-half the normal degree of compression forces between the true vocal folds during phonatory efforts. These data suggest a mildly hypofunctioning laryngeal mechanism.

Figures 6–51A and 6–51B illustrate the appearance of the vocal folds and subglottic region using videostroboscopy. Note the appearance of a large, granular, yellow-tan colored mass emanating from the lower lip of the posterior one-third of the left true vocal fold, seen only on deep inhalation. This mass interferes only marginally with the vibratory behaviors of the ipsilateral fold, with some irregularity in the mucosal wave due to load effects. Also noted are mild erythematous mucosal changes consistent with reflux laryngitis.

The clinical diagnosis: the patient was taken to the operating room for an excisional biopsy of the subglottic mass. The lesion was noted to be firm to palpation and approximately 1 cm in greatest diameter. It was removed in its entirety from the left subglottic region and undersurface of the true vocal fold. Histologic analysis confirmed a diagnosis of granular cell tumor.

## DISCUSSION

Granular cell tumors are uncommon benign lesions of the head and neck, occurring most often in the tongue or soft tissues. Laryngeal involvement is rare, accounting for less than 5% of head and neck presentations.

Patients with laryngeal involvement will typically complain of hoarseness. The lesion usually appears as a firm, yellowish mass deep within the laryngeal musculature. It may also present as a granular appearing tumor on the surface of the true vocal fold, typically located over the posterior two-thirds of the cord. These lesions may also emanate from the arytenoid cartilage or subglottic region.

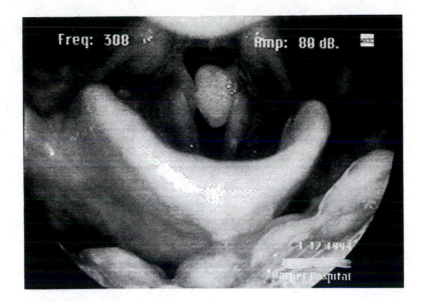

**FIGURE 6–51A.** This photograph was obtained from a young man with the diagnosis of granular cell tumor emanating off of the undersurface of the vocal process of the arytenoid on the left side. The patient's voice is only mildly affected by this growth.

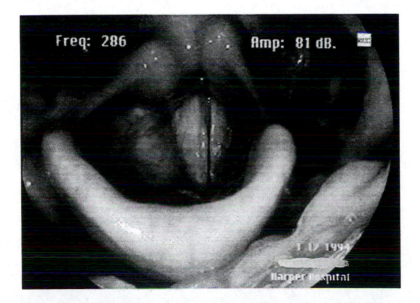

**FIGURE 6–51B.** This illustration was obtained from the same patient during the closed phases of vibration associated with voice. The tumor is essentially hidden from view and does not interfere with glottal competency. The rest of the mechanism is unimpaired in its anatomical and physiological characteristics.

The tumor is thought to be of Schwann cell origin. Histologic analysis will reveal large, uniform cells with pink granular cytoplasm. The cytoplasmic granules will stain positive for the periodic acid-Schiff reaction. Pseudoepitheliomatous hyperplasia of the overlying epithelium may mimic squamous cell carcinoma. However, the lack of epithelial dysplasia will confirm the benign nature of this disease.

Treatment for this lesion includes excision of the entire mass using microlaryngoscopic technique. Tumors that are incompletely removed may recur. The patient described here had a normal appearing larynx and good voice quality postoperatively. Subsequently he was lost to follow-up.

# APPENDIX

# A

# *Additional Cases With Voice Samples*

This section contains brief background descriptions of patients whose voice samples have been added to CD 2 after the last **voice** segment for Case 51 in Chapter 6. It can be assumed that these audio vignettes were obtained prior to phonosurgery unless otherwise indicated.

# CASE 52
## *Psychogenic Muscle Tension Dysphonia*

**CD 2**
**Track 19**

Female, age 37 years. Nurse by profession. Denied use of tobacco or alcoholic products. Admitted extreme emotional despair associated with a failing marriage. No clinically significant medical history. Normal laryngeal anatomy. The voice disorder had persisted for 4 months, despite eight sessions of voice therapy. Refused consultation with psychologist.

# CASE 53
## *Generalized Dysplasia of Vocal Folds*

**CD2**
**Track 20**

Male, age 73 years. Retired auto worker. Heavy user of both cigarettes and alcoholic beverages. Admitted to chronic voice abuse, coughing, and throat clearing. Hypertension, cardiomyopathy, and mild emphysema. Voice disorder persisted for 18 months. Disseminated ulcerative lesions on covers of both vocal folds. Biopsies revealed bilateral dysplasia.

# CASE 54
## *Unilateral Vocal Fold Leukoplakia*

**CD2**
**Track 21**

Female, age 55 years. Elementary school teacher by profession. Thirty-five year history of cigarette smoking, at 1 pack per day. Admitted chronic voice abuse behaviors, including smoker's cough. Voice disorder persisted for 7 months. Focal white-patchy lesion on middle third of left vocal fold. No biopsy performed to date.

# CASE 55
## *Idiopathic Bilateral Abductor Vocal*
## *Fold Paralysis with Laryngospasms*

**CD2**
**Track 22**

Male, age 42 years. Police officer by profession. History of clinical depression with chronic use of neuroleptic drugs. Sudden onset of dyspnea, bilateral vocal fold paralysis, and laryngospasms, which persisted for 14 months. Patient refused tracheotomy or laryngeal surgery for airway maintenance.

## CASE 56
### *Unilateral Vocal Fold Submucosal Cyst*

Male, age 68 years. Evangelical minister by profession. Active participant in church choir for more than 50 years. Admitted to voice abuse patterns, both at home and in his ministry. Dysphonia progressively worsened over course of 4 months. Submucosal cyst identified on middle third of right true vocal fold.

**CD2**
**Track 23**

## CASE 57
### *Supraglottal Laryngectomy with Dyspnea*

Male, age 54 years. Diagnosed with T4N1 squamous cell carcinoma of the supraglottis. Underwent supraglotal laryngectomy and postoperative radiation therapy 6 months prior to taping. Remained tracheotomy dependent because of dyspnea associated with chronic inflammation and mucositis of the glottic and subglottic regions. Used Passy-Muir valve for verbal communication purposes.

**CD2**
**Track 24**

## CASE 58
### *Hyperkinetic Dysarthria: Meige's Syndrome (Oromandibular Dystonia)*

Male, age 52 years. Construction worker by profession. Long history of heroin and ETOH abuse. Developed progressively worsening symptoms of oromandibular dystonia 2 years prior to taping. Underwent bilateral Botox injections into the masseter, internal pterygoid, temporalis, and orbicularis oris musculature 3 months prior, with minimal symptomatic relief. Predominant dysfunctioning of the articulation subsystem, with secondary dysphonia and dysprosodia.

**CD2**
**Track 25**

The first audiotape segment was obtained prior to the introduction of a putty bite block appliance. The second **voice** sample was collected during use of the bite block (18 X 30 mm), placed unilaterally between the upper and lower bicuspid teeth, to inhibit hypermandibular activity.

# CASE 59
## T4N2 Transglottic Squamous Cell Carcinoma: Prelaryngectomy Exam

**CD2**
**Track 26**

Male, age 46 years. Auto mechanic by profession. Heavy smoker at 3 packs per day for 30 years. Developed hoarse voice 6 months earlier, which progressed into whispered phonation 6 weeks prior. Massive transglottic lesion, with laryngeal cartilage invasion and fixed vocal folds. Large neck mass. Scheduled for total laryngectomy, bilateral neck dissections, and postoperative radiation therapy.

# CASE 60
## Presbylaryngis: Vocal Fold Bowing

**CD2**
**Track 27**

Female, age 82 years. Retired librarian. Denied use of tobacco or alcoholic products. Began experiencing progressively worsening hoarse vocal quality 12 months prior. Unremarkable medical history. Bilateral bowing of the vocal folds, with elliptically shaped glottal chink.

# CASE 61
## Bilateral Dysplasia of Vocal Folds

**CD2**
**Track 28**

Male, age 70 years. Attorney by profession. Heavy cigarette smoker at 2 packs per day for 50 years. Episodic hoarse voice over previous 10 years. Chronic throat clearing and coughing behaviors. Hypertension under control with medications. Shortness of breath and transient chest pains. White patchy lesions on the anterior and middle thirds of the vocal folds, with generalized erythema of the free edges. Biopsies revealed bilateral, moderate grade, vocal fold dysplasia.

# CASE 62
## Neurapraxia of Phonation

**CD2**
**Track 29**

Female, age 62 years. Suffered a left CVA 2 months prior, with residual right hemiplegia and mild aphasia. Predominant involvement of the phonation subsystem. No previous voice, speech, or language difficulties.

# CASE 63
## *Postradiation Therapy Dysphonia*

Male, age 65 years. Underwent 7000 cGy radiation therapy for T2N0 glottic squamous cell carcinoma; treatment was completed 4 months prior. Persistent dysphonia, moderately more severe than pre-RT level. Widespread mucositis involving vocal folds, arytenoid cartilages, aryepiglottic folds, and epiglottis. Severely reduced mucosal wave features, bilaterally. Mild glottal incompetency. Profound recruitment of the ventricular folds during phonation efforts.

**CD2**
**Track 30**

# CASE 64
## *Bilateral Reinke's Edema*

Female, age 32 years. Mother of four young children. Did not work outside of the home. Admitted to chronic voice abuse behaviors since her own childhood years. Suggested that she has had a hoarse voice since grade school. Unremarkable medical history. Nonsmoker and nondrinker. Bilateral Reinke's edema, with moderate anatomical irregularity of the free edges of the vocal folds. Retarded mucosal wave dynamics and persistent incompetency across the posterior half of the glottis during phonation. Intermittent recruitment of the ventricular folds.

**CD2**
**Track 31**

# CASE 65
## *Total Laryngectomy with T-E Puncture*

Female, age 56 years. Underwent total laryngectomy and tracheo-esophageal puncture surgical voice restoration 12 months prior. Wore an *In-Health* 20 Fr. low pressure voice prosthesis; used finger-to-stoma valving technique for vocal communication.

**CD2**
**Track 32**

# CASE 66
## *Bilateral Vocal Fold Edema*

Male, age 9 years. Forcefully cleared his throat more than 20 times per hour. Admitted to chronic voice abuse behaviors at home, play, and school. Hoarseness persisted for 16 months and had recently worsened. Began aspirating thin liquid material in prior few weeks. Bilateral, irregular swelling of the anterior two-thirds of the vocal folds, with associated chink in the posterior half of the glottis during all phonation efforts.

**CD2**
**Track 33**

# CASE 67
## *Infectious Laryngitis*

**CD2**
**Track 34**

Female, age 32 years. Longstanding symptoms of gastro-esophageal reflux disease. Moderate relief with antacid medication. Recurrent bouts of sinusitis and postnasal drainage. Underwent fiberoptic endoscopic sinus surgery 13 months prior. Recent episode of upper respiratory infection with severe dysphonia. Bilateral erythema and irregular free edge anatomy of the vocal folds. Erythema of the apexes of the arytenoids, ventricular folds, epiglottis, and aryepiglottic folds.

# CASE 68
## *Webbing of the Anterior Commissure*

**CD2**
**Track 35**

Female, age 23 years. Chronic voice abuser. Underwent bilateral vocal fold nodulectomy 5 months prior. Developed a web in the anterior commissure region postoperatively. Moderate mechanical tether of the anterior half of the vocal folds during voice production.

# CASE 69
## *Hypothyroidism: Vocal Fold Myxedema*

**CD2**
**Track 36**

Male, age 63 years. Suffered from slow thyroid gland functioning for 9 years. Developed low-pitched, harsh voice in previous 2 years. Diabetic with daily insulin injections for 13 years. Hypertension under control with medication. Triple coronary artery bypass surgery 14 months ago. Generalized thickening of the vocal folds, with moderately retarded mucosal wave dynamics. Dry, sticky mucosa of the laryngeal inlet.

## CASE 70
### *Idiopathic Ventricular Dysphonia*

Male, age 59 years. Plica ventricularis began suddenly about 4 months prior. Admitted to extreme emotional tension and stress associated with loss of employment last year. Tap-and-die machinist by profession. Relatively unremarkable medical history. Normal vocal fold anatomy. Severe recruitment of the ventricular folds during most phonatory efforts.

**CD2**
**Track 37**

## CASE 71
### *Hyperkinetic Dysarthria:*
### *Palato-Pharyngeal-Laryngeal Myoclonus*

Male, age 49 years. Experienced brainstem CVA 9 months prior. Moderate degree of resting myoclonus @ 3 Hz, involving velum, pharynx, and vocal folds. Undetectable during connected discourse. Most evident on vowel prolongation. Trace degree of hypernasal resonance. Thought to be a hyperkinetic, involuntary movement disorder, due to damage to the Guillain-Mollaret triangle in the posterior brainstem.

**CD2**
**Track 38**

## CASE 72
### *Unilateral Vocal Fold Paralysis*

Female, age 44 years. Underwent goiter surgery 2 years prior. Recently hospitalized for surgical treatment of esophageal diverticulitis. Mild hoarseness persisted since the goiter surgery, but became exacerbated because of recent intubation anesthesia. Right vocal fold paralyzed in the median position, enabling the left fold to make adequate compensatory contact at the midline of the glottis. No signs of aspiration. Patient was on a normal diet. Only mild dysphonia evident. Trace degrees of vocal fatigue with prolonged phonation.

**CD2**
**Track 39**

# CASE 73
## *Spastic Dysarthria*

**CD2**
**Track 40**

Female, age 66 years. Suffered bilateral, subcortical CVA with consequential pseudo-bulbar palsy and spastic dysarthria. Predominant strained-strangled phonatory features, with less severe articulatory imprecision and hypernasality. Normal anatomy of the vocal folds. Abnormal prolongation of the closed phases of vibration, with intermittent recruitment of the false vocal folds. First **voice sample** obtained 3 months post-stroke, and prior to Botox injections into the thyroarytenoid musculature bilaterally. Second **voice sample** obtained 3 days postinjection.

# CASE 74
## *Psychogenic-Muscle Tension Dysphonia*

**CD2**
**Track 41**

Female, age 59 years. Persistent dysphonia began 2 months prior. Episodic history of laryngitis. Hypertension, asthma, and allergic rhinitis successfully managed with various medications. Admitted to high strung personality and bouts of depression. Normal anatomy of the vocal folds. Profound recruitment of the ventricular folds, with tight anteroposterior squeezing of the entire laryngeal inlet during most vocal efforts. First **voice sample** obtained prior to experimental voice therapy.

Second **voice** sample collected 10 minutes after brief muscle relaxation, yawn-sigh phonation, strap muscle massage, humming, and pitch excursion exercises.

# APPENDIX

# B

# *Index to Cases with Voice Samples*

# INDEX

# W